Nursing Research and Statistics: Generating Evidence

Nursing Research and Statistics: Generating Evidence

by

Dr. Swati Kambli
Former Principal and Professor
Institute of Nursing Education
JJ Hospital
Mumbai
Former Principal
DY Patil School of Nursing
Navi Mumbai

Contributors

Dr. Nancy Fernandes
Principal
LT College of Nursing
SNDT Women's University
Mumbai

Dr. Pradnya Wakpainjan
Professor
SNDT Women's University
Churchgate
Mumbai

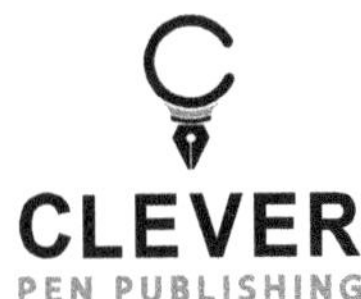

First Edition: 2022

Published by:

Clever Pen Publishing
D-2 Neelkanth Business Park Co-op. Premises Society Ltd.
Nathani Road
Vidyavihar (West)
Mumbai 400086
Mob.: 09867214519

Email:

cleverpen9@gmail.com

ISBN 978 93 92215 37 7

Printed & Bound in India

Dedicated
To
My loving family without whom the book would have been completed twice as quickly, but would have been less than half as much fun. I also dedicate this book to the teachers who love to teach and encourage other minds to grow... They are the purest breed!

Preface

Nursing is a profession. To attain optimum level of professionalism, there is a need to have an autonomous body of knowledge, which can be acquired through rigorous research projects conducted in the field of nursing. Research process helps in the advancement of knowledge leading to evidence based nursing practice. Nursing students at undergraduate level are budding/neophyte researchers. They need to have basic & clear understanding of research process. Educators & senior nursing personnel can motivate & become role model as producer & consumer of research, to these budding researchers helping to conduct research projects which can contribute for evidence based nursing practice. Having the research books in simplified form makes the task easier for the students to learn & understand the contents efficiently & effectively.

Coverage of the topics that are included in this book are commonly included in various nursing curricula of various universities & it is based upon Indian Nursing Councils recently revised Undergraduate & Postgraduate courses syllabi. Also to keep pace with advancing world, & considering the need of the hour, certain topics are added like use of an artificial intelligence in search of review of research literature, developing systematic reviews etc. Recent definitions of important terms including research, nursing research & qualitative research, data analysis soft wares are added in the contents of the book. To develop accurate definitions of variables in measurable terms, new process of concept analysis also is included in this book. This book will help nurses at various levels to understand research in more effective manner so that they will motivate & guide nursing students to develop research proposals & dissertations/thesis effectively. Also it will help in clear understanding of published research articles & communicating research conducted to the society by publishing it. Several topics covered in this book will take care of the gap between theory & practice like meta-analysis, meta-synthesis & systematic reviews, which will enhance the process of evidence based nursing practice.

Through the use of this book, I expect that these efforts will help the nursing personnel to be an active producer & consumer of research by genuinely developing interest for the research process.

Swati Kambli

Foreword

We all possess the vital instinct of inquisitiveness for anything happening around us. When the unknown confronts us, we wonder and our inquisitiveness makes us probe and attain full and fuller understanding of the unknown. This inquisitiveness is the mother of all knowledge, which humans employ for obtaining the knowledge of whatever is unknown, and it can be termed as research. Research, a scientific method is an orderly and systematic process and its results are based on the empirical evidences.

The upgradation of any profession including nursing depends upon the continuous research efforts, dissemination of newly acquired knowledge and utilizing the best evidence in its practice. The practice based on the best evidence will definitely enhance the quality of nursing care that would go a long way in meeting global standards of health care, which is the need of the hour.

The scientific base of nursing practice is strengthened through the promotion of research studies and the dissemination of findings – particularly the findings that are readily integrated into practice. Only through research can nursing truly be recognized as a profession because, credibility of any profession depends upon its research; and nurses therefore, must take research seriously. Research has become a major force in nursing and knowledge generated from research is changing practice, education and attitude of nursing community. Nursing research has now become an integral part of nursing curricula at all levels from diploma (GNM) to masters and of course at doctorate level.

This book, titled, "Nursing Research: Generating Evidence", authored by Swati Kambli, Nancy Fernandes and Pradnya Wakpainjan, has been written with a purpose to make research process easy to comprehend by the students. Language used is simple and clear yet scientific, giving all necessary details of content needed for undergraduate and post graduate students pursuing to learn about different aspects of research and also to conduct research projects of their interest. The content is comprehensive and has been explained well with examples to make it interesting. Several special features also have been added to make this book very 'student friendly' such as appropriate illustrations, summary at the end of each chapter and inclusion of content from information technology, use of artificial intelligence in review of literature for conducting research, new concept like conceptual analysis for accuracy in defining various concepts involved in research and latest trends in collection of data and data analysis and many more. How to write a research proposal? 'How to promote research utilization and dissemination of the research work and how to write a research based article for publication' is another special feature of this book that would motivate and help the research scholars to share their research work with their colleagues and general public. Several important topics covered in this book also will take care of gap between theory & practice like meta-analysis, meta-synthesis & systematic reviews which will enhance Evidence Based Nursing Practice.

I commend the authors, for bringing out this much needed textbook that has general content on research with new features which will be very useful in the field of nursing research. The book would cater to the needs not only of U G and P G students, but also nursing faculty and other healthcare professionals.

Dr Usha Mullick Ukande
RNRM, PhD(N)
Former President
Nursing Research Society of India

Acknowledgements

- I would like to acknowledge the extraordinary support of my family, my son Sagar, my daughter-in-law Charushila, my daughter Prajakta, my granddaughter Anahita and my son-in-law Aashish.
- I am grateful to Dr Usha Ukhande, former president of Nursing Research Society of India, who has spared her valuable time to review & write the foreword for this book.
- This book could not have been completed without the cooperation & support of Dr Nancy Fernandes and Dr Pradnya Wakpainjan, who have shared their expertise via writing chapters in this book. Their contribution will benefit every reader of this book.
- I am eternally grateful to all my teachers, who have always inspired me to persevere. I would especially like to thank Dr Naina Potdar and Madam Bakul Tambat for cultivating me into the person that I am today.
- I owe my editorial team **Mr. Rajesh Bhalani & Mr. Rushabh Bhalani and Mrs. Harsha Shah** from **Clever Pen Publishing** along with the DTP typesetter, who has helped edit this book with expert skill, warmth and precision & helped us in realizing what sort of textbook will be appropriate & best suited for the readers.
- Offering special thanks to Mr D Vilas Jadhav, Deputy Librarian, SNDT Women's University, 1 NT Road, Mumbai, 400020, for helping out for plagiarism check of this book.
- It would be unfair to not give a shout out to my students and colleagues who have always pushed me to better myself, either through positive encouragement or via reverse psychology, by telling me that 'I wouldn't be able to do it'.

Swati Kambli

Contents

SECTION I - RESEARCH & NURSING RESEARCH

SECTION II - STATISTICS

Section I

Research & Nursing Research

CHAPTER

1 Introduction to Research, Nursing Research & Evidence Based Practice (EBP)

Swati Kambli

RESEARCH
"CREATIVITY IS THE POWER TO CONNECT THE SEEMINGLY UNCONNECTED."
Creativity & Novelty of Research helps in the Provision of Quality Care to Mankind & Attainment of Highest Level of Professionalism in Nursing

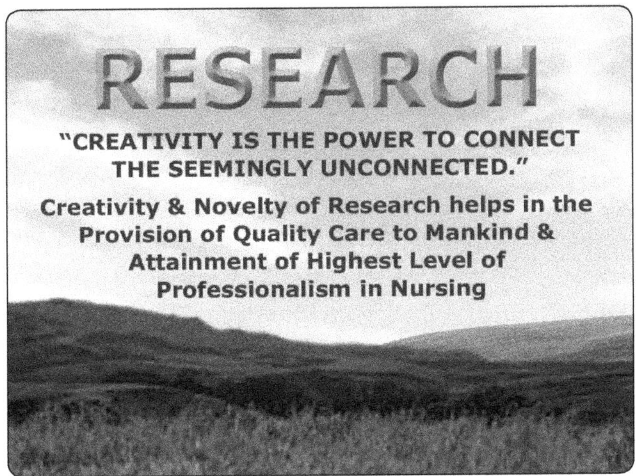

Learning Objectives

This chapter helps the reader to –

- understand the concept & define Research & Nursing Research.
- identify the sources of acquiring knowledge in Nursing.
- acquire knowledge of problem solving & scientific method.
- identify needs, purposes & scope of Nursing Research.
- discuss areas of Nursing Research i.e. practice, service, administration & education, health & social research.
- explain development of Research in Nursing.
- describe & implement the concept of Evidence Based Practice.

INTRODUCTION

Nurses play a vital role in providing quality health care to all individuals of all ages, families, & sick or well, in all settings. Nursing is a Profession. To attain the highest level of professionalism, nursing need to develop autonomous body of knowledge. There are various sources of knowledge & the accurate & best knowledge is derived only from ongoing research. In order to provide quality healthcare, nurses need to incorporate an evidence based practice. Nurses should use best clinical evidence in making patient care decisions; such evidence comes from research. Over the past few decades there has been remarkable growth in relation to Nursing Research. Still many questions remain to be answered about Nursing Research.

Definition of Research & Nursing Research

The word research is derived from the Middle French "reserche" which means to go about seeking, the term itself being derived from old French term "reserchier" or "searcher", meaning "search". The earliest recorded use of the term, was in 1577.

- Research is a logical & systematic search for new & useful information on a particular topic. It is an investigation of finding solutions to scientific & social problems through objective & systematic analysis. **Rajasekar et al (2006)**
- Research is defined as the creation of new knowledge &/or the existing knowledge in a new & creative way so as to generate new concepts, methodologies, & understanding. This could include synthesis & analysis of previous research to the extent that it leads to new & creative outcomes. **Western Sydney University. Jan., 2020**
- Research is an investigation/experimentation aimed at the discovery & interpretation of facts, revision of accepted theories or laws in the light of new facts, or practical application. **Meriam Webster, https:// www'meriamwebster.com. Sept., 2020**

As per the advancement of knowledge, nurses are facing tremendous changes & challenges in relation to nursing practice. In order to cope with changes & to meet challenges, Evidence Based Nursing practice will help in providing quality care to the society.

- Nursing research is defined as a systematic search for knowledge about issues of importance to nursing. (**Polit & Hungler, 2001**)
- Nursing research is a scientific process that validates & refines existing knowledge & generates new knowledge, which directly & indirectly influences nursing practice. (**Burns & Groove, 2005**).
- Nursing research is a scientific, systematic & orderly process to find out solution for problems concerned to nursing or generating & refining the

nursing knowledge to improve quality of nursing care, nursing education, & nursing administration. (**S.K. Sharma, 2005**).

- Nursing research is a systematic approach to gathering information for the purpose of answering questions & solving problems in the pursuit of creating new knowledge about nursing practice, education & policy. (**Heck & Moule, 2006**).
- Nursing research is research that provides evidence used to support nursing practices. Nursing as an evidence based area of practice, has been developing since the time of Florence Nightingale to the present day, where many nurses now work as researchers based in universities as well as in the health care setting. **(Wikipedia, the free encyclopedia 2013).**

Through the abovementioned definitions of **Research, Nursing Research,** various experts emphasize on solving problems in the pursuit of creating knowledge about nursing practice, education, & administration. Also direction is given to **analyze, & synthesize previous research,** which has impact on **Evidence Based Nursing Practice,** which will contribute to provide quality nursing care to the society.

Characteristics of Good Research

Nursing research is progressing faster & continues with it in future focusing on taking care of research practice gap & enhancing Evidence Based Nursing Practice (EBNP).

- Based on current health/professional issues & involves a quest for answers to unsolved problems. For growth of the profession, current health or professional issues need to be considered, so that unsolved problems can be taken care of.
- Contribution toward EBNP - Research conducted should be beneficial to the population under study. It should take care of research practice gap, & implemented as EBNP.
- Orderly, logical, systematic process - There are certain scientific principles & steps to be followed in research, so that process becomes more accurate.
- Begins with clear, specific, achievable objectives, which are related with each step when study is conducted.
- Helps in developing, refining & expanding professional knowledge. Nursing as a profession, need to develop its own autonomous body of knowledge. Thus nursing research helps in developing new knowledge & refining existing knowledge & expanding body of professional knowledge.

- Directed towards development or testing theories. Theory development & testing follows scientific principles so a good research helps to take care of it.
- Use of appropriate methodology - selection of a methodology in any research depends on a methodology related several factors, because each variable & research has unique features. Therefore a good research always employs the most appropriate & suitable methodology.
- Use of appropriate, valid & reliable data collection tools - A tool prepared for data collection should be valid & reliable to generate evidences from it, which can lead to successful conduct of research.
- Conducted on representative sample - Generalization of research findings is only possible if study is conducted on a larger size & representative sample, which has characteristics similar to the population of the study.
- Research involves gathering of data from primary/first hand source/ existing data for a new purpose. Most of the research studies data collection is done from primary or first hand source. Sometimes research study like meta-analysis, data is collected from existing sources so that stronger evidence is generated.
- Carefully recorded & reported - to generate quality empirical evidences recording & reporting of study should be done carefully.
- Adequately & appropriately analyzed research - Research findings are important part of research process. Objectives of the study cannot be achieved unless gathered data is appropriately analyzed using standardized & accepted methods of data analysis.
- Unhurried activity - conducting research study carefully requires a lots of time & patience. Success of research depends upon patience & endurance of the researcher.
- Researcher's expertise, motivation & courage - Good knowledge of the research topic helps in the harmony & success of doing research study. Researcher should have genuine interest & courage to do it. In the absence of these attributes among researchers, good outcomes of the research are not possible.

SOURCES OF ACQUIRING KNOWLEDGE IN NURSING

- There is a widespread support that nursing practice should rely more heavily on evidence from research.
- There are various sources of evidence for nursing practice.

1. **Tradition/Authority**
   - Many questions answered/decisions made by tradition. It is believed that many nursing interventions are based on tradition, customs & 'culture' rather than on sound evidence.
   - **Authority** - Another common source of information is an authority, i.e. a person with specialized expertise & recognition for that expertise. As a source of evidence, authority has shortcomings. Mostly there is no update in knowledge.
2. **Clinical experience, trial & error & intuition.**
   - **Clinical experience** is familiar & functional source, but each nurse's experience may be too narrow to be generally useful. Also perception of events may differ for each nurse.
   - **Trial & error** - This method alternately tried successively until a solution to a problem is found. Method is haphazard. Evidence is not recorded & inaccessible in subsequent clinical situations.
   - **Intuition** - Cannot be explained on the basis of reasoning. It is difficult to develop policies & practices for nurses on the basis of intuition.
3. **Logical reasoning**- Solutions to many problems are developed through logical thought processes.
   - Combines experience, intellectual faculties, & formal systems of Thought i.e.
   - **Inductive reasoning**- It is the process of developing generalizations through specific observations.
   - **Deductive reasoning**- It is the process of developing specific predictions from general principles e.g. separation anxiety in children, we predict child will develop separation anxiety in hospital, if parents do not attend child. Validity is based upon accuracy of information.
4. **Assembled information**- Various data which is available of local, national, international aspects & it is used in practice.
   - It provides no mechanisms for determining whether improvements in patient outcomes are a result of use of this data.
5. **Problem solving**- It is more systematic than the abovementioned methods. When a problem solving method is used to take care of a particular situation, same interventions may be used to solve same problem in future in other similar situations.

6. **Disciplined research**- Research is considered to be more formal, systematic & scientific process for the purpose of developing or refining a professional body of knowledge.

PROBLEM SOLVING

- Process has series of steps.
- Problem definition- Most essential step is to define problem.
- Problem analysis- Next step is to analyze how the problem affects the researcher & his/her current situation & the other people involved in the situation. Factors affecting problem determined. Further analysis helps in the confirmation of the problem to be answered.
- Generating possible solutions- At this stage focus is identifying & generating all possible solutions for a problem.
- Analyzing the solutions- In this section, various factors about each solution are analyzed.
- Selecting the best solution- The best solution is selected out of various solutions, based on accuracy of data & critical analysis of data available of specific problem.

SCIENTIFIC APPROACH

- Most advanced objective means of acquiring knowledge.
- System of logical & orderly elements.
- Directs formal structured inquiry process in the effort to obtain knowledge.
- Research is accepted as scientific approach to knowledge generation.
- Process is used in research.
  - adheres to principles of logic.
  - uses standards for data collection & analysis.
  - there is absence of investigators bias.
  - rules governing generalizability or universality of findings.

Polit & Hungler (1991) describe character of scientific approach.

1. Systematic/orderly
2. External factors can be controlled, which can affect study.
3. Forms basis for discovering new knowledge.
4. Knowledge gained in the process is applied generally.

5. Helps in testing/developing theories for advancement of knowledge.

   Research has all this characteristics & uses scientific method.

Assumptions of scientific approach-

- Basic principles are accepted on faith/assessed to be true without proof/verification
- Its a scientific belief that antecedent factors relating to all phenomena exist & can be discovered. e.g. heart disease caused due to smoking, sedentary lifestyle etc.

Purposes of scientific approach

- To observe in order to know
- To know in order to predict
- To predict in order to control
- To control in order to practice & prescribe in a professional manner.

Limitations of the scientific approach

Scientific approach is the highest form of attaining knowledge. There are certain limitations.

- Moral/ethical problems
- Human complexity such as uniqueness of human beings, personality, environment, mental abilities, values, culture, lifestyle may affect knowledge generation.
- Measurement problems- tools such as biological/physiological functions are more precise/accurate than tools related to psychological dimension of human activity.
- Control of external variables- Certain variables may not be under direct investigator's control, specially when dealing with human beings.

Relation of scientific method & Research

Following are the similarities in scientific methods & research

- Both are determined by logical considerations & there are attempts to achieve an ideal.
- Relies upon empirical evidence.
- Utilizes relevant concepts.

- Committed to only objective considerations.
- Presupposes ethical neutrality.
- Results are based upon probabilistic predictions.
- Methodology is known to all.
- Conclusions are tested through replications.
- Aiming at formulating theories.

NEED FOR RESEARCH IN NURSING

Research in nursing helps updating knowledge in the areas of Nursing Education, Nursing Administration & Practice, so it should be an integral part of all these areas. It also promotes Evidence Based Practice which will help in providing cost effective quality care to the society.

- It moulds nurses' attitudes, intellectual competence & technical skills.
- Helps in filling up the gaps in knowledge & practice.
- Fosters commitment, accountability to clientele.
- Provides basis for professionalism & professional accountability.
- Identifies a role of a nurse in changing society.
- Discovers new measures for nursing practice.
- Helps to take prompt decisions by the administration to related problems.
- Helps to improve the standards in nursing education.
- Refines the existing nursing theories & discovers new theories.

PURPOSES OF NURSING RESEARCH

- Finding answers to questions & solution to problems.
- Discovering, interpreting new facts.
- Testing theories to revise accepted theories or laws in the light of New facts.
- Formulating new theories.

  Considering implementation of new educational policy, much more changes are expected in relation to nursing practice, education, administration & health systems. To keep pace with advancing world, ongoing research is needed in all the abovementioned areas. The scope of nursing research may be classified in the following broad categories

- Clinical nursing practice
- Nursing education
- Nursing administration
- Health systems & outcomes of care

Research in clinical nursing practice

Nurses working in the hospital & community are well prepared by various nursing educational courses at various levels of education. Nurses are prepared well to provide comprehensive & quality health care to the individuals & society. To keep pace with advancing world, nurses need to update their knowledge & this is only possible with the help of ongoing research in relation to following aspects-

- All levels of prevention in relation to communicable & noncommunicable diseases.
- Nursing process approach focusing on individualized care in the hospital & community considering social, cultural, religious, traditional & family practices.
- Geriatric problems & related care.
- Health of vulnerable, minority groups & marginalized communities.
- Development of systematic reviews & promote Evidence Based Practice.
- Genetic testing & therapeutics.
- Palliative & end of life care.
- Nurses working environment.
- Home care & community health nursing care practices.

  However research can be conducted on any of the topics that fall in the nursing care domain.

Research in Nursing Education

The main aim of nursing education is to prepare nurses as bedside nurses, community health nurses, administrators & researchers in nursing. It helps in the development of leaders also in the above areas. As new educational policy to be implemented soon emphasizing more about research centric, learners' need based curriculum, the existing curricula of different nursing courses need to be updated with the help of research in the following areas-

a. Testing the effectiveness in relation to participative & other learner centric teaching & learning methods at UG & PG level courses.

b. Curriculum & learning experiences of nursing students at UG & PG level of courses.

c. Practicing nursing process approach & effectiveness of care given & various nursing procedures performed at the bedside.

d. Improvement in the evaluation methods & techniques at various levels of learning.

e. Effectiveness of information technology used in teaching learning process.

f. Enhancement of learners, teachers & other stakeholders feedback.

g. Managing problems of absenteeism, lack of motivation, slow learning & enhancing student support systems.

Research in Nursing Administration

There are several issues & problems related to nursing administration, those require solutions, may be obtained through research. Common areas which require research are as follow-

- Developing new knowledge/refining existing knowledge regarding nursing administration process
- Organizational structure, span of control. Communication, staffing pattern, wages, benefits, performance appraisal practices.
- Taking care of burnout syndrome, turn over of staff, absenteeism among employees.
- Recruitment procedures, retention & motivation of nursing personnel in providing quality nursing care.
- Developing & testing different administrative models to enhance administration.

Research in Health systems & outcomes of care

This is an important area for research. Effectiveness of existing healthcare systems & outcomes can be identified with research in relation to this area. Common aspects requiring research are as follow-

- Existing new health problems of rural & urban areas & developing cost effective & accessible healthcare models.
- Effectiveness of digital techniques to provide healthcare services from tertiary care centers to the remote & outreach areas.
- Evaluate the effectiveness of national healthcare policies, programs for healthcare of people.

Problems in Nursing, Health & Social Research

- Slow development of systematic reviews in India & other developing countries which can help in generating strong evidence to be implemented. Less numbers of meta-analysis & meta-synthesis is being done which contributes for developing systematic reviews.
- It is not possible to conduct true experimental studies in nursing, health & social sciences. As research is conducted on human beings, it is not possible to conduct research studies in laboratory.
- There are less numbers of qualitative research studies in nursing, health & social sciences. Also there is significant dearth of experts equipped with the knowledge of qualitative research.
- Lack of interest among the researchers-

  Mainly research is conducted as a requirement of fulfilment of UG & PG degrees or as a compulsion for promotions, salary increment etc.
- Ethical constraints- As per ethical guidelines given by ICMR (Indian Council of Medical Research) risks & benefits of the study need to be weighed. That sometimes becomes constraint to conduct a study. Also when studies are conducted on the human beings where safeguarding their rights become an important issue. Several problems cannot be studied only because of ethical constraints.

EVIDENCE BASED NURSING PRACTICE (EBNP)

Nursing Research began with Florence Nightingale but developed slowly until its rapid acceleration in 1950s. Since 1970s nursing research has focused on problems relating to clinical practice. Nursing practices based on research evidences will help in providing scientific & quality care to the patients. Also Evidence Based Practice will help in providing cost effective safe practices.

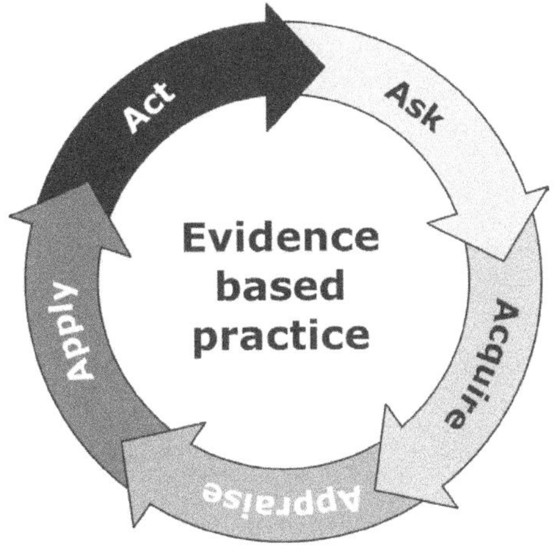

As per Schuster et al., 1998, Grol 2001, a knowledge practice gap is identified presently in nursing.

It is estimated that 30-45% of patients are not receiving care according to scientific evidence.

Also it is observed that 20-25% of care provided is not needed or potentially harmful.

Definitions of EBP

1 EBP is a problem solving approach to the delivery of healthcare that integrates the best evidence from studies & patientcare data with clinician expertise & patient preferences & values. **Fineout Overholt. E. 2010.**

2 EBP is the practice of healthcare in which the practitioner systematically finds, appraises & uses the most accurate & valid research findings as the basis for clinical decisions. **Mosby.**

3 EBNP is the process of shared decision making between practitioner, patient & significant others, based on research evidence, the patient experiences & preferences, clinician's expertise & the robust sources of information. **STTI, 2007.**

4 Evidence Based Nursing Practice also means that nurses make clinical decisions based on the best research evidence, their clinical expertise & the healthcare preferences of their patients. Although EBNP may be based on factors other than research findings such as patient preferences & the expertise of clinicians, the aim of EBNP is to provide the best possible care based on the best available research. To back up the importance of EBNP, Sigma Theta Tau International Honor Society of Nursing & Blackwell Publishing initiated a new journal in 2004 titled Worldviews on Evidence Based Nursing. It's a quarterly peer reviewed journal.

Purposes of EBNP

EBNP helps in improvement of patient outcomes with large amount of research & information that exists in nursing. It helps nurses in learning the skills of EBNP, allowing to search for, assess & apply the literature to their clinical situation. Following are the essential purposes of EBNP in nursing-

EBNP helps

- To identify an evidence that there may be scope for a practice & rating it according to patient outcomes.
- To provide high quality & most cost effective nursing care possible.
- For better patient outcomes.
- To focus nursing practice away from other unstructured sources of knowledge than research, also eliminating unsound or risky practices.

- For contribution to highest level of professionalism in Nursing.
- To keep practices current & relevant.
- To increase confidence in decision making.
- In increasing patient satisfaction.

Development of EBNP

Evidence Based Nursing Practice has shown progress as follow-

- Term research utilization emerged in 1980s. It is a narrower term comparing to EBNP.
- Michigan Nurses Association has conducted 5 years project termed as CURN (Conduct & Utilization of Research in Nursing). Main objective of project was to increase use of research in nurses daily practices.
  - It helped in implementation of innovations & enhancing collaborative clinical research.
  - A research practice gap was identified.
  - As a result of implementation of this project, patient care improvements were seen.
  - During 1990s, EBNP movement has superseded RU & there was a push for EBNP.
  - As the EBNP movement progressed there was development of Cochrane center in Oxford during 1993.
  - Development of international collaboration globally & dozen location centers were established.
  - During this move of EBNP, clinical decisions were based on preparing maintaining & disseminating systematic reviews of the effects of healthcare interventions.
  - Dr. David Sackett- pioneer of EB medicine developed strategy in 1996 & concept shifted from RU to EBP, & thus best evidence was selected & used by all healthcare practitioners & multidisciplinary team approach was followed.

Sources for EBNP

- Systematic Reviews (SR) - This is methodical, scholarly inquiry & follows same steps like primary studies. SR includes meta-analysis & Meta-synthesis.

- Meta-analysis is based on quantitative research studies.
- Meta-synthesis is based on qualitative research studies.

Further development of SR includes CDSR (Cochrane Database SR)

- AHRQ- Agency for Healthcare Research & quality. Reports of these database have shown improvements of the quality, effectiveness & appropriateness of clinical care.
- Simultaneously there was development of database in various countries such as-
    - DARE- Database of Abstracts of Reviews of Effects was developed in UK, by University of York.
    - Development of SR in nursing & other health fields in Australia by Adelaide University.
- CATs- are Critically Appraised Topics. These are brief critical synopsis of high quality studies & SR for effective teaching & learning tool for EBNP. A software was developed to generate CATs.
- Also Clinical Practice Guidelines were developed which combined synthesis of research evidence & specific recommendations for clinical decision making.

Models & Theories for EBNP

A number of different models & theories of EBNP & Research Utilization (RU) have been developed. These models offer frameworks for understanding the EBNP process & for planning & implementing an EBNP project in a practice setting. Some models focus on the use of research from the perspective of individual clinicians (e.g., Stetler Model), whereas some focus on institutional EBNP efforts (e.g., lowa Model). Models that offer a framework for launching an EBNP or RU effort include the following:

1 Center for Advanced Nursing Practice Model (Soukup, 2000).

2 Iowa Model of Research in Practice (Titler et al., 2001)

3 Stetler model of Research Utilization (Stetler, 2001)

4 Johns Hopkins Nursing EBP Model (Newhouse et al., 2005)

5 Advancing Research & Clinical Practice Through Close Collaboration (ARCC) Model. (Melnyk & Fineout-Overholt. 2005)

Although each model offers different perspectives on how to translate research findings into practice, several of the steps & procedures are similar across the models.

Steps of EBNP

- Process of EBNP involves 5 steps.
- EBNP project can be individual/institutional/organizational.

1. Framing a clear answerable clinical question. Selection of final question requires good brain storming about ideas obtaining consensus among the team. A multidisciplinary team approach to approve final question is needed. Priority of the topic must be considered while formulating a clear question. A **PICO** model as follows can be used.

   P - Patient/population.

   I - Potential intervention.

   C - Comparison intervention/control group.

   O - Desired outcome.

2. Search for current relevant literature review should be done for best available evidence. It is better to review high level of evidences such as systematic reviews of randomized control trials. Extensive review of literature is to be done. Current & fresh information/evidences are considered more/weighted than the older one.
3. Appraising & analysing evidence for validity of study findings.
   - Use of rating systems to determine the quality of the research is very important to the development of EBNP. There are several rating systems available online. The national guidelines clearing house is a database of published EBP guideline abstracts at http:// www'guideline.gov.
4. Implementing useful findings in clinical practice & integrating evidence with other factors.
   - Implementation of evidence is to be weighed for costs & risks. Patient preferences, value need to be considered during the process. Utility & importance of evidence in clinical situation is to be assessed. Before implementation, pilot testing is to be done.
5. Evaluating efficacy & outcomes of evidences through a process of self reflection, audit or peer assessment is done.

BARRIERS IN EBNP

It is being observed that there is slow movement or less progress in developing highest level of evidence in India, i.e., Systematic Reviews & implementation of EBNP. There is a great need to bridge a gap of research & practice. There are still many barriers to promote EBNP. Some of the significant barriers in EBP are discussed below-

Barriers: Nurses

- Lack of professional ability to critically appraise research i.e., research evaluation skills, access to library books & journals, lack of time to carry out EBNP, workload pressures, & completing priorities of patient care.
- There are no updates in the knowledge of research methodology. Lack of continuing education programs for nurses in India specially for bedside nurses.
- Resistance towards change.
- No autonomy to the nurses to implement newer evidences in the clinical practice.

Organizational barriers

- Lack of understanding of importance of on the part of EBNP for quality patient care, so un-cooperation for implementation of EBNP.
- No funds are available to implement EBNP.
- Very old organizational policies which are outdated.

Nursing Profession related barriers

- Lack of mentors to support & motivate nurses for EBNP.
- Lack of co-ordination between nursing education & Nursing Administration.
- No role models among nursing leaders. Lack of initiatives among nursing leaders & managers to enhance move of EBNP.

SUMMURY

- Research is a systematic & orderly process for search of new & useful knowledge on a particular theme. It is scientific in nature & follows problem solving approach.
- Nursing Research is a systematic approach to gathering information & providing evidence, used to support nursing practices, nursing education, & nursing administration.
- Various sources for acquiring knowledge in nursing are tradition, trial & error, personal experience, intuition, logical reasoning, assembled information & disciplined research.

- Nursing research encompasses problem solving approach, which has definite steps & there are similarities between nursing research & problem solving process.
- Nursing research is also accepted as scientific approach to knowledge generation.
- Purposes of nursing research are to find answers to questions, discover new knowledge, theories & test existing theories.
- The four major areas for nursing research are nursing practice, nursing education, nursing administration & health systems.
- The main problems of the nursing, health & social research are- slow development of SR & meta-analysis. Inability to conduct true experimental studies in nursing.
    - Less amount of qualitative research & lack of experts.
    - Due to ethical constraints there are limitations to undertake several topics for research study.

BIBLIOGRAPHY

- Burns N., Groove S. (2011) The Practice of Nursing Research: Conduct, Critique & Utilization. 5th edn. Philadelphia: W B Saunders co.
- Creswell J. W., (2008) Educational Research: Planning & Conducting, & Evaluating quantitative & qualitative research. 3rd edn, Upper Saddle river. Pelarson.
- Dempsy P.A., Dempsy A.D. (2000) Using Nursing Research: Process, Critical Evaluation, & Utilization. (2000) 5th edn, Philadelphia, Lippincott Williams & Wilkins.
- DiCenso, A., Guyatt, G., & Ciliska D. (2005) Evidence Based Nursing: Some misconceptions. 1, 38 – 40.
- Fee E., Garo falo M.E. (2010) Florence Nightingale & the Crimean War. A M J Public Health, 100 (9): 1591.
- Heck G., Moule P. (2006) Making sense of Research: An introduction for Health & Social Care Practitioners, 3rd edn, London: Sage.
- Jacelon, C.S., O'Dell, K.K. (2005) Case & Grounded theory as qualitative research methods. Urologic Nursing, 25, 49-52.
- Jadad, A.R., Haynes, R.B. (1998) The Cochrane Collaboration. Advances & challenges in improving evidence based decision making, 18, 2-9.
- Machee, C.L. (2004). Understanding nursing research: Reading & using research in practice. 1st edn. Philadelphia, PA: Lippincott Williams & Wilkins.
- Melney B.M., Fineout Overholt, E. (2005) Evidence based practices in nursing & healthcare: A guide to best practice. Philadelphia, PA: Lippincott Williams & Wilkins.
- More. J.M. (2005) Evolving trends in qualitative research: Advances in mixed method design. Qualitative Health Research, 15, 583-585.

- Munhall, P.L. (2005) Nursing Research: A qualitative perspective, 3rd edn, Boston: Jones & Bartleft.
- Nieswiadomy R.M. (2008) Foundations of Nursing Research. 5th edn, New Delhi, India Dorling Kindersley.
- Polit D.F., Beck CT. (2007) Nursing Research: Principles & Methods. 7th edn, Philadelphia. Lippincott Williams & Wilkins.
- Sacket D.L., Rosenberg W., Gray J. A.M., Haynes, R.B. (1996). Evidence based medicine: What it is & what it isn't. BMJ, 312, 71-72.
- Scott K., McSherry, R. (2009) Evidence based nursing: Clarifying the Concepts for nurses in practice. J of Clinical Nursing., 18 (8). 1085-1095.

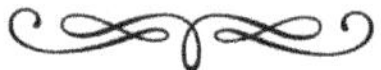

CHAPTER

2 Overview of Nursing Research & Nursing Ethics

Swati Kambli

Learning Objectives

This chapter helps the reader to –

- Understand the development of research in nursing.
- Describe overview of qualitative research process.
- Discuss overview of quantitative research process.
- Follow the concept & importance of ethics in nursing research.
- Recognize the importance & develop informed consent format for data collection of human subjects during research process.

Development of Research in Nursing

Other Countries

1800s

- 1859 - Nightingale's notes on nursing were published.

1900s

- 1900 American Journal of Nursing (AJN) begins publication.
- 1923 Columbo University establishes first doctoral programme for nurses.
- 1930s AJN publishes clinical case studies.
- 1936 Sigma Theta Tau awards first nursing research grant in U.S.
- 1944 Brown publishes report on inadequacies of Nursing Education.
- 1952 The Journal of Nursing Research begins publication.
- 1955 Inception of the American Nurses Foundation to sponsor Nursing Research.
- 1957 Establishment of Nursing Research center at Walter Reed Army Institute of Research.
- 1963 International Journal of Nursing studies begins publication

- 1965 American Nurses Association (ANA) begins sponsoring nursing research conferences.
- 1969 Canadian Journal of Nursing Research begins publication.
- 1971 ANA establishes a Commission on Research.
- 1972 ANA establishes its Council of Nurse Researchers
- 1976 Stetler & Marriam publish guidelines on assessing research for use in practice.
- 1978 The Journals: Research in Nursing & Health & advances in Nursing Science begin publication.
- 1979 Western Journal of Nursing Research begins publication.
- 1982 The conduct & Utilization of Research in Nursing (CURN) project publishes report.
- 1983 Annual Review of Nursing Research begins publication.
- 1985 ANA cabinet Nursing Report establishes research priorities.
- 1986 National Center for Nursing Research (NCNR) is established within US National Institutes of Health.
- 1987 The Journal Scholarly inquiry for Nursing Practice begins publication.
- 1988 The Journal Applied Nursing Research & Nursing Science Quarterly begins publication. Conference on Research Priorities is convened by NCNR.
- 1989 US Agency for Healthcare Policy & Research is established.
- 1992 The Journal Clinical Nursing Research begins publication.
- 1993 NCNR becomes a full institute i.e. The National Institute of Nursing Research (NINR).
    - The Cochrane collaboration is established.
    - The Journal of Nursing Measurement begins publication. AHCPR
- 1994 The Journal Qualitative Health Report begin publication.
- 1995 The Joanna Brig's Institute an International EBP collaborative is established.
- 1997 Canadian Health Services Research Foundation is established with federal findings.
- 1999 AHCPR is renamed as Agency for Healthcare Research & Quality.

2000s

- 2000–2004 NINR issues funding priorities. Annual funding exceeds $100 million. The Canadian Institute of Health Research is launched. The Journal Biological Research for Nursing begins publication.

- 2004 The Journal Worldviews on EBN begins publication.
- 2005 Sigma Theta Tau International issued a position paper on Nursing Research priorities from all international Nursing Organizations.
- 2005–2006 NINR launched a roadmap for the opportunities & gaps In research & issued strategic plan for 2006–2010.
- 2011 NINR released its history book titled 'NINR' - Bringing science to life & issued a new strategic plan.
- 2013 NINR published a report on trends in end of life & palliative care research published during the last 14 years, titled as 'Bridging Momentum': the science of End of life & Palliative care: A review of research trends & findings from 1997–2010.
- 2016 NINR released its new strategic plan, 'Advancing Science, improving lives: A Vision of Nursing Science'.
- 2017 ICMR has released revised policy on Research integrity & publication ethics.

Major Milestones of Nursing Research in India

Many developments have taken place in India, including emergence of associations, growth of educational institutions, & efforts of prominent leaders of Nursing in areas of education, administration, to directly or indirectly adopt scientific approaches. Some of the milestones in relation to nursing research in India are as follows –

1900s

- 1910 Trained Nurses Association of India (TNAI) published the first issue of a scientific Research Journal titled as The Nursing Journal of India during the first scientific nursing conference of T.N.A.I. held at Banaras, U.P.
- 1946 Bhore Committee (1943) submitted a report which included recommendations for improvement of various aspects of Nursing Profession, Nursing Education, Nursing Research, working conditions, Nursing services in both hospitals & community, sending nurses for higher education abroad.
- 1954 TNAI established a standing committee for Nursing Research under chairwoman of Ms. Margaretta Craig to promote the Nursing Research in country.

- 1960 First program of M. Sc. Nursing started by RAK College of Nursing, New Delhi, which included Nursing Research as a full subject with a thesis work on nursing topics.
- 1963 A study of health services was carried out in connection with revision of syllabus of General Nursing & Midwifery by Indian Nursing Council (INC). The study provided valuable insights into the trends in the health services & implications for nursing.
- 1966 TNAI established a research section under the chairwoman Ms. Margaretta Craig.
- 1976 Dr. Marie Farrel & Dr. Aparna Bhaduri, of RAK College of Nursing, New Delhi conducted seminars on nursing research for educationist at Delhi, Mussoorie (Uttarakhand) & Yereand (Tamil Nadu) to strengthen the nursing research in India.
- 1980 Indian Council of Medical Research (ICMR) issued the policy statement on ethical considerations involved research on human subjects.
- 1982 During October, first national conference titled Nursing Research in India: prospect & retrospect in relation to research was held at college of nursing Bangalore & certain recommendations were made.
- 1986 The Nursing Research Society of India (NRSI) was established to promote research within & related to nursing. Dr. Mrs. Inderjit Walia was Founder President, & Mrs. Uma Handa was its first secretary. NRSI conducted research conferences every year.
    - For the first time M.Phil. program in nursing started at RAK college of nursing, New Delhi.
    - Introduction of nursing research was done in B. Sc. Nursing curriculum by INC.
    - Ph.D. in nursing first time started in college of nursing, PGIMER Chandigarh, however later it was discontinued. Later on in south India, some private institutes started Ph.D. nursing program.

2000

- 2005 National consortium for Ph.D. Nursing has been constituted by INC in collaboration with Rajiv Gandhi University of Health Sciences, Bangalore.
- 2009 Central Institute of Nursing & Research was brought into existence under the control of TNAI in New Delhi.
- 2012 NRSI has started an initiative to create database of thesis abstracts for

nursing research conducted by nurses during PG & Doctoral level nursing education. Several private universities started offering Ph.D. degree in nursing through distance mode in India.

- 2013 Six institutes started Ph.D. program in nursing at Bhopal, Bhubaneswar, Jodhpur, Patna, Raipur & Rishikesh.
- 2015 Partially funded Post-Doctoral fellowship program was started by NRSI to promote research among young doctoral nurses.
- 2017 ICMR released revised national ethical guidelines for Biomedical & Health research involving human subjects, which can be used for public health research, social & behavioral sciences research for health including nursing.
- NRSI has also developed the standard guidelines for conducting research.
  - Nursing research is thus progressing faster & continuing with it in future focusing on EBNP.

OVERVIEW OF NURSING RESEARCH

Quantitative Research Process: Overview

In quantitative research study variables are preselected & defined by the researchers, data collected during research process is quantified & then statistically analysed often with the view to establish relationship between independent, dependent & other variables included in the study. The research process starts with the identification & formulation of the research problem & ends with the dissemination of research findings. There are phases/steps to be followed. Five phases are to be followed for conducting research, i.e. assessment, diagnosis, planning, implementation & evaluation.

Assessment phase

- Identification of a researchable problem in nursing.
  - A current problem on priority should be selected with good review of literature. Review of literature should focus on unanswered questions. From a general topic a specific researchable problem to be identified. A good review of literature in relation to the topic will identify a gap in the existing knowledge & justify the need to conduct a research in relation to the topic selected.
- An important step in quantitative research approach is to define the concepts & variables. Conceptual definitions are derived from standard

& medical dictionary, & then converted into operational definitions for accurate quantification of variables under study.

Diagnostic phase

Review of literature, & preparation of research proposal

This phase involves the following-

Another important step is formulating research proposal. It's a summary of steps stating what is to be done, how to do it & who will do it.

A proposal is to be presented to the guide & later on to the research committee. A needed refinement in the research proposal is to be done whenever expected till finally it is approved by guide, research & institutional ethical committee.

- Stating objectives which are clear, achievable, specific & measurable. Based on the objectives hypotheses are to be developed. Hypotheses predict relationship between two/more variables under study. It is a statement of expectations of a researcher concerning relationship of variables under investigation.
- Development of research design should take care of ethical principles like autonomy, beneficence, respect for human dignity & non maleficence i.e. doing no harm to the subjects participating in the study. Institutional ethical committee (IEC) should approve the research proposal. An informed consent format to be approved by IEC. All human rights like participants' decision to participate or not in the study should be protected & taken care of. Also participants have full right to know about all important aspects of research study.
- A good research & non research type of review is very essential to progress of research process so that outcome of the research is good. Once problem area is decided more critical review is to be done focusing on strengths & weaknesses of the study.
- Identifying theory, assumptions & limitations. An explanation of research based on a specific theory is to be done to thoroughly understand about interrelationship of variables among phenomena which is to be investigated.
    - Most of the relevant recent research articles usually help in specifying theory or assumptions upon which the study is based.
    - Delimitations are the aspects of the research which will not be studied. Theoretical or conceptual framework is to be developed & written down.

Planning phase

Plans for sampling, data collection & analysis of data

- A blueprint of the research study is to be developed i.e. describing research design. It is overall planned to obtain an answer to questions which are to be studied. A research approach need to be specified i.e. whether it is quantitative/qualitative approach. Research methods are to be selected.
- Describing research methods - it includes methods of sampling, sample size is selected appropriately so that study findings are generalized, also it involves plans for data collection, analysis & interpretation. A valid & reliable tool is to be developed.

Implementation phase

Data collection process

- Well organized research plan prevents or keeps to a minimum, the unanticipated problems from designs, method & data analysis.
- Ethical guidelines given by regulatory bodies need to be followed & human rights are to be protected during this phase. Depending upon the study, type of sample is to be selected. Size of the sample calculated as per the population for which the study findings are applied. Permission is obtained from institutions where data collection process is to be carried out. There after pilot study is to be conducted following same data collection procedure like actual study. It is worth to conduct pilot study as problems or errors may prove costly during actual study, which can be identified earlier & taken care of. All principles of data collection process thoroughly followed which will influence the process of data analysis. Once data collection process is completed, the evaluation phase of research begins.

Evaluation phase

Data analysis & communication of research study

Once data collection process is completed, next step is to examine raw data for completion & accuracy. Then the data is coded, numbered & entered into master table to bring different category of data together. Then as per the classification of data, it is entered into specific tables. Frequency, percentage is used to summarize the data of demographic variables. For inferential statistics specific statistical tests are used to analyze the data. In relation to inferential statistics the population parameters are estimated & null hypotheses are tested. Based on objectives of research study analysis is being done. Based on research study findings & analysis recommendations are made for nursing practice, education, administration & further research. An abstract of research is prepared. Finally research report is to be communicated. All steps of research study are to be communicated. Graphs & tables included in the report gives clarity & meaningfulness of report. Report should be organized well. Skillful writing skills needed for clarity, precision & meaningfulness of research report. Length, amount of detail required varies depending on topic selected, type of study, & readers of written report & audience during presentation of research report. Upon completion of the report, plagiarism check is being done. Later on research report can be published in peer reviewed journal.

QUALITATIVE RESEARCH: OVERVIEW

Qualitative research is a method of inquiry carried out in many different academic disciplines traditionally in the social sciences. Researchers aim to gather an in-depth understanding of human behavior & the reasons that govern such behavior. Process is less formally planned, where planning & execution of research moves hand in hand. Steps of qualitative research are slightly different from that of quantitative research.

Assessment phase

Initially a broad research area is identified, & then the focus is narrowed down as the researcher gets more familiarity & experience in research setting. e.g. effect of covid-19 on psychological & social status of persons affected with covid-19 infection from Pune city.

Planning phase

- **Formulating broad study objectives** - in qualitative research only broad objectives may be planned which can later be modified based on the need of the research.
- **Review of literature**- will help the researcher to gain some amount of prior information to have an effective planning & execution of research project.

Diagnostic phase

- **Entry in research setting-** Researcher may not always be aware about population & phenomenon, & thus this is an important step for further planning & execution of the research process. Entry in research setting requires prior permission from competent authorities as well as contacts with key persons who are important sources of information about the phenomenon & subjects under study.

- **Selecting research approach/design-** Designs used in qualitative research are phenomenology, grounded theory, ethnography, case study, historical research, action research. Choice of a research design in qualitative study depends on the nature of phenomenon under study.
    - **Phenomenological design-** It is about description of experiences of people.
    - **Ethnographic design-** Involves the collection & analysis of data about cultural groups.
    - **Grounded theory-** collecting data about special experiences of people undergoing any crisis situation.
    - **Case study-** in this there is in depth examination of people, objects, or institutes.
    - **Historical -** involves with identifying, locating, & synthesizing data from the past.
    - **Action research -** concentrating on problem & its solution.
- **Selecting a small sample-** Generally qualitative studies are in depth studies so a quite small sample (10–15) subjects selected for the study. There are no definite rules for it but the principle of data saturation is used to decide sample size.
- **Establishing ethical considerations -** ethical guidelines by regulatory bodies are to be followed like quantitative research but it is more important in qualitative research because of more intimate nature of the relationship between researcher & subjects.
- **Tools -** used for qualitative research are mostly open ended.

Implementation phase

- **Collecting data -** very important in qualitative research & is time consuming process. Interview & observation are two most common types of data collection methods used. Data collection is done through video, tape recording, focus group interviews, photographs, field notes, diaries etc

Evaluation phase

- **Organizing data for analysis -** Data organized for analysis & interpretation is done by following techniques-
    - Listing

- Categorizing
- Comparing
- Laddering

- **Analysis & interpretation of data** – analysis of data in qualitative research usually understands & analyses the words rather than numbers. Large amount of data is in the form of narrations which could be large numbers of pages of notes so it remains challenging task. Qualitative research data analysis is divided into 5 categories.
    - **Content analysis** - Process of categorizing verbal/behavioral data to classify, summarize & tabulate the data.
    - **Narrative analysis** - the formulation of stories presented by respondents taking into account context of each case & different experiences of each respondent.
    - **Discourse analysis** – naturally occurring talk & all types of written text.
    - **Framework analysis** - a more advanced method that consists of several stages as familiarization, identifying a thematic framework, coding, charting, mapping & interpretation.
    - **Grounded theory** - Analysis of single case to formulate a theory & then additional cases are examined to see if they contribute to theory.

  Qualitative data analysis follows 3 steps.

  1. Developing & analyzing codes - for categorization of data.
  2. Identifying themes, patterns, & relationships.
  3. Summarizing the data.

- **Communication of research findings-** research findings may be communicated by writing thesis, article, or presenting an oral report at scientific professional conferences.

ETHICS IN NURSING RESEARCH

The term ethics is derived from the Greek word "Ethos" meaning character & defined as "moral principles" that govern a person's or group's behavior.

Historical background of nursing & medical ethics

The nursing code of ethics is suggested to have been found in 1893 & named as the "Nightingale Pledge" after Florence Nightingale, the founder of modern nursing. The Nightingale Pledge has been recited by nursing students at graduation & candle lighting ceremony for first year UG & GNM candidates. The formal code of ethics was developed in 1950s by American Nurses Association (ANA) & has undergone numerous modifications since. The most recent change was in 2015 when 9 interpretative statements of provisions were added to the code of ethics to help guide nursing practice in a more definitive way. The four principles described were similar to medical ethical principles i.e. autonomy, beneficence, justice & nonmaleficence. In the early 1960s, most notably in U.S. instances of unethical medical research was reported over the volunteers of especially those who were terminally sick, were treated with disrespect & exposed to significant risks or harm. Following are some of the examples of unethical medical practices.

1. At the Willobrook home for children with mental retardation, the children were deliberately infected with hepatitis C, not only raised serious concerns in public, but it had defamed the medical profession.
2. In 1996, Henry Beecher's article, 'Ethics & clinical research', in the New England J. of Medicine, reported 22 examples of medical research which included suboptimal ethical treatment of human subjects.
3. From 1932–1972, for nearly 40 years the U.S. National Health Services conducted a research named the "Tuskegee study of untreated syphilis in the South African males". Around 600 South African males participated in the study, of whom 399 had syphilis. The subjects were never informed that they were involved in a research study, & no informed consent was obtained. Such unethical incidents necessitated the dire need of informed consent from participants & researchers' responsibility towards weighing risks & benefits of research study, so later on a number of treaties & declarations have been reported in the literature, which have addressed fundamental principles of ethical conduct in biomedical research. Principles have been emphasized specifically to protect human subjects from harm & to demonstrate respect for their autonomy. The two comprehensive & pioneering documents about research ethical issues are considered to be the **Nuremberg code & the declaration of Helsinki in 1975** is considered as a document of ethical principles for medical research involving human subjects including research on identifiable human material & data.

   Indian Council of Medical Research (ICMR) is the apex body in India for the formation, co-ordination & promotion of biomedical & health related research, is one of the oldest & largest medical research bodies in the world. ICMR in October 2017 issued revised version of the National Ethical Guidelines for Biomedical & Health research involving human participants. The purpose of these guidelines is to safeguard the dignity, rights, safety & wellbeing of the human. ICMR has also developed revised version of Policy on Research integrity & publication ethics in 2019, which has emphasized that the quality & availability of research is dependent on integrity of researchers who have a significant social responsibility to abide by the standards prescribed for their professions & by their institutions & also to be guided by the applicable regulations & guidelines. It is further mentioned in the policy that responsible conduct of research involved components such as planning & conducting research, reviewing & reporting responsible authorship & publication of research work. The research team should maintain highest standards to uphold the fundamental values of research. The four basic principles of research ethics mentioned in the policy are autonomy (respect for persons), beneficence (to do good), nonmaleficence (to do no harm), & justice (concept of fairness irrespective of caste, creed, region or religion etc). It was emphasized that these principles must be followed for safeguarding the dignity, rights, safety & wellbeing of research participants & for maintaining research integrity.

- **Nursing research ethics are based on Nightingale Pledge**, in doing no harm & aimed to protect the individuals who are cared for.
- **Indian Nursing Council (INC)** has published the code of ethics for nurses in India in the year **2006.** When nurses are dealing with human beings including nursing research they need to follow ethical principles as it represent values, rights, & relationships. The code of ethics for nurses in India involves the respect for the uniqueness of & individual rights, as partners in care, & helps in making informed choices, individual's right to privacy, maintaining confidentiality, & sharing information judiciously. The nurse maintains competence to render quality nursing care, & obliged to practice within the framework of ethical, professional & legal boundaries. The nurse is obliged to work harmoniously with members of the health team. The nurse commits to reciprocate the trust invested in nursing profession by society.
- Thus all the abovementioned ethical principles are to be followed by nurse researchers to protect the rights of research subjects who are vulnerable & research proposal must explain how subject's rights are protected.
- Definition of Ethics in Nursing Research- ethics in nursing research that concerns with activities following moral principles while conducting nursing research to ensure rights & welfare of individual, group, or society under investigation.

- Ethical principles incorporated in nursing research are similar to medical ethics such as beneficence, autonomy, human dignity & non maleficence.

Importance of ethics in nursing research

Following are the important reasons to support importance of ethics in nursing research.

1. Ensure the respect, dignity, privacy, disclosure of information, & fair treatment to human participants.
2. Establish the risk/benefit ratio for human participants.
3. Protect vulnerable group & other participants from harmful effects of the experimental interventions.
4. Protect the rights of the individuals for decision making in participation in study & to have access to informed written consent for participation in research study.
5. Maintain integrity by following ethics throughout the research study, so that the unethical practices like plagiarism & other can be prevented.

Code of ethics in Nursing Research

As per the ANA, INC & Medical Research Ethics, the principles of nursing research are to be followed throughout the research study.

Beneficence - this can be followed by -

- Weighing risk/benefit ratio, where the risk of research should not exceed expected benefits for participants from knowledge generated by research activity.
- Participants should be protected from any physical, psychological, & socially any harmful effects of research study, e.g. any sensitive issues giving rise to psychological disturbances, or affecting any social relationships, etc.
- Research must be conducted by a well qualified & experienced expert to avoid any undue discomfort or distress to subjects.
- Dignity, respect & individuality of human participants to be taken care of.

Principle of justice

- This principle takes care of certain human rights like fair treatment & maintenance of privacy/confidentiality of data shared by subjects. Can be taken care as follows-

- Fair & nondiscriminatory selection of participants as per inclusion criteria of study & following process of randomization.
- Respecting decision of participants to decline to participate or later on to withdraw after agreeing to participate.
- Anonymity of participants & confidentiality of information must be maintained.
- Information collected from study participants should not be used for any other purposes than research.
- Vulnerable subjects like children, pregnant women, geriatric group, mentally ill, physically disabled must be protected from overuse & undue use for research study.

Principle of respect of human dignity

- As per this principle, participants decision for participation/nonparticipation in the study need to be respected.
- It is the participants' right to have any kind of information about research study, they are participating in.
- An informed consent should be obtained from participants. In case of fetus & all age group of children, or physical, psychological, neurological inability to give consent, this can be obtained from parents or legal guardians. In case of children aged between 7 & 18 years an assent may be obtained.

Principle of nonmaleficence

During research study, there is possibility that participation in study may be inadvertently harm them in some unintended way. This may include the following-

- Physical harm- During the course of study any kind of physical harm is to be avoided. e.g. any hot applications during course of study may cause burns to participants, if the temperature of application, or its duration is not taken care of.
- Psychological harm- use of language or certain words in relation to sensitive issues like homosexuality, positive status of HIV test may cause emotional disturbances in subjects.
- Social harm - e.g. disclosure of positive results of sexually transmitted diseases like syphilis may lead to discrimination or stigmatization of persons in the society.

Informed consent

Majority of nursing research studies involve human participants. To protect participants' freedom of choice & respect individual's autonomy, an informed consent must be obtained. It is the responsibility of the investigator to prepare an informed consent document (ICD), which includes a) Participant Information System (PIS) b) Informed consent form (ICF) & get it approved by Ethical Committee (EC). After sharing all information with participants written consent should be obtained from all participants, before the data collection process begins. If participant is not capable of giving voluntary consent, it must be obtained from a legally acceptable or/authorized representative (LAR). While obtaining consent from an illiterate participant, the presence of an impartial literate witness is mandatory during consent process. The two parts of informed consent i.e. PIS & ICF, which is discussed as below-

Participant Information Sheet

A complete information of research study must be provided to participants. Informed consent must be sought only after the participant has read & understood the information provided in PIS. Contents of the participant information sheet must include the following-

- Study title & name of institute/persons conducting the study.
- An invitation paragraph including data provided voluntarily by participants will be used in study.
- Study purposes/objectives of the study & methods of research study.
- Name of sponsoring agency.
- Benefits to participants & community.
- Expected duration & frequency of data collection in study.
- Information about participant selection.
- Foreseeable risks/discomfort & inconvenience to the participants.
- Anonymity/confidentiality of information.
- Reimbursement & incidental expenses to be given to participants.
- Provision of free treatment & or compensation for the participants in case of research related injury.
- Consent as a voluntary process or freedom for decision to withdraw any time during course of study.
- Contact details of the research team for any queries

- Some additional information may be included in PIS as an alternative procedure/course of treatment, risk of stigmatization, insurance coverage related to research, foreseeable extent of information on possible current & future uses of data to be generated from research.
- At the end, expression of gratefulness for participants co-operation & should sign documents.

Informed Consent Form (ICF)

ICF is a part of informed consent document, has declaration that participant has read carefully & he/she is being asked to participate in a study. Also participants have had the opportunity to ask questions & have had answered to their satisfaction, so they have voluntarily agreed to participate in the research study. They are not giving any legal right by signing forms. They will be given a copy of the ICF form. In the end, the form has signature lines for participant & researcher. PIS & ICF can be two different sheets, however a single document can be there.

Online/Electronic consent

Electronic media can be used to provide information as in the written informed consent documents.. Online consent may be obtained in research studies, which involves sensitive data like use of sanitary pads by girls during menses etc. Investigators must ensure that privacy of participants & confidentiality of related data is taken care of.

- Researchers' responsibility in obtaining informed consent.
  - Researcher should use only the institutional ethical committee approved version of informed consent documents.
  - It is mandatory to all researchers to provide all necessary information to the participants.
  - There should not be any coercion to participants on the part of researcher to obtain informed consent.
  - If participant cannot provide consent, a legal acceptable/authorized representative (LAR) may give consent on behalf of participant.
  - Where participant or LAR are illiterate, a neutral literate person, not connected to research, should be present as a witness while obtaining informed consent.
  - Differently abled persons, appropriate methods are to be used. e.g.

blind participant etc.

- All queries/questions of the participants in relation to research are to be satisfied.
- A re-consent or a fresh informed consent must be obtained from participants under following circumstances-

• New development in the study & changes in risk/benefit ratio.
• Unconscious person regaining consciousness.
• Developing of an insight by mentally ill person.
• Child attaining an adulthood during the course of study.
• Research requires extension.
• Change in the independent variables, research methods etc

- Any compensation for research related injury over & above medical management by investigator/institution as the case may be.
- A person's decision to withdraw participation at any time during the course of study to be permitted.
- The details of confidentiality to be conveyed to participants.
- A permission for conducting study should be obtained from Head of Institution, where research will be conducted.
- After obtaining informed consent, participants should be given a copy of informed consent documents. If participant is not accepting it, then it should be recorded.

Institutional Ethical Committee (IEC)

As per the ICMR ethical guidelines (2017) every health related research project must be scientifically & ethically reviewed by ethical committee (EC)/IEC to safeguard the dignity, rights, safety & wellbeing of participants. The institutes may have their own ethical committee or they may utilize the service from EC of another institute. Ethical committee must have a written Standard Operating Procedure (SOP) based on the ICMR guidelines which must be updated based on changing needs. SOP should mention scope, tenure, & renewal policy of the EC. The ethical committee should be registered with the relevant regulatory authorities.

The IEC will take care that all important principles of research ethics i.e. autonomy, beneficence, non-maleficence & justice are taken care of in research protocols. For this purpose, it will look into the aspects of informed consent process, risk benefit ratio, distribution of burden & benefit & provisions for appropriate compensation whenever required. It will review the proposals before start of the studies as well as monitor the research throughout the study until & after completion by examining the annual reports & final reports.

Composition of IEC

1. Chairperson: from outside the institute.
2. A basic scientist
3. Two clinicians
4. Experts or members from clinical specialties
5. A lawyer
6. A social scientist
7. A philosopher
8. A lay person
9. Member secretary

Ethical responsibilities of a nurse researcher

Following are essential ethical responsibilities of nurse researcher.

1. All four cardinal ethical principles i.e. autonomy, human dignity, beneficence, non-maleficence throughout research study by all researchers are to be taken care of.
2. Informed consent by participants should be a voluntary process.
3. During research study optimum balance between risk benefit ratio is ensured by minimizing harms & maximizing the possible benefits for all subjects participating in the study.
4. The confidentiality & anonymity must be promised & protected during entire study period.
5. Nurse researcher should be competent in identified research area & proficient in research methods.
6. There should be adequate protection of vulnerable group in study i.e. children, pregnant women, elderly, mentally ill patients, disabled, terminally ill & institutionalized people etc.
7. Research integrity to be maintained throughout study.
8. The researcher has to give appropriate credit to all parties' contribution to the research.

SUMMARY

- Quantitative research is orderly, systematic process which explores phenomena by collecting numerical data that is analyzed by using statistical methods. The five phases to be followed in this approach are assessment, diagnosis, planning, implementation & evaluation. The research process starts with the identification & formulation of research problem & ends with the dissemination of research findings.
- Qualitative research is a method of inquiry carried out in many different academic disciplines, traditionally in the social sciences. Researcher aims to gather an in-depth understanding of human behavior & the reason that govern such behavior. Process is less formally planned where planning & execution of research moves hand in hand. Steps vary in qualitative research than quantitative research process.
- Ethics in nursing research can be divided as research activities based on moral principles that researcher has to follow throughout research study to ensure safety, & welfare of individuals, groups or society under study.
- Various ethical guidelines developed by nursing regulatory bodies & other bodies like ICMR should be followed in designing & conducting research study which are based on four cardinal principles i.e. beneficence, justice, respect of human dignity & non-maleficence.
- An informed consent to be obtained voluntarily from each study participant & there should be approval of each research study by IEC, which consists of 8–12 members from across disciplines & levels & chairperson should be from outside the institute.

BIBLIOGRAPHY

- Caelli K, (2003) The changing face of phenomenological research: traditional & American phenomenology in nursing. Qualitative Health Research, 10 (3), 366-377.
- Code of ethics & Professional conduct. (2006) Indian Nursing Council.
- DeSantis I., Ugarriza, D.N. (2000) The concept of theme as used in quantitative nursing research. Western J of Nursing Research, 22, 351-372.
- Indian Council of Medical Research (2017) National Ethical Guidelines for Biomedical & Health Research involving human participants. (p1-170). New Delhi.
- Kader P. (1997) Nursing research: Principles, process & issues. New York: Palgrave Macmillan Publishers.
- Polit F.D., Beck C.T. (2008) Generating & assessing evidence for nursing practices. 8th edn. Philadelphia, PA.: Lippincott Williams & Wilkins.

- Saini R., Singh S. Clinical trials in India: need for bioethics. The Tribune, Chandigarh, Monday, August 9, 2010; 130;219:11.
- Nuremberg Military Tribunal (1996) The Nuremberg code. J of the American Medical Association. 276,1691.
- World Health Organization. (2000) Operational Guidelines for Ethics Committees that Review Biomedical Research. Geneva: World Health Organization.

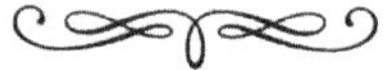

CHAPTER

3 Stating of Research Problem

Swati Kambli

Learning Objectives

This chapter helps the reader to –

- Define research problem.
- Identify the sources of research problem.
- Understand the criteria for selecting a good research problem.
- Develop skills in formulation of research problem.
- Identify different variables & classify them.
- Explain about importance of operational definitions in research.
- Describe characteristics, needs & types of research objectives.
- Develop skills in formulation of research objectives

Many scientists owe their greatness not to their skill in solving problems but to their wisdom in choosing them.

—Wilson

This section discusses the formulation & development of research problems. It is the beginning to generate new evidence. Identification & formulation of research problem is the first step of research process & most important requirement of research process.

- Considered as one of the most challenging & difficult phases of any research project.
- A researcher should ensure that selected problem has high significance & implications for nursing profession.
- It requires a lots of time to select a good research problem.
- For a neophyte researcher it remains a difficult task to identify a good research problem.

I) Definitions

1. A research problem is a statement about an area of concern, a condition to be improved, a difficulty to be eliminated, or a troubling question that exists in scholarly literature, in theory or in practice that points to the need for meaningful understanding & deliberate investigation in some discipline. **(www.scriblr.com)**
2. A research problem is a specific issue, difficulty, contradiction, or gap in knowledge that researcher aims to address in her/his research. Researcher looks for practical problems aimed at contributing to change or theoretical problems aimed at expanding knowledge. (**Shona Mc Combes).**
3. According to **Kerlinger,** 'A problem is an interrogative sentence or statement that asks what relation exists between two or more variables. The answer to questions will provide what is having sought in the research'.
4. **R. S. Woodworth** defines problem as 'a situation for which we have no ready & successful response by instinct or by previous acquired habit. We must find out what to do', i.e., the solution can be found out only after an investigation.

Importance of research problem

When topic is selected for research it is interesting & lots can be said about it, but this isn't a strong basis for academic research. Without a well defined research problem, one is likely to end up with an unfocused & unmanageable project. Research problem statement is needed to do research that contributes new & relevant insights. While writing a research proposal the research problem is the first step towards knowing exactly what's to be done & why it should be done.

- The type of research problem to be selected depends on broad topic of interest & type of research to do.
- Considering the research problems & research approaches, some research problems are better suited to qualitative versus quantitative approaches. Quantitative studies usually involve concepts that are fairly well developed about which there is an existing body of literature, & for which reliable methods of measurement have been (or can be) developed.
- Qualitative studies are often undertaken because some aspect of a phenomenon is poorly understood, & the researcher wants to develop a rich, comprehensive, & context bound understanding of it. Thus the

nature of the research question is closely related to research type & research approach.

II) Sources of research problems

At the most basic levels, research topics originate with researcher's interests. Because research is a time consuming enterprises, curiosity about & interest in a topic are essential to a projects success.

- Generally a broad area is selected & then a broad topic is delimited or narrowed down to a specific one sentence statement of the problem.
- The ideas a researcher collects to identify a research problem are influenced by variety of sources.

The common sources from which a researcher may find ideas to identify & formulate a research problem are as follows–

1. **Critical review of literature**- When a researcher identifies an area of interest like high risk newborn care, tries to identify about research studies about it, or reads more about recent neonatal care books, journals articles, dissertations etc. Critical appraisal of review of literature, helps researcher to narrow down the topic to be selected for research study, e.g. neonatal thermoregulation & related care.
   - Once a topic is identified then gaps in the previous literature are identified to justify the need for research study to be conducted.
   - Also certain previous studies where sample size is small can be replicated on another sample, & another settings to generalize the findings.
   - Sometimes a need is identified to extend or refine existing knowledge e.g. post-surgery pain management etc.
   - Further refinements may be made in the experimental treatments, or more appropriate outcome measures may be identified.
2. **Cultural practices** - There are certain food practices of low socio-Economic group where children are prohibited to consume certain foodstuff like peanuts, as it is believed that it may cause cough & cold in children. Another common belief is that consumption of sugar may lead to worm infestation in children.
3. **Practical experience**- During practical experience, several observations are noted by nurses e.g. Glasgow coma scale may vary when verbal stimuli is applied by close relatives of patient than a nurse. That is how nurses get plenty of ideas to formulate research problems from their enriched clinical experience.

4. **Theory development & testing**- Research is a process of theory development & testing. Generally a part or parts of the theory are subjected to testing in the clinical area or through qualitative research study a new theory can be developed.
5. **Through planning & implementation of various health related programs** there is an emphasis on improving standards of health. e.g. during pandemic of Covid-19, certain guidelines were prepared & implemented by central & state government i.e. the type of masks to be used & how to use the masks effectively, social distancing norms, criteria for home quarantine of affected person etc. Implementation of national health programs may open new avenues to conduct various research studies. e.g. multi drug resistant tuberculosis etc.
6. **Global health problem related priorities**- Global & national health problems related priorities are identified by **World Health Organization** & various governmental agencies like ICMR, academic regulatory bodies like UGC or various non-governmental organizations working for health related problems. There will be several significant areas to conduct a research study e.g. Covid 19 pandemic etc.
7. **Brain storming sessions**- Brain storming sessions which occurs during research proposal presentations or various academic meetings; it is observed that these sessions are good techniques to find new questions, or ideas for research studies. Also ideas may emerge from reviewing research priorities by having brain storming sessions with other nurses, researchers or nursing faculties.
8. **Consultations with experts**- Experts are believed to have enriched experience in their respective field. They can help in suggesting significant problem for research study or refine/modify any topic for research study.

III) Criteria for selecting a good research problem- There are many factors to be considered while deciding a significance of a particular research question for a scientific investigation. Every problem must satisfy the following criteria - a Significance to nursing profession - Following questions are to be satisfied by the research problem selected for research study.

- Is it important to nursing profession? A research problem selected for research study, should be significant to nursing profession, when it is directed to develop or refine the professional knowledge.
- Is the problem selected for study original or novel? Research should not be mere repetition of previous topics. It should be based on current professional or health related problems of the society which can

contribute for growth of the existing body of knowledge of profession.

- What are the benefits to patients, nurses, society, health care fraternity through research study?
- How far the outcomes or results of the study will help to improve clinical nursing practice?
- Do research findings lead to theory development or challenging untested theory?
- Is it providing solutions to current nursing practice problems? Is it generating information to get practical implications for nursing profession?
- **Feasibility of research study should be checked against the following considerations.**
    1. Regarding study design whether appropriate selection is there for Selected research study?
    2. Access to organizations & subjects or respondents - Whatever research study is to be conducted whether getting a permission from the organization for study should not be a problem.
    3. Sample to be studied should be available as per the inclusion criteria of the study.
    4. Tool used for the study should be valid & reliable so all the procedures of tool validity & reliability are to be taken care of.
    5. Method of collecting data- Data collection procedure should remain same for all subjects or respondents. Required facilities should be available in the institute where data collection is being done.
    6. The types of variables involved - If the study requires dependent & independent variables, it should be accurately operationally defined, so while conducting a study there will be no chaos, & it also should be checked that all extraneous variables should be under control.
    7. There should be appropriate selection of statistical methods to carry out descriptive & inferential analysis & selected methods should be relevant to the study objectives.
    8. Time required - As per the plans research study should be completed in time. Time is always a factor to be considered. It's wise to allow more time than seems to be needed because unexpected delays frequently may occur.

9. Cost of everything - Everything should be well planned, i.e. the budget for the study. The researcher must consider realistically the financial resources available & prepare a plan.

- **Interest -** A researcher should have a genuine interest to conduct a research study. Researcher's interest in doing a research will motivate fully so that research is conducted with full enthusiasm & not merely to complete task.
- **Current -** A research study should be based on current problems & needs of a profession, so the subjects or respondents will be benefitted. It should contribute for evidence based nursing practice.
- **Experience & creativity -** Enriched field experience is conducive to original thinking. Gives an insight into scientific process of planning & execution of research study. Lots of creativity is needed to plan & execute research study.
- **Ethical considerations -** Any research conducted should follow ethical guidelines by regulatory & research related Government bodies. Ethical committee should approve research study & guide further till completion of the research study.
- **Researcher's competence -** A researcher should be competent enough to conduct a research project, so that research objectives can be achieved fully.
- **Administrative & peer support -** Financial as well as psychological support from administration is very much essential & can be a very powerful motivating force. Thorough brain storming interactive sessions help in developing many research ideas. A climate of shared interest in nursing research is essential among the members of the nursing profession.

A wise choice of problem comprises originality, initiative to do good to the subjects, profession & society. Ingenuity without so many personal expectations like salary hike, promotions etc & foresight to contribute for **Evidence Based Nursing Practice** is very much essential.

IV) Formulation of final statement of the problem

Forms- A statement of research problem could be in **declarative** or **interrogative** format.

- **Declarative format-**

- A descriptive study on prevalence of urinary tract infection among post-operative patients with urinary catheter with urological disorder.
- An exploratory study on factors influencing thermoregulation in normal neonates.

- In declarative format a research problem is stated in declarative statement.

- **Interrogative format –**
  - In interrogative format, a research problem is stated in question form e.g.
    - What is the effect of selective nursing interventions on intracranial pressure of patients undergone neurosurgery?
    - What is the effect of giving bath to a neonate on his/her thermoregulation?

  The choice of either of these two types of formats for formulation of research problem depends on the researcher's preference & institutional policies, however, declarative format is more popular among the researchers. However both the formats can be combined.

- **A good problem statement** has 4 characteristics-
  - Research problem is clearly & precisely stated.
  - It clearly states the variables, population, & research setting under study.
  - Variables are expressed in measurable terms.
  - The type of study also may be included in the research problem statement. Example of a well formulated research problem as follow-

- An exploratory study on factors influencing neonatal infections in NICU of Jerbai Wadia Children's hospital, Parel. Mumbai.

  It is an example of declarative form of the statement of problem, where it is precisely stated & includes most of the required components of a research statement. Some of theses components are listed below-

- Research study design- non-experimental- exploratory`
- Two research variables- factors influencing is an independent variable but not manipulated & neonatal infections is dependent variable.
- Population – neonates admitted in NICU.
- Research setting – Jerbai Wadia Children's hospital, Parel, Mumbai.

VARIABLES

Variables are something that has quantity & quality that varies.

Definition – A variable is any qualitative or quantitative characteristic that can change & have more than one value such as age, height, weight & gender etc.

- Variables are broadly categorized into –
  - Independent
  - Dependent
  - Control

Table 3.1: Type of variables, definitions & examples

Type of variable	Definition	Example
Independent (stimulus)	It is the variable that influences other variables	Any planned interventions/Actions
Dependent (response)	The dependent variable is the outcome of influence of the independent variable	Research study How refined CHO affect the health of human being?
Independent variable- refined CHO, dependent variable- health of human beings. Manipulation of the consumption of refined CHO in human participants is done & levels of consuming processed CHO can be measured.		
Control	Control variables are variables that are not changed & kept constant throughout the experiment	Natural environment of participants etc.

Types of variables based on the types of data- A data is referred to as Information & statistics gathered for analysis of a research topic. Data is broadly divided into two categories, such as-

- Quantitative/numerical data - associated with the aspects of measurement, quantity & extent.
- Categorical data is associated with groupings.
- Quantitative data further divided into continuous & discrete
- Categorical data is divided into ordinal & nominal.

Table 3.2: Types of continuous & discrete variables

Type of variable	Definition	Example
Continuous variable	A continuous variable is type of quantitative variable that can take a value between two specific values	Income & age scale: interval & ratio
Discrete variable	A discrete variable is quantitative variable whose attributes are separated from each other	literacy rate, gender, & nationality scale- nominal & ordinal

Categorical variables - The categorical variables include measurements that vary in terms of categories such as types of names but not in terms of rank or degree. It means one level of a categorical variable cannot be considered as better or greater than another level. The categorical variable is further categorized into three types **(Table 3.3)**.

Table 3.3: Types of categorical variables

Type of variable	Definition	Example
Dichotomous (binary) variable	This variable is with two possible results (yes/no)	Alcoholic (yes/no)
Nominal variable	This variable can take the value that is not organized in terms of groups, degree, or rank	Eye color, religion gender, brand
Ordinal variable	This variable can take value that can be logically ordered or ranked.	Size of clothes (small, medium, large, extra large etc.) level of seniority in college students (fresher, junior, senior)

Sometimes an ordinal variable also acts as quantitative variable. Ordinal data has an order, but the intervals between scale points may be uneven.

Other types of variables

It's important to understand the difference between independent & dependent variable & know whether they are quantitative or categorical variable to choose the appropriate statistical test. There are many other types of variables to help to differentiate & understand them.

Table 3.4: Other types of variables

Type of variable	Definition	Example
Confounding	This is a hidden variable produces an association between two unrelated variables because the hidden variables affect both of them	There is an association between difficulty in understanding a subject like Microbiology for 1st year B. Sc. Nursing Students & low scoring in the tests (the confounding variable could be difficulty in understanding lectures in English & attempting answering the tests in English)

(Continued...)

Type of variable	Definition	Example
Latent variable	These variables cannot be observed or measured directly	Self confidence & motivation cannot be measured directly, still they can be interpreted through other variables such as achievements, perception & lifestyle of the person.
Composite variable	It is a combination of multiple variables. It is used to measure multidimensional aspects that is difficult to observe	Survey questionnaire in which nursing students asked to indicate the purpose of using computers. They could score multiple categories such as—Entertainment, online education, accounting, database management, storage, retrieval etc.
Moderator variable	Affects the cause & effect relationship between the independent & dependent variables. As a result, there is influence of the independent variable in the presence of moderator variable.	Gender, race & class
Outcome variable **Criterion variable**	It is a presumed effect of predictor variable in non-experimental study.	Consumption of tobacco leads to mouth cancer.
Predictor variable	It is a presumed cause, observed in natural setting without manipulation in non-experimental studies to see effect on outcome variable.	High blood cholesterol leads to coronary artery disease.

Research studies may have one, two or many variables under study, research studies are called univariate study (one variable is studied), bivariate study (two variables are studied), & multivariate study (more than two variables are studied.

- **Univariate study**- In descriptive & comparative studies, generally a single variable is studied. This variable is called research variable.
- **Bivariate studies**- Correlational, experimental, pre-experimental & Quasi-experimental studies include two variables in research e.g. A prospective

cohort study on tobacco consumption & oral cancer among adults in urban slum of city Mumbai. This correlational study is bivariate study as it included two variables, one independent (tobacco consumption) & the other dependent (oral cancer).

- **Multivariate studies**- When more than two variables in research are studied together, called as multivariate studies. Qualitative research studies are usually multivariate studies. e.g. A study on factors contributing to non-adherence of treatments among patients with A.I.D.S. in selected urban communities of slum area, Mumbai, Maharashtra.

Table 3.5: Examples of the statement of research problems & variables in Quantitative research studies.

Type of study	Example of research problem statement	Variable
Descriptive	A descriptive study on prevalence of diarrhoea among infants in selected villages of district Raigarh, Maharashtra.	Prevalence of diarrhoea research variable
Exploratory	An exploratory study on contributing factors of coronary artery disease, among adults in Mumbai, Maharashtra.	Contributing factors of coronary artery disease research variable
Correlational	A prospective cohort study on smoking & lung cancer among slum dwellers of Mumbai city, Maharashtra.	Predictor variable – smoking; outcome variable - lung cancer
Comparative	A comparative study on mental health problems among rural & urban older people of Gulbarg Karnataka.	Research variable – mental health problems
Experimental	A randomized control trial on efficacy of oral Remdesivir in management of patients diagnosed as Covid-19, admitted in hospitals at Delhi	independent variable - oral Remdesivir; dependent variable - patients diagnosed as Covid-19.
Quasi Experimental	A quasi-experimental study of needle gauge on pain perception among patients receiving intra-muscular injections in O.P.D. of Christian Medical College & Hospital, Vellore, Tamil Nadu.	independent variable - needle gauge; dependent variable - pain perception during Intra-muscular injection

(Continued...)

Type of study	Example of research problem statement	Variable
Phenomenological	A phenomenololgical study on lived experiences of flooding due to heavy rain in selected villages of Andhra Pradesh.	Research variable lived experiences
Ethnographical	An ethnographic study on the features, critical attributes, processes & benefits of self help groups of women with domestic violence in selected villages of U.P.	Research variable features, critical attributes, processes & benefits of self help groups of women
Grounded	A study on response & adaptation process **theory** of patients diagnosed with chronic renal failure on dialysis in Nehru hospital, PGIMER, Chandigarh.	Research variable response & adaptation process
Case study	A case study on availability & utilization of services of Covid-19 centers at Ujjain, Madhya Pradesh.	Research variable availability & utilization of services of Covid-19 centers
Historical study	A historical study on experiences of ward facilities for nurses working in ICUs during 1960 & 1970 in KEM hospital,	Research variable experiences of ward facilities for nurses
Action	A study on practicability of integration of service & education in selected premier nursing nursing administration, institutions of India.	Research variable practicability of integrating nursing administration, Service & education in selected premier institutions of India.

The main type of variables used in nursing research are independent variable, dependent variable, research variable, & extraneous variable.

Operational Definitions in Research

One of the keys to successful research, in addition to careful planning, is the use of operational definitions in measuring the concepts & variables we are studying or the terms we are using in our research documents.

It is critical to operationally define a variable in order to lend credibility to methodology & to ensure the reproducibility of the result of the study.

- The operational definition is different from the dictionary definition, which is often conceptual, descriptive & consequently imprecise.

- In contrast, an operational definition gives an obvious, precise, & communicable meaning to a concept that is used to ensure comprehensive knowledge of the idea by specifiying how the idea is measured & applied within a particular set of circumstances.
- Operationalization is the process by which a researcher defines how a concept is measured, observed, or manipulated within a particular study.

Definition

Operational definition refers to a precise statement of how a conceptual variable is turned into a measurable variable. **Ana Safaya**.

An operational definition serves following purposes-

1 It establishes the rules & procedures the researcher uses to measure the variable.

2 It provides unambiguous & consistent meaning to terms/variables that otherwise can be integrated in different ways.

3 It makes the collection of data as well as analysis more focused & efficient. (iEdunote.com)

Research Objectives

- Clearly defined research objectives are very important to conduct a research study.
- Research objectives enlighten the way in which the researcher has to proceed.
- Well written objectives are important features of good research study.
- It gives good direction for successful outcome of research study.
- Research findings are evaluated for full achievement of stated objectives, otherwise validity of research remains questionable.

Also well stated objectives facilitate scientific findings.

- Objectives in quantitative & qualitative studies are similar. In qualitative studies objectives are broad & include complex & abstract variables.
- Relationship between variables are clearly identified by objectives.
- Objectives of research project summarize what is to be achieved by research study.

Characteristics of Research Objectives

- A well worded objective will be **SMART** i.e. specific, measurable, attainable, realistic & time bound.

Research objectives

- Should be relevant, feasible, logical, observable & measurable.
- Summarize what is to be achieved by the study.
- Give clear specific directions for what is to be achieved by the study.
- Include clear solutions for problems included in research study & help for testing of hypotheses.

Need for research objectives

Objectives will help the researcher to-

- Focus on the study. Give clarity for what is to be achieved.
- Avoid the collection of data not necessary.
- Helps in organization of research study in a clearly defined parts/phases.
- Give directions for facilitation of development of research methodology, & helps in the collection, analysis, interpretation & utilization of data.

Method of stating objectives

- Precise
- Relevant
- Logical
- Operational terms to be used about what researcher is going to do, where it should be done, & for what purpose it should be done?
- Realistic
- They use action verbs that is specific enough to be evaluated.
- Examples of action verbs- to assess, to identify, to find out, to determine, to compare, to verify, to calculate, to describe, to analyze, to establish etc.

- Throughout research project, objectives are evaluated & correlated with each stage of research project & finally results are compared with objectives.
- A critical component of a successful research engagement is a set of clearly defined objectives narrow & focus the research & ensure that the findings relevant to evidence based nursing practice.

SUMMARY

- A research problem is a specific issue, difficulty, or gap in knowledge that researcher aims to address in research. Researcher looks for practical problems aimed at contributing to change or theoretical problems aimed at expanding knowledge.
- Some research problems are suited to qualitative versus quantitative methods.
- Various sources of research problem are critical review of literature, popular conceptions, practical experience, theory development & testing, political concerns, global & national health related priorities, brain storming session during professional & academic meetings, consultation with experts etc.
- The criteria for selection of good research problem are significance & importance to nursing profession, originality, novelty, outcome results of the study, theory development & testing, implications to nursing practice, ethical & relevant, interesting topic, cost, time requirement, researcher's competence etc.
- Good problem statement will have characteristics as
    1 clear identification of variables
    2 expresses variable relationship with each other.
    3 specifies the population.
    4 empirical testing.
- Formulation of research problem consists of
    - selection or broad research area
    - reviewing literature & theory
    - specifying research topic
    - identification of significance of research study
    - formulation of final problem statement.
    * A variable is any qualitative or quantitative characteristic that can change & have more than one value such as age, gender, height, weight etc. Different types of variables are independent, dependent, control, variables are based on data like quantitative, qualitative, categorical, confounding, latent, moderator & outcome variable.
- Conceptual definition is based on dictionary meaning but operational definition refers to a precise statement of how conceptual definition is turned into a measurable variable.

- A research objective is clear, concise statement which provides direction for successful outcome of research study & findings which are evaluated for achievement of stated objectives. Relationship of variables are clearly identified by objectives.
- The characteristics of research objectives are SMART i.e. Specific, Measurable, Achievable, Realistic & Time bound. Research objectives are also relevant, feasible, logical & observable.

BIBLIOGRAPHY

- Creswell J. W. Educational Research: Planning, Conducting, & Evaluating quantitative & qualitative Research. 3rd edn, Upper Saddle River, Pearson.
- Dona Van DeWater, September,17,2020. www.lipmanearne.com/how-to-define-good-problem-statement.
- Kahn, C.R. (1994) Picking a research problem: The critical decision. The New England J of Medicine, 330 (21), 1530-1533.
- Polit D.F., Beck C.T. (2007) Nursing Research: Principles & Methods. 7th edn, Philadelphia. Lippincott Williams & Wilkins.
- Shona McCombes, (April 15,2019) revised on (June,19,2020) www.scribbr.com/research process/problem statement accessed on 14-2-2021.
- Shruti Datt & Priya Chetty, July,18.2016. How to write problem statement in research paper. projectguru.in/write-problem-statement-research-paper. Accessed on 14-2-2021.
- Henri Bwisa. March, 15, 2018.www.editage.com/insight/the basics of writing a statement of the problem for your research proposal. Accessed on 14-2-2021.
- Libguides.usc.edu/writing guide/variables. January,21,2021. Accessed on 14-2-2021.

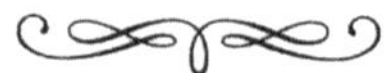

CHAPTER

4 Review of Literature

Swati Kambli

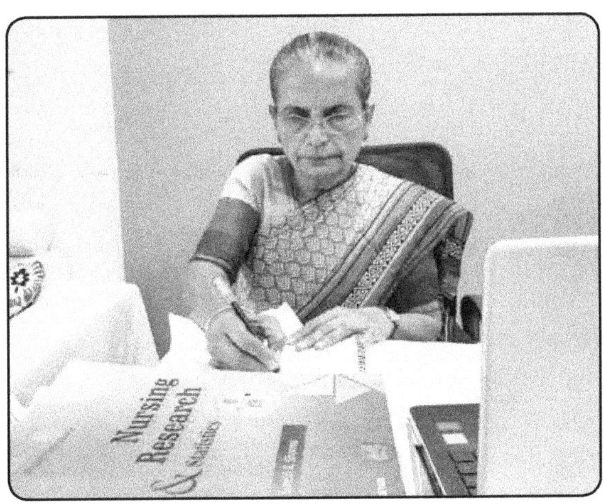

Learning Objectives

This chapter helps the reader to –

- Define the concept of literature review
- Understand the importance of literature review
- Identify the purposes of literature review
- Explain the types of literature review
- Mention the sources of literature review
- Discuss the steps for conducting literature review
- Describe well written literature review
- Develop skills in writing the annotated bibliography

INTRODUCTION

Review of literature is the step in research process. Research is a continuous process. Any investigation is based on previous research studies. A literature review is a broad, comprehensive in depth, systematic, critical review of scholarly publications, unpublished scholarly print materials, audio-visual materials, & personal communications.

- After selection of research problem literature review further helps in refinement & finalization of problem area selected for the study.
- Research makes a contribution for new knowledge, insight, & general scholarship of researches.
- Literature review helps in developing conceptual framework of the study, analysis & interpretation of the results, & making judgments about application of new knowledge in nursing practice.

Definitions

- A literature review is a body of text that aims to review the critical points of knowledge on a particular topic of research. **(ANA, 2000)**
- A literature review summarizes & synthesizes the existing scholarly research on a particular topic. Literature reviews are a form of an academic writing commonly used in the sciences, social sciences, & humanities. However unlike research papers, which establish new arrangements & make original contributions. Literature reviews organize & present existing research. **(www.thoughtco,com/literatureresearch Aug. 5,2019)**
- A literature review is a survey of scholarly sources (such as books, journal articles, & theses) related to a specific topic or research question. It is often written as a part of thesis, dissertation or research paper, in order to situate work in relation to existing knowledge. **(www,scribbr.com/dissertation/literaturereview2020)**
- A literature review surveys books, scholarly articles, & any other sources relevant to a particular issue, area of research, or theory, & by so doing, provides a description, summary, & critical evaluation of these works in relation to the research problem being investigated. **(Robert Labaree, Nov.,2020)**

Importance & Purposes of Literature Review

- It helps in generating research questions, & also helps known & unknown aspects of research area.
- Determines how well theory & research developed in the study.
- Helps in clearly operationally defining the concepts.
- Examines research design, methods, scales, instruments, measures & techniques of data collection & analysis used by others.

- Identify a study for replications/comparison.
- Examine difficulties reported by others.
- Define ethical implications of similar studies &
- Identify a guide to use in writing the research report.
- Describe the relationship of each study to other studies under consideration.
- Identify new ways to interpret & shed light on any gaps in previous research.
- Resolve conflicts amongst seemingly contradictory previous studies.
- Develop general explanation for observed variations in a behavior or phenomena.
- Identify potential relationships between concepts & identify researchable hypothesis.
- Identify data sources that other researchers have used.
- Place one's original work (thesis or dissertation) in context of the existing list.
- Review of literature helps in many ways for development of new research projects/study as following-
  - In selection & formulation of problem
  - Providing conceptual framework for research study
  - Assess practicality of research study
  - Providing methodology
  - Comparison with other studies & replication of study
  - Avoiding obstacles & making generalizations

Types of Literature Review

On the basis of purposes & methodologies, literature review would be broadly classified in following categories-

1. **Traditional or narrative literature review-** This type of literature review presents summary of literature & draws conclusions about the topic in question. The primary purpose of traditional literature review is to offer a comprehensive background of subject under study to understand subject area, identify gaps, inconsistencies in body of knowledge & highlighting the significance of new research. It is very useful in identifying topic for research & till completion of research project. It helps in development of

objectives, hypothesis, theoretical framework, methodology, analysis, & interpretation of data. Narrative literature may also be carried out for non-research purposes like-

- an academic assignment,
- to update knowledge & practice in a field
- to develop & refresh the practice guidelines, specific procedures & policies

2. **Systematic reviews -** The main aim of systematic review is to find the answer for well focused questions of clinical practice. Method used to develop systematic review is similar to be followed for any research study, i.e.—

   A) formulation of research problem

   B) inclusion & exclusion criteria for doing systematic review

   C) selection & access of the literature

   D) criteria to assess the quality of literature reviewed

   E) analyze, synthesize & disseminate the findings

   The systematic review uses explicit & rigorous criteria to identify, critically evaluate, & synthesize all the published & unpublished literature available on particular topic of interest.

3 **Meta-analysis** - It is one of the advanced form of systematic review, which includes a large body of findings from quantitative studies & computes the statistical analysis in order to draw integrated & cumulative inferences & conclusion. Forest plot is used as a means of graphically representing results of meta-analysis of randomized control trials (RCTs). Meta-analysis is used to improve the quality of evidences in a particular area of research, which can be served as the highest level of evidence for generating evidence based practices for the discipline.

4 **Meta-synthesis** - It is a non-statistical technique used to integrate, evaluate, & interpret the findings of multiple qualitative research studies. Findings from phenomenological & ethnographic studies may be integrated & used. Such studies may be combined to identify their core elements & themes. It also involves analyzing & synthesizing important elements in each study, with the aim of transforming individual findings into new conceptualizations & interpretation.

Uses of literature review - can be used for both research & non-research activities.

- **Qualitative approach-** use depends upon selected designs, types & phases.
  A) **Phenomenological-** findings are compared with information from review of literature.
  B) **Grounded theory-** constantly there is comparison of data with literature review.
  C) **Ethnographic-** literature used is more conceptual than data based & provides framework for research study.
  D) **Historical**- review of literature becomes a source of data.
  E) **Action research**- review of literature is being used to identify alternative & final selection of alternative to solve a problem.
  F) **Case study-** uses detailed intensive knowledge about a 'single' or a small number of related cases.

Quantitative designs- The review of literature is used for all designs/levels. It is a step of the research process & used in developing all the steps of research process as follow-

A) Problem finalization

B) Justification/need to conduct study

C) Development of hypotheses, assumptions

D) Development of conceptual or theoretical framework

E) Research design/methodology

F) Specific instrument (testing of validity & reliability)

G) Data collection methods

H) Analysis & interpretation of findings

I) Simplification of findings & comparison with other studies

J) Recommendations based on findings

Use of review of literature: non-research purpose: academic purpose

Major non research focus of the literature reviewed is on uncovering knowledge for use in educational & clinical practice settings.

- Used by students to develop academic scholarly papers & to prepare oral presentations/debates of a topic, problem/issue.
- Used by faculty to develop & revise curricula & to develop theoretical papers for presentations/publications.

Use of review of literature: Nursing practice

I. Evidence based nursing practice

II. Hospitals: development of specific nursing protocols/policies related to patient care

III. Development & substantiate hospital/specifically quality assurance, continuous quality improvement/total quality management projects/ protocols.

IV. Literature review used by professional organizations/government agencies for developing policies & standards for clinical practice & also to develop evidence based practice guidelines.

Sources of Literature Review

To have good literature review, many sources should be tapped to draw together the information about a particular subject under study. These are generally described as primary or secondary sources.

Primary sources - These are original, peer reviewed, & published research journal articles reported by original researchers. So primary sources are research reports, written by researchers who conducted them. Most primary sources are found in published literature e.g. a nursing article. Mainly primary sources are used in most of literature sources.

Secondary sources - These are description of studies prepared by someone other than the individuals who developed the theory or conducted the research. The secondary sources include the comments & summaries of multiple research studies on one topic e.g. systematic reviews, meta-analysis, meta-synthesis etc. The main sources from literature can be searched are electronic database, books, journals, conference papers, theses, encyclopedia, dictionary, research papers, magazines & news papers.

- **Books -** Are acceptable & important source of information. Books should be evaluated on the basis of current date of publication, authors & publishers.
- **Journals** - Professional journals are most valuable resource for researchers. Can be national or international. Bibliography or references section of useful article can help in identifying further meaningful & important sources of literature needed for a particular study. A journal which is referred should be a peer reviewed journal.
- **Conferences -** Papers presented during conferences could be useful for getting the information regarding the topic of research. If the conference is

exactly on the same topic of the research, a lot of information on different dimensions regarding the topic may be obtained.

- **Reports -** Reports from government & other organizations are also useful sources of information.
- **Theses & dissertations -** These are also an excellent source of literature, because each research study includes recommendations for further research.
- **Online sources of literature -** Electronic sources are one of the most important sources of literature searches. The computer databases facilitate access to an enormous quantity of information. It can be retrieved more easily & quickly than a manual search. These databases can be accessed through the internet free of charge in case the library of a college, university, or institute has subscribed these databases. However, many databases ask the private users a fee for downloading an article on a personal computer. A commonly used databases are as follow-
    - **Cumulative Index to Nursing & Allied Health Literature (CINAHL) -** It is the complete source for nursing & allied health journals. It provides full text for more than 580 journals. It provides scholarly journal articles about nursing & allied health. It is accessible at http://www.cinahl.com, it contains citations of nursing literature published after 1988. It also has a paid webpage.
    - **MEDLINE** – (Medical Literature Analysis & Retrieved system online) It is another electronic source of literature review commonly used by nurses. The National Library of Medicine provides free access to MEDLINE through Pubmed, available at www.pubmed.com or http://www.ncbi.nih.gov/entrez/queri.fcgi.

      Generally, abstract of research articles are provided free of cost;

      Some of the full text copies are also freely available & some others are paid services. Medline Plus is the national library of medicines websites for consumer health information available at http://www.medlineplus.gov.
    - **Pub-med -** is a way to access MEDLINE, & can be used to search research abstracts, available at http://www.medlineplus.gov. New citations are added weekly. Pub-med is more current than MEDLINE via EBSCO. The most important feature is that it is freely available.
    - **Registry of Nursing Research -** Sigma Theta Tau International Honour Society of Nursing makes this database available through its Verginia Henderson International Nursing Library. Access to this database is redesigned & made easier for nurses to obtain evidence & scientific

findings from more than 2200 research articles & conference abstracts. Free access to database may be found at http://www.nursinglibrary.org.

- **Cochrane database of systematic reviews -** The Cochrane Library is named after the Scottish doctor named Archie Cochrane. Cochrane Library is a collection of Cochrane reviews that represent the highest level of evidence on which to base clinical treatment decisions. It also conducts & disseminates systematic literature reviews on health care issues. The database is available at http://www.cochrane.org.
- **PsycINFO-** The PsycINFO database belongs to American Psychological Association & covers literature from psychological or related disciplines. It may be searched at http://www.psycinfo.com. It includes journal articles, dissertations, books, technical reports from over 45 countries in more than 30 languages.
- **Scopus -** Elsevier is SCOPUS is the largest abstract & citation database of peer-reviewed literature comprising of scholarly journal articles in the field of science, technology, medicine & social sciences, arts & humanities. Scopus features h-index to track, analyze & visualize research thereby measuring the number of citations of the published work of a researcher.
- **Proquest -** It is an Ann Arbor (a city in US), Michigan based global information content & technology company. Today it provides tools for discovery & citation management & platforms that allow library users to discover, manage, use & share research gained from reliable content. The various contents include dissertations, theses, e books, newspapers, periodicals, historical collections, governmental & cultural archives, & other aggregated databases. Content is accessed most commonly through library internet gateways. Renowned abstracting & indexing makes this information easily navigable, while content tools, including instant bibliography & citation generators, simplify management & sharing of research.

A free Artificial Intelligence powered research tool- Semantic Scholar, a research tool for scientific literature is being developed. The creators of a scientific search engines have unveiled software that automatically generates one sentence summaries of research papers, which they say could help scientists to skim read papers faster. **The free tool, which creates TLDRs (Too Long Didn't Read)** was activated for search results at Semantic Scholar, a search engine created by the non-profit Allen Institute for AI2 in Seattle, Washington. Beginning, the software generates sentences only for ten million computer science papers covered by Semantic Scholar, but papers from other disciplines should be getting summaries within few months. **(Jeffery M. Perkel & Richard Van Noordan 23 Nov., 2020) (nature.com/articles/041586-020-03277-2)**

Characteristics of Relevant Review of Literature

Written summary & critique of each reviewed source of information of particular research project reflects original thinking & scholarly writing content satisfies the following criteria-

1. Purposes of review of literature are met.
2. Summary is adequate representing reviewed source.
3. Objective critical evaluation of literature reviewed reflects proper
4. Literature review uses only primary source & current sources.
5. Sufficient number of sources of literature are used.
6. Summary of reviewed literature is done in a logical manner with conclusion/ synthesis of the reviewed material, which reflects why research study was undertaken.

Skills needed for literature review

- First stage review - to finalize research problem will be general, which can help in focusing from a broader aspect to specific one.
- Second stage review will be more critical to support the research study undertaken.

  While critically analyzing the existing knowledge in the literature, it is essential for the investigator to use his/her critical thinking & reading skills to comprehend the research articles.

Steps of Literature Review

Literature review is a systematic & orderly process, which is undertaken for various reasons such as a step of research process or obtaining information for various other purposes like developing policies & evidence based nursing practice. There are many questions in the mind which can be answered by following appropriate steps of literature review.

Step 1: Understanding the concepts of research problem & identifying the key search terms. The key search terms serve as the foundation for the overall search of literature. These key terms are the important concepts/variables that appear in the research problem.

Step 2: Identifying the relevant sources after identifying the key search terms, a researcher has to locate the relevant sources of the literature review. Electronic literature sources are most commonly preferred sources for literature review because of quick & easy access of vast amount of research database than manual search. Thus it is very essential to judiciously decide the relevant electronic database for literature search.

Step 3: Searching the literature - Traditional methods include searching hard copies of current journals, specially related to the topic of interest. This is slow & tedious task but often a rewarding way of searching a literature. Nowadays searches are undertaken most commonly using a computer or electronic database on search engines. Therefore, identifying & use of key words is the most critical act in literature review. It is very important to consider all the possible keywords, including synonyms & alternative terms, that are related to research topic. The alternative keywords with similar meanings might bring out further information. Another strategy is using 'Boolean Operators' when keywords are combined to facilitate the search. The most commonly used 'Boolean Operators' are 'AND', 'OR' & 'NOT'. They are presented as follow-

Table 4.1: Boolean Operators

Command	Purpose	Example
AND	Look for articles that include all the identified keywords	Abdominal distension/acute abdomen
OR	Look for articles that include any of the identified keywords	Painkillers/analgesics
NOT	Exclude articles that contain the specific word	Lobar pneumonia NOT interstitial pneumonia

It is a common question of this stage how much old literature must one review for a particular study. Generally 3–5 years old literature is ideally included in literature search. Sometimes it may be extended upto ten years, if it is significant & relevant to the research undertaken.

Step 4: Analyzing & synthesizing the literature. After collecting the relevant literature, next step is to analyze & synthesize the reviewed literature. The most popular & simple method is referred to as the preview, question, read, & summarize (PQRS) system. This system facilitates easy identification & retrieval of the relevant literature.

A. **Preview/overview**- It is done through an abstract/summary of articles, given at the beginning of each article, so there is an understanding about article whether it is worthy of inclusion for further reading.

B. **Question, read & summarize -** In this stage the questions are asked of each article under review. An indexing/summary can be used, or a combination or both can be used. Generally the criteria for indexing & summary include the authors year of study, title of article, purpose & methodology of study, main findings & outcome of study. It is also important to include important comments of reviewer of reviewed article. A source & reference is written down.

Step 5: Writing the literature review -

- It is a final step of literature review after completing the adequate appraisal of literature while writing literature review. One need to take care as follow-
  - Essential to avoid long confusing words & jargon & sentences should be precise with one clear message
  - Spelling & grammar must be taken care of
  - Organization of literature should be done in objective manner
  - Approaches can be followed like thematic i.e. dividing literature into themes/categories. Chronological presentation, theoretical vs methodological & theoretical vs empirical organization should be done.
  - The format for writing review should include introduction, body & conclusion of each study. It is more relevant to summarize similar or contrasting studies under a particular theme in a single paragraph.
  - To have a quick look at the reviewed literature a summary table of reviews can be prepared.
  - In conclusion points to be taken care of as follows-
- Main contribution of studies to the body of knowledge for a particular topic under study.
- Specify the gaps, findings, inconsistencies in methodologies, theories, & procedures of literature reviewed.

Step 6: Referring & reviewing final draft of literature. Last step in which the final draft of literature is reviewed for completeness, accuracy & relevance of the content. Specific style of referring to be followed like Vancouver, American Psychological Association etc.

Annotated Bibliography - Annotated bibliography is a list of citations of books, research articles & documents & to each of these citations are followed by a brief description about content & evaluation about its usefulness. (about 150–200 words) as annotation.

Purposes of annotated bibliography-

- To inform readers about the relevance, accuracy & quality of source cited in a particular paper.
- Serve as a guide for other researchers about its usefulness of cited literature to them.
- Helps researchers to comprehend the content of a particular source of literature so that they can include the particular literature in their paper.

Components of annotated bibliography –

Annotated bibliography comprises the following components.

1 Citation - First component is to make citation of article, book or document using prescribed style of bibliography writing such as Vancouver, American Psychological Association (APA), Modern Language Association (MLA), Chicago & so on.

2 Annotation – This is to briefly write the summary of content in approximate 4–7 sentences or 150–200 words, which can vary from university to university based on local policies. Following information is included in annotated bibliography.

   A. Author's background & authority for content.
   B. Central theme of article, book or document
   C. Methodology (if research paper)
   D. Strengths, weaknesses & justification on usefulness of contents
   E. Comparison with other studies on topic
   F. Conclusion about content & source

Process of writing Annotated Bibliography

It requires various academic & intellectual skills like literature search strategies, critical appraisal, & better understanding.

1. Literature source identification relevant to particular topic under study like journals, books, other documents etc.
2. Critical review & appraisal of content for relevance, accuracy, & quality of particular content in the literature source.
3. Choosing relevant content to particular topic from variety of domains & perspectives.

4. Citation of source - prescribed style of bibliography writing to be used like Vancouver, American Psychological Association (APA), Modern Language Association (MLA), Chicago & so on.
5. Annotation writing - brief summary of content for its central theme, strengths, weaknesses, conclusion & evaluative sentence about usefulness of the topic (as brief as 4–7 sentences or 150–200 words).

Example of use of annotated bibliography

Kambli S.V., Mane Nisha, Mistry M.A. - Identification of knowledge of mothers in relation to effect of use of home remedies for diarrhea among infants from Navi Mumbai. The authors are nursing faculties from D. Y. Patil university, Navi Mumbai, & research study was conducted on the topic of identification of knowledge of mothers in relation to effect of use of home remedies for diarrhea among infants from Navi Mumbai. Knowledge of mothers about home remedies easily available at home & used were assessed, observational check list was used to assess diarrheal status among infants. It was identified that certain home remedies like banana, buttermilk were identified in use & control of diarrhea among infants. Other available studies reported similar results.

SUMMARY

- Literature review is very important step in research process. A literature review refers to an extensive, exhaustive & systematic examination of publications & other literature sources relevant to research project undertaken. It provides description, summary & critical evaluation of the works in relation to the research problem being investigated.
- The main type of literature reviews are traditional or narrative, systematic, meta-analysis & meta-synthesis.
- The sources of literature review are primary & secondary. Mostly primary sources are used in most of the literature sources. The original research published in peer reviewed journals categorized as primary sources & literature source written other than original researcher is categorized as secondary source. e.g. meta-analysis, meta-synthesis, systematic reviews & so on.
- The main sources of literature review are electronic database, books, journals, conference papers, theses, dissertations, papers.
- Literature review consists of systematic & orderly steps i.e.
    i. understanding concept of research problem & identification of keywords,

ii. identifying relevant sources
iii. searching literature
iv. analyzing & synthesizing literature
v. writing literature review
vi. referencing & reviewing final draft of literature.

- A list of citation of books, research articles & documents is called as Annotated Bibliography. Also it includes a brief description about content & evaluation about its usefulness (about 150–200 words) as annotation.

BIBLIOGRAPHY

- Carnwell R., Daly w. (2001) Strategies for the construction of critic review of literature. Nurse Education in Practice, 1,57-63.
- Colling J. (2003) Demystifying the clinical nursing research process: The literature review. Urologic Nursing.23 (4), 297-299.
- Coughlan M., Cronin P., Ryan F. (2008) Undertaking a literature review: a step by step approach. British J of Nursing, 7 (1), 38-43.
- Hek G., Langton H. (2000) Systematically searching & reviewing literature. Nurse Researcher, 7 (3), 40-57.
- Libguides.usc.edu/writing guide/literature review. Accessed on 14-2-2021.
- Olivia Valdes. (5,2019) thoughtco.com/literature-review-research-1961252# Accessed on 14-2-2021.
- Timmin F., McCabe C. (2005) How to conduct an effective literature search. Nursing Standard, 20 (11):41-47.
- Patrick L.J., Munro S. (2004) The literature review: Demystifying the literature search. The Diabetes Educator, 30 (1),30-38.
- Younger P. (2004) Using the internet to conduct a literature search. Nursing Standard, 19 (6), 45-51.

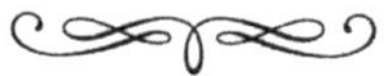

CHAPTER

5 Hypothesis, Assumptions & Delimitations

Swati Kambli

Learning Objectives

This chapter helps the reader to –

- Define assumption, hypothesis & delimitations.
- Identify & enumerate the sources of hypothesis, compare & differentiate.
- Recognize the importance & characteristics of hypothesis.
- Develop skills in formulation of hypothesis, assumptions & delimitations.
- Define delimitations, understand its types & uses.

HYPOTHESIS

Formulation of hypothesis in research is an essential task in the entire research process. A hypothesis is a formal tentative statement of the expected relationship between two or more variables under study. It is a tentative solution to a research problem or question. The research hypothesis is the first step & basis of all research endeavours. The research hypothesis shows the direction to the researcher conducting the research. It states what the researcher expects to find from the study. It is a tentative answer that guides the entire research study.

Hypothesis in Quantitative Research

Consists of one independent & one dependent variable & the hypothesis mentions the expected relationship between both variables.

- When both variables are used in continuous nature, then it is easy to describe negative or positive relationship between both of them. In case of categorical variables, the hypothesis statement indicates about which category of independent variables are associated with which group of dependent variables.
- The null hypothesis also be used between two variables which state that there is no relationship between the variables. The null hypothesis is the basis of all types of statistical research.

Hypothesis in Qualitative Research

Hypothesis in qualitative research is rarely used or many times not used at all in qualitative types of research studies. Role of hypothesis is different as compared to its role in quantitative research.

- The hypothesis is not developed at the beginning of research due to inductive nature of qualitative research. Hypothesis is introduced during data collection process & interpretation of data.
- The hypothesis helps the researchers consider more questions & find out answers for disconfirming evidence.

Hypothesis is being defined by various experts as follows-

Definitions

- **Walter R. Bory** states that hypothesis reflects the research workers' guesses to the probable outcomes of their experiment. It places clear & specific goals before the researchers & provide them with a basis for selecting samples & research procedures to meet these goals.
- **Polit & Beck** define hypothesis as a statement of researcher's expectations about the relationship between the variables under study.
- **Hitesh Bhasin (Sept.2020)** defines hypothesis as a clear, specific & predictive statement that states the possible outcome of a scientific study. The result of the research study is based on previous research studies & can be tested by scientific research.

  The abovementioned definitions of hypothesis emphasize about outcomes of research study, development of clear & specific goals, basis to follow accurate research methodology, to achieve set goals for research study. These definitions also focus on prediction of relationships between variables under study & scientifically testifying the results of research study undertaken.

Importance of Hypothesis in Research

Research works are developed to verify hypothesis so a researcher of course, would understand the meaning, nature & importance of hypothesis in order to formulate & test it. The important characteristics given below will help researcher to formulate the hypothesis for study accurately.

- Hypothesis helps the researcher to investigate objectively new areas of discovery.
- To use it as powerful tool for the advancement of knowledge.
- To get clear direction to conduct research.

- To set clear specific goals for research undertaken, so that it becomes a basis for selection of sample & procedures to achieve these goals.
- It provides a link between theories & actual practical research & bridges a gap between theory & reality.
- It helps in identifying & following the type of research which is likely to be most appropriate.
- It helps in stimulating the thinking process clearly in understanding about what to expect from the results & drawing conclusions of a research study.

Characteristics of a Good Hypothesis

Good, specific & clear hypothesis must be written in declarative statements, using present tense. It has 3 elements i.e. variables, population under study & relationship between variables. Also it should be relevant to the phenomena under study, so that it can be easily tested. Following are the characteristics of good hypothesis-

- It has conceptual clarity by clearly defining concepts.
- It must have empirical basis from the area of inquiry. Hypothesis must be based on concepts that are empirically tested.
- Hypothesis facilitates objectivity in data collection process & keeps research activity from researcher's value, judgment or bias. So there is clarity about what to measure.
- It should be specific & not too broad or general & clearly explains relationship between variables.
- It should be relevant to the research problem under study & objectives of the study.
- It should clearly state the manipulable independent variable & measurable dependent variable in a specific population, giving clear idea of an interventional protocol how dependent variable is accurately measured in the study. Hypothesis is tested through inferential statistical tests to identify the effect of independent variable on dependent variable.
- It should be consistent with existing body of theories & knowledge, research findings & other hypothesis of the study.
- It should be written in simple language & understandable terms.
- A good hypothesis can be verified in practical terms.
- It should have profound effect upon a variety of research variables.
- It should be economical in terms of requirement of manpower, money & material etc.

Sources of Hypothesis

Hypothesis are generated from variety of sources, such as theoretical or conceptual frameworks, previous research findings, real life experiences & academic literature.

Research study is based upon a **specific theory**, so the hypothesis should be relevant to the theoretical or conceptual frameworks for testing them e.g. a study is based upon theory of Emogene King, where a hypothesis can be drawn from a concept of theoretical mode that teaching specific neurological interventions to mothers of children with hydrocephalus & ventriculoperitoneal shunt will maintain intracranial pressure at normal level in children.

- **Previous research findings** - Findings of previous studies may be used for development of hypothesis for another study. e.g. in a small sample descriptive study it is identified that persons affected with cerebrovascular accident had history of hypertension. In another research study a researcher may use findings to develop hypothesis as 'persons with hypertension are at risk for development of cerebrovascular accident,
- **Real life experiences** – Also contribute in the forming of hypothesis for research studies. e.g. domestic violence in women may lead to depression in women.
- **Academic literature** - It is based on formal theories, empirical evidences, experiences, observations & conceptualizations academicians, so literature may serve as a good source for developing hypothesis for research studies.

TYPES OF HYPOTHESIS

Simple & Complex

Simple hypothesis – Statement reflects the relationship between two variables. e.g. The higher the blood glucose levels, more chances for developing various infectious diseases among persons diagnosed with diabetes.

Complex hypothesis – In which the statement reflects relationship between more than two variables. e.g. Incidence of psychiatric illnesses are lower among persons performing yoga & physical exercises regularly than persons following only physical exercises.

Associative & Causal Hypothesis

Associative hypothesis - It states the relationship between variables that occurs or exists in natural settings without manipulation. Mainly used in correlational studies. e.g. Lower the low density lipoprotein blood levels, lesser the risk of developing coronary artery disease among obese individuals.

Causal hypothesis - It predicts cause & effect relationship between two or more independent & dependent variables in experimental or interventional studies where independent variable is manipulated by the researcher to examine the effect on dependent variable e.g. Effects of planned instructions and demonstrations about precautionary measures like use of mask, frequent hand washing and social distancing on occurrence of Covid 19 infections in adults from Mumbai city.

Directional & Nondirectional Hypothesis

Directional hypothesis – It specifies not only the existence, but also the expected direction of the relationship between variables. It states the relationship between two or more variables like positive or negative or no relationship. The directional terms are used to state hypothesis as positive, negative, less, more, increased, decreased, greater, higher, lower etc. e.g. There is a positive relationship between educational status of nurses & quality care provided by them to patients.

Nondirectional hypothesis - It reflects the relationship between two or more variables but it does not specify the anticipated direction & nature of relationship as positive or negative. It shows only the existence of relationship between the variables. e.g. There is a relationship between educational status of nurses & quality care provided by them to patients.

Null & Research Hypothesis

Null hypothesis (Ho) - It is also known as statistical hypothesis & is used for statistical testing & interpretation of statistical outcomes. It states the existence of no relationship between the independent & dependent variables. e.g. There is no relationship between consumption of gutkha & occurrence of oral cancer among human beings.

Research hypothesis - also known as alternate hypothesis. It states the existence of relationship between two or more variables. e.g. there is a relationship between consumption of gutkha & occurrence of oral cancer among human beings.

A research hypothesis can be simple, complex, associative, causal, directional & nondirectional. However, commonly recommended to use directional hypothesis.

Formulating a hypothesis - Hypothesis usually formulated in quantitative studies, which investigate the relationship between independent & dependent variables such as experimental & correlational studies. While in other studies use of hypothesis is not is not much effective. The formulation of hypothesis is one of the most difficult steps in the entire scientific research process. Therefore, certain steps to be followed in the formulation of hypothesis are as follows–

1. **Define variables** - First step is to define variables. Important concepts or variables are to be clearly defined. Variables should be quantifiable & measurable, which will guide for effective outcome or results of research study.
2. **Study the variables in depth** – An in depth study, rigorous questions will make researcher to confirm hypothesis. Independent & dependent variables are to be specified.
3. **The nature of relationship of variables to be specified.** Relationship between variables to be identified.
4. **Study population to be decided** - Entire population may not be participating in the study, so accessible population to be identified to participate in the study.
5. **It should be made sure that variables are testable** – If variables are not testable then the hypothesis will be worthless. Testable variables can only be accepted or rejected.

Steps of Hypothesis Testing

1. State hypothesis in null (Ho) & alternate (Ha) hypothesis. Several research experts argue that it is more desirable to state hypothesis in directional form. As these hypothesis clarify the study framework & demonstrate that researchers have thought critically about the phenomena under study.
2. Data collection should be done in a way designed to test hypothesis.
3. Inferential statistical tests to be used to test the hypothesis.
4. It is to be decided whether null hypothesis is supported or rejected. It is very clear that when null hypothesis is rejected, research hypothesis is accepted & vice a versa. Ideally hypothesis should be restricted to six or less as more numbers of hypothesis will lead to chaos.
5. Analyze & interpret the findings of the study.

Criteria for evaluation of research hypothesis

1. Statement evaluation - check for clarity, precision, whether in declarative form & use of present tense.
2. It should be relevant to research problem, objectives, variables, operational definitions & relevant theories.
3. Whether independent & dependent variables are included.
4. Population under study is included.

5. Empirical testing is possible or not?
6. Is there a single prediction of relationships of study variables?
7. Setting of level of significance for testing hypothesis.

Assumptions

An assumption is a belief which does not have empirical evidences to support it. Assumptions provide a basis to develop theories, research instruments etc & therefore, influence the development & implementation of research process. Assumptions are an essential & integral part of the research.

Definitions

- **W. Pol Vogt** defines an assumption as a statement that presumed to be true, often only temporarily or for a special purpose, such as,
  a) building a theory,
  b) the conditions under which statistical techniques yield valid results.
- Assumptions are statements that are taken for granted or are considered as true, even though they have not been scientifically tested.
- Assumptions are principles which are accepted as being true based on logic or reasons, but without proof or verification.

Table 5.1: Differences between assumption & hypothesis

	Hypothesis	Assumption
Definition	is a tentative prediction or explanation of the relationship between two or more variables	principles that are accepted as being true based on logic or reasons
Testing	tested through statistical methods & then accepted or rejected	not tested through statistical but helps in formulation of hypothesis
Reasoning	supported by logical reasoning	may be supported by logical reasoning
Uses	Primarily used in experimental & correlational studies	used in descriptive, exploratory, explanatory & qualitative research

Uses of Assumption in Research

- Forms a ground or basis to progress in research study.
- Guides research questions, evidence investigation, conclusion & generalization of research study.
- Becomes good sources of hypothesis.
- Assumptions found to be true through research studies help in the advancement of professional knowledge.

Delimitations & Limitations

- **Delimitations** are restrictions identified by the researchers before starting of the study & these are mentioned in the initial chapter of the dissertation or thesis. Many times delimitations & limitations are interchangeably used by the researchers.
- **Limitations** are the challenges or difficulties faced by the researcher during the course of the study & mentioned in the last chapter of the dissertation or thesis, which are necessary to inform the readers about drawbacks on credibility of the evidences generated through this particular research.
- The concept of **delimitations** may be clearly understood from the following points-
  - Delimitations are boundaries set by researcher to control range of a study. They are thought about before commencement of the research study; may be sometimes seen to unnecessary, or not related to research study.
  - There are certain inclusion & exclusion criteria decided like region, study setting, sample size, the variables studied, the theoretical perspectives, the instruments, the generalizability etc.

Uses of Delimitations

Delimitation is used to make the study better & more practical. It also identifies restrictions of research study which is not within the control of researcher. Delimitation helps the researcher to-

- Define the boundaries of selected study parameters like region or area, age, gender, population characteristics, sample size, instrument used for study & other considerations.
- Identify constrains before starting study so that strengthening of evidences generated through study may be determined.
- Mention of delimitations in the study, can give an idea of credibility & generalizability of the research findings.

How to Write Delimitations?

The researcher should take care as follows–

- Write delimitation with reasons for not considering certain parameters in the research study.
- Describe delimitation clearly but in concise form.
- Identify & mention the intended impact of each delimitation in relation to the overall findings & conclusion of the study.

SUMMARY

- The research hypothesis is the first step & basis of all reseach endeavours. It shows direction to the researchers conducting the research. A hypothesis is a statement about the relationship between two or more variables. Researchers set the variables to prove or disprove. Hypothesis essentially includes three elements. i.e. variables, population & relationship between variables.
- In quantitative studies research hypothesis consists of an independent & dependent variable & mentions the expected relationship between the two variables. It is a trend to use directional hypothesis as a research hypothesis. The null hypothesis is the basis of all types of statistical research.
- Role of research hypothesis in qualitative research is different as compared to its role in quantitative research. Hypothesis in qualitative research is introduced during the process of data collection & interpretation phase.
- Hypothesis directs researcher in setting clear goals, bridges gap between theory & practical, directs researcher throughout research study.
- A good hypothesis has characteristics like it has conceptual clarity, facilitates objectivity in research study & keeps research activity from researchers value, judgment & bias. Hypothesis should be specific, relevant to phenomena to be studied, testable etc.
- Hypothesis is generated from variety of sources like theoretical or conceptual frameworks, previous research findings, real life experiences & academic literature etc.
- Types of hypothesis are simple & complex, associative & causal, directional & non-directional & null & research hypothesis. A research hypothesis can be simple, complex, directional, non-directional, associative, causal. However commonly recommended to use directional hypothesis in research.
- An assumption is a belief which does not have empirical evidences to support it. Assumptions provide a basis to develop theories, research instruments etc & therefore influence the development & implementation of research process. Assumptions are essential & integral part of the research.
- The main difference between hypothesis & assumption is that hypothesis is tested statistically, then accepted or rejected. Assumptions are not statistically tested. Hypothesis is used commonly in experimental & correlational studies. Assumptions are used in descriptive, exploratory & qualitative research.
- Assumptions form a basis for progress of research study.
- Delimitations are restrictions identified by researcher before starting of the study & they are mentioned in the initial chapters of the dissertation or thesis. There is difference between delimitations & limitations as limitations

are challenges or difficulties faced by the researcher during the course of the study & mentioned in the last chapter of the dissertation or thesis.

BIBLIOGRAPHY

- Iedunote.com/research-hypothesis-accessed on 15-2-2021.
- Shona McCombes. Revised on 22-10-2020.scribbr.com/research-process/hypotheses. Accessed on 15-2-2021.
- Durek Jansen, June, 2020. What is a Research Hypothesis? gradcoach.com/what-is-a research-hypothesis? Accessed on 15-2-2021.
- Researchprospect.com/how-to-write-a-hypothesis? Accessed on 15-2-2021.
- Readingcraze.com/index.php/what-is-research-hypothesis? Accessed on 15-2-2021.
- William G. Wargo. (August,19, 2015) Identifying Assumptions & Limitations for your dissertations. Academicinfocenter.com/identifying-assumptions-&-limitations-for-your-dissertation.html. Accessed on 15-2-2021.

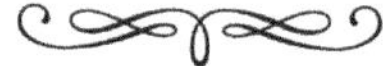

CHAPTER

6 Developing a Theoretical or Conceptual Frameworks in Nursing Research

Swati Kambli

Learning Objectives

This chapter helps the reader to –

- Define specific terms related to theoretical & conceptual framework.
- Describe characteristics of theoretical & conceptual framework.
- Explain the role of theoretical & conceptual framework in nursing research.
- Understand the concept of theory testing & theory development.
- Develop skills in formulation of conceptual & theoretical framework to guide the research work.

A high quality research study always have a high level conceptual or theoretical integration. This means, the research questions are appropriate for the chosen methods & strategies & also conceptual rationale, as a guide for progress & successful outcome of research study. Theories, concepts, models & frameworks are the primary mechanisms by which researchers organize the whole study into a broader conceptual context. The connection of conceptual context for research has several terms such as conceptual map, schematic diagram, model, framework & theories. Theory describing a phenomena under study should be integrated with research. This chapter discusses theoretical & conceptual contexts for nursing research problems.

THEORY

Classically scientists have used theory to refer to an abstract generalization of a phenomenon. This type of theory is referred as descriptive theory as this theory can account for a single phenomena. Descriptive theory plays an important role in qualitative research. Sometimes descriptive theories may become the foundation for the generation of predictive & explanatory theories. Development of theory is fundamental to the research process where it is necessary to use theory as a framework to provide perspective &

guidance to the research study. Theory can also be used to guide the research process by creating & testing the phenomena of interest. To improve nursing profession's ability to meet the societal duties & responsibilities, there need to be a continuous reciprocal & cyclical connection with the theory, practice & research. This will help connect the perceived "gap" between theory & practice & promote theory guided practice.

DEFINITIONS

- Theory is a belief, policy or procedure proposed or followed as the basis of action. It refers to a logical group of general propositions used as principles of explanation. Theories are also used to describe, predict or control phenomena.
- Theory is often defined as an abstract generalization that explains how phenomena are interrelated. As classically defined, theories consist of two or more concepts & a set of propositions that form a logically interrelated system, providing a mechanism for deducing hypotheses **(www.nurselabs.com/nursing theories, December 2020)**
- A theory is a set of interrelated concepts, definitions & propositions that present a systematic view of phenomenon by specifying relations among variables with the purpose of explaining & predicting the phenomenon (**Kerlinger 1973).**
- A theory is a statement that purports to account for or characterize some phenomenon & that it pulls out the salient parts of phenomenon so that one can separate the critical & necessary factors or relationships from accidental unessential factors (**Barnum, 1990).**

  The abovementioned definitions given by specially the www.nurselabs.com & **Kerlinger,** are comprehensive definitions of theory, emphasizing systematic view of phenomena with the help of interrelationships of concepts of phenomena, helping for deducing of hypotheses of research study undertaken.

CLASSIFICATION OF NURSING THEORIES

There are different ways to categorize nursing theories. They are classified depending on levels of abstraction or goal orientation & various other ways. **By Abstraction-** There are three major categories when classifying nursing theories based on their level of abstraction: **grand, middle range & practice level or micro theories.**

Grand Nursing Theories

- They are abstract, broad in scope & complex, so require further research for classification.
- Do not provide guidance for specific nursing interventions but rather provide a general framework & ideas about nursing.
- Theorists develop their works based on their own experiences.
- Address the nursing metaparadigm components as: person, environment, health & nursing.
- In addition, grand theories may provide the foundation for middle-range theories.
- Some of the **grand theories** of nursing are-
  - **Florence Nightingale**: Nightingale's environmental theory. (1860)
  - **Rosemarie Rizzo Parse**: Theory of human becoming. (1981-1992)
  - **Verginia Henderson**: Theory of nursing needs. (1960)
  - **Dorothy Johnson**: The behavioural system model. (1990)
  - **Martha E Rogers**: Nursing: A science of Unitary Human Beings. (1970,1990)
  - **Dorothea Orem**: The self-Care Deficit Nursing Theory. (2001)
  - **Callista Roy**: Roy Adaptation Model. (2009)
  - **Parse:** Human Becoming Paradigm. (2014)

Middle Range Nursing Theories

These theories are limited in scope & present concepts & propositions at a lower level of abstraction. They address specific phenomena in nursing.

- Nursing scholars proposed using this level of theory.
- Most of the theories are based on the works of grand theorists. But can be conceived from research, nursing practice, or theories of other disciplines.
- Some of the examples of middle range theories are-
  - Theory of unpleasant symptoms. **(Lenz et al, 2009)**
  - Theory of holistic comfort. **(Kocaba, 1994.2009)**
  - Theory of Flight Nursing Expertise. **(Reimure & Moore, 2010)**
  - Theory of post-partum depression. **(Becks, 2012)**

- Theory of Health Promotion Model. **(Pender & colleagues 2006, 2016)**

Practice Level/Micro Theories

These theories are situation specific, narrow in scope & focus on specific patient population at a specific time.

- These theories describe, explain or provide understanding of the patient's experiences of specific phenomena.
- They provide frameworks for nursing interventions & suggest outcomes or the effect of nursing practice. They are also known as prescriptive theories.
- They are interrelated with concepts from middle range theories or grand theories.
- Some examples of situation specific theories in nursing are–
  - Theory of Caucasian cancer pain experience. **(Im, 2010)**
  - Theory of Heart Failure Self care. **(Riegel & Dickson, 2008)**
  - Theory of Asian Immigrant Women's Menopausal Symptom experiences in the USA, **(Im, 2010)**

Classification of theories by Goal Orientation-

These theories can be classified based on their goals, can be descriptive & prescriptive.

Descriptive Theories

- This is the first level of the theory development. They describe the phenomena & identify its properties & components in which it occurs.
- They are not action oriented or attempt to produce or change a situation.
- **There are two types of descriptive theories: Factor isolating & explanatory theory.**
- **Factor isolating theory is also known as category formulating or labelling.**
- These theories describe the properties & dimensions of phenomena. e.g. Theory of unpleasant symptoms **(Lenz et al, 2009)**
- **Explanatory theory -** Describe & explain the nature of relationship of certain phenomena to other phenomena. e.g. Asian Immigrant Women's Menopausal symptom experiences in USA **(Im 2010)**

- **Prescriptive theory** - Addresses the nursing interventions for a phenomenon, guide practice change & predict consequences.
  - Includes propositions that call for change.
  - Used to anticipate the outcomes of nursing interventions.
  - Example of prescriptive theory is 'Theory of Heart Failure Self-care, **(Riegeland Dickson, 2008)**

Building Blocks of Theories

The nursing theories have five basic building blocks; these are **concepts, constructs, conceptual definitions, relational statements & conceptual models.**

Concepts - A concept is an idea, especially an abstract idea or notion. It has been evolved from Latin word conceptum i.e. ' something conceived'. They are primarily the vehicles of thought that involve images. Concepts need to be defined within the context of their use to be understood. Concept can be classified as abstract of concrete concepts. An example of concrete concept is nursing competency & example of concrete concept is an intra-muscular injection.

Construct - The meaning of word 'construct' is to make or to create. It is to build, to create a story, a theory or a sentence by systematically arranging/ organizing number of simple elements such as ideas, terms, words etc. Constructs are defined as the building blocks of theories that help to describe the phenomenon. They help to explain different components of theory. The constructs can be observed/measured directly & indirectly. Directly measured constructs are height, weight, blood pressure etc. Indirectly measured constructs are satisfaction, happiness etc.

Conceptual definitions - Concepts may have more than one definition so it is necessary to have a clear & accurate definition of concept used in a particular theory or research is explicitly defined at the outset even if the concept seems to be very basic & uncomplicated. Thus conceptual definitions are clearly stated meanings of the abstract idea.

- In recent years, concept analysis has become an important enterprise among students & health scholars. Several methods have been proposed for undertaking a concept analysis & clarifying conceptual definitions **(e.g. Walker & avant, 2011).** Efforts to analyse concepts of relevance to nursing should facilitate greater conceptual clarity among nursing researchers. Here is an example of developing a conceptual definition. **RamZani & colleagues (2014) used Walker & Avant, (2011) eight step concept analysis** to conceptually define spiritual care in nursing. They searched & analyzed national & international databases & found 151 relevant articles & books. They proposed the following definition.

The attributes of spiritual care are healing presence, therapeutic use of self, intuitive sense, exploration of spiritual perspective, patient centeredness, meaning centered therapeutic intervention & creation of spiritually nurturing environment.

- **Relational statements -** Relational statements enable the theorist to state the expected relationship among the concepts. Relationship statements can be described as the positive or negative relationship, direct or indirect effects or linear or nonlinear associations among concepts.
- **Conceptual model -** A conceptual model broadly presents an understanding of group of phenomena in which interrelated phenomena are linked together for interpretation. In other words, conceptual model is a careful description of the concepts & the relationships among them. Models may be simple, representing only a small number of concepts & relationships, or may be quite complex & multifaceted; & when they are tested through research, they give rise to theory. Two types of models used in research contexts are **schematic & statistical models**.
- **Schematic** or conceptual models visually represent relationships among phenomena & are used in both qualitative & quantitative research. Concepts & linkages between them are depicted graphically through boxes, arrows or other symbols.
- **Statistical models** are equations that mathematically express relationships among a set of variables & that are tested statistically.

MODELS & FRAMEWORKS

Models - Models are representations of the interaction among & between the concepts showing patterns. They present an overview of the thinking behind the theory & may demonstrate how theory can be introduced into practice.

Frameworks - A framework is the conceptual underpinning of a study. Not every study is based on theory or model but every study has a framework. In a study based on theory, the framework is called theoretical framework. In a study that has its roots in a conceptual model, the framework may be called the conceptual framework. However, the terms conceptual framework, conceptual model & theoretical framework are often used interchangeably.

- In qualitative research within a tradition, the framework is part of that tradition. e.g. ethnographers generally begin within a theory of culture. Grounded theory researchers incorporate sociological principles into their framework & approach. The research question selected for qualitative study inherently reflect certain theoretical formulations. The research studies are being done either to develop or test theory.
- Thus conceptual or theoretical frameworks are required in research studies for following purposes.
  - Helps to stimulate research & extent of knowledge.
  - Useful in clarifying concepts, variables & their relationship.
  - Helps in formulating research questions & hypotheses.
  - Provides structure for examining a research problem.
  - Helps to guide in research process like planning, developing strategies, selecting tools, in an implementation process.
  - Developing interventions to promote Evidence Based Nursing Practice.
  - Allows easier generalization of the knowledge gained by the research endeavour.

USING THEORY IN RESEARCH

Stewart & Klein (2016) identified that theories can be applied at many stages of research process, including providing justification for the research study, formulating research questions; methodology, data collection methods/tools & procedures & framework for data analysis & interpretation. However use of theory in research is done three ways i.e. theory testing, use of theory as a framework & theory development as an outcome of the research.

Use of Theory in Quantitative Research

- Used mainly for testing or verifying, which provides explanation for a research question
- Well integrated with whole research study.
- It is suggested by eminent researchers that theory used must be included as an entirely separate section in the research proposal, so that researchers explicitly understand the use of theory in research.

Use of Theory in Qualitative Research

- Qualitative research like grounded theory, the final outcome of research is the development of a new theory.
- In other qualitative research studies like ethnography research, theory is used in the beginning, which provides guidance for research question, hypotheses & methodology of the study.
- Use of theory in mixed method research could be both as the testing & theory generating, or it can guide the whole research study.
- **Silvia (1986)** identified three different ways in which nursing theories were incorporated in nursing research, as follows-
    - Some studies there was minimal use of theory. Theoretical framework was used but no incorporation of theory in the studies was observed.
    - Second approach, concepts from theories were used to organize the research usually for descriptive rather than theory testing purposes.
    - In third way, adequate use of model for theory testing is characterized by explicit indication of model use along with a study purpose for determining the model's validity. Hypotheses are tested in appropriate manner & research findings are analysed in a manner that they offer support for or against theory & or possible revision of theory.
- It is being observed that there is minimal use of theories in nursing research studies & theory is explicitly identified research framework but minimally integrated into research study.
- Theory also can be used to guide research process by creating & testing phenomena of interest.
- To improve nursing profession's ability to meet the societal duties & responsibilities, there need to be a continuous reciprocal & cyclical connection with theory, practice & research. This will help connect the perceived 'gap' between theory & practice & promote the theory guided practice.

TESTING & DEVELOPING THEORIES

Theory testing is being done deductive reasoning approach, where researcher proceeds from general (theory) to specific (empirical findings), while theory development is accomplished by inductive reasoning process, where researcher proceeds from the specific (empirical findings) to the general (theory).

- Theory testing is done through quantitative research studies.
- Qualitative research studies like grounded theory research considered as theory generating research.
- Theory testing is relatively easier than theory generating.

Theory Testing

Quantitative research studies are theory testing or theory verifying research studies, where theories are tested through deductive reasoning approach.

Following Steps are followed for Theory Testing

- Identification of research question & hypotheses from theory to be tested.
- Variables derived from theory are defined & operationalized.
- In data collection process variables are observed & measured.
- Hypotheses are tested to confirm/disconfirm of theory. (Results & conclusion of the study)
- **Evaluation of theory testing research Acton, Irvin & Hopkins (1991)** built a theory based on **Silvia's** work by suggesting 15 specific criteria useful to evaluate theory testing research studies. These criteria are listed below-
    1. The statement of purpose specifies theoretical testing.
    2. The researcher makes the underlying theory explicit & summarizes it appropriately.
    3. Concepts or construct is defined in terms of theory.
    4. Prior studies based on selected theoretical framework are included in the literature review or are derived from the concepts that are clearly shown in current study.
    5. The researchers use the tenets of the theory to logically arrive at their research questions.
    6. By using very specific hypotheses, the theory can be approved or disapproved or refined.
    7. The operational definitions of the study are clearly generated by terms of the theory.
    8. The theory & research design are philosophically congruent.

9. Instruments used to test the theory have adequate reliability & validity.
10. The choice of sample selected for the study is guided by theory.
11. Researchers should use strongest statistics into the study.
12. In data analysis, the researchers should offer support for or against & or possible revision of the theory.
13. Analysis with interpretation of findings related to theory must appear in the research report.
14. The research report considers the impact of theory on nursing.
15. The researchers offer suggestions for the revision of the study & more studies based on their theoretical findings.

Theory Development Process

A theory is an explanation or model based on observation, experimentation & reasoning, especially one that has been tested & confirmed as a general principle helping to explain & predict natural phenomena. Theory development in nursing is an essential component in nursing scholarship for professional knowledge advancement. The legitimacy of any profession is built on its ability to generate & apply theory **(McCrae 2011).** Nursing theories that clearly set forth understanding of nursing phenomena i.e. self care, therapeutic communication etc. guide scholarly development of science of nursing through research. Scientific evidence accumulates through repeated rigorous research that supports or refutes theoretical assertions & guides modifications or extensions of theory. Nursing theory development is a scholarly endeavour pursued systematically. Rigorous development of nursing theories is a high priority for the future of the discipline & nursing practice.

Theory components - Development of theory requires understanding of selected scholarly terms, definitions & assumptions so that scholarly review & analysis may occur. Attention is given to terms & defined meanings to understand theory development process that was used. Therefore, the clarity of terms, their scientific utility & their value to the discipline are important considerations in the process. It is a systematic & rigorous process; which is accomplished through some of the qualitative research studies as grounded theory research. **Hage (1972)** identified six theory components & specified the contributions they make to theory development process.

Table 6.1: Theory components & their contribution to theory

Theory components	Contribution to theory
Concept & definitions	
Concept	Describe & classify phenomena
Theoretical definitions of concept	Establish meaning
Operational definitions of concepts	Provide measurement
Rational statements	
Theoretical statements	Relate concepts to one another, permit analysis
Operational statements	Relate concepts to measurements
Linkage & ordering	
Linkage theoretical statements	Provide rationale of why statements are linked:add plausibility
Linkage operational statements	Provide rationale of how measurement variables are linked: permit testability
Organization of concepts & definitions into primitive & derived terms	Eliminates overlap (tautology)
Organization of statements & linkage into primitive & derived hypotheses & equations	Eliminates inconsistency

Three categories of theory components are presented as a basis for understanding the function of each element in the theory building process.

- Theory development process begins with analysing & clearly defining the concepts. Theoretical definitions are essential to explicitly define the concepts & to avoid any ambiguity in understanding the concepts. Then conceptual definitions are converted into operational definitions which provide observable & measurable definitions of concepts.
- Next step of theory development is to identify relationship between two or more concepts through theoretical & operational statements. Concepts must be connected with one another in a series of theoretical statements to devise a nursing theory.
- Linkage & orderly statements are vital for logical understanding. Then, concepts & statements are organized to eliminate the possibility of overlapping & inconsistency. Thus, the first step of theory development is to build a conceptual model or framework to understand & define phenomena of interest & second step is to build relationship between

related concepts with linkage. Finally, the relationship statements or propositions are developed to develop a theory.

Evaluation of Theory Development Research

Silvia & Sorrell (1992) proposed the following evaluation criteria for the theory development research studies.

1. The purpose of the studies is to verify the relationship of described personal experiences to philosophical beliefs & assumptions that underline the development of nursing theory.
2. Identification of the research questions (s) is based on an attempt to provide elaboration of concepts related to the development of nursing theory.
3. The primary data sources include sufficient in-depth description of personal experiences to capture the essence of phenomena under investigation.
4. Simplicity, ethical integrity & aesthetic presentation are integral characteristics of the described personal experiences.
5. Analysis of data incorporates a sense of wholeness of the described personal experiences
6. Formative hypotheses and/or theories are derived inductively from qualitative analysis of the described personal experiences.
7. Multiple personal experiences of individual & or similar personal experiences of several individuals about a particular phenomena are used to validate the derived hypotheses.
8. Analytic procedure of data analysis & generated concepts of the personal experiences provide indirect evidence of the validity of the developed nursing theory.
9. Findings are discussed in terms of how they are related to the theories developed & tested inductively; both the developing & existing theories must be internally consistent & congruent with one another.

Developing Conceptual or Theoretical Framework & Models

Developing an effective theoretical/conceptual framework: steps to be followed—

Identification of general concepts

- Examining research problem which forms the basis from which framework to be constructed.

- Identification of key variables in research. Also assessing factors contributing to the presumed effect.

Gathering relevant information

- Review of literature is done to find out how research scholars have addressed the research studies similar to the study undertaken.
- Relevant nursing theories are reviewed & selected which can best explain the relationships between the key variables in the study.

Formulation of general scheme of relevant concepts

- Variables to be grouped as independent & dependent category.
- Assumptions & propositions of selected theories need to be stated focusing on their relevance to the research study under investigation.

Development of logical construct

- After establishing the logical relationship between two variables, the researcher develops a final construct. Construct term is used to indicate a phenomenon that cannot be directly observed but must be inferred by certain concrete or less abstract indicators of the phenomenon.
- Connections or linkages are to be shown between different related & relevant concepts with the help of arrows & should be related to the desired outcomes. A good diagram helps in quicker visualization & identification of the interdependency between the various concept/variables. The end point of the conceptual framework should reflect desired outcome of the research undertaken.
- There is no universal rule or procedure to draw a conceptual framework. It should be simple with minimum data but getting maximum understanding while viewing it.

Evaluation & revision

Concepts & constructs act as the building blocks for the framework, which later evaluated for their relevance & relationship to conclude or generalize the facts. After the evaluation, revisions may be made before development of a framework. Following criteria is used to evaluate the theoretical framework.

- Consistency of framework with the research question, design, variables & interpretation of the study.

- Identification & defining of major concepts.
- Description of relationship among concepts within model.
- Concepts whether help in testing & generation of theory.

Establishment of the congruity

Once a framework is developed, it is important to establish the congruity between conceptual model & its components, the research problem, hypotheses, the description of operationalization concepts & the selection of research design. In the real sense, congruity of framework may only be established if most of the research decisions & interpretations of the study findings are based on the framework.

Conceptual models developed by experts in nursing

Several experts in nursing have formulated conceptual models representing explanations of what the nursing discipline is & what the nursing process entails. As **Fawcett & DeSanto Madeya (2013) have noted four concepts which are central to models of nursing: human beings, environment, health & nursing.** The various conceptual models define these concepts differently, link them in diverse ways & emphasize different relationships among them. Moreover, the models emphasize different processes being central to nursing.

Other alternative models used in nursing (nursekey.com)

Several alternative models have gained prominence in the development of nursing interventions to promote health enhancing behaviours & life choices. Non nursing theories have frequently been used in nursing studies as follow-

- **Bandura's social cognitive theory 2001**
- **Prochaska et al: Transtheoretical model of stages of change 2002.**
- **Becker: The health belief model 1974.**
- **Ajzen: Theory of planned behaviour.**
- **Theories from other related disciplines like social behavioural sciences are also used in nursing.**

Example of conceptual or theoretical framework

A study to develop skills of caregivers in providing home care to maintain thermoregulation in preterm neonates.

The conceptual framework of the abovementioned is based on 'Bertalanffy's General System Theory model which was given by **Ludwig Von Bertalanffy (1969).**

System: According to Bertalanffy "a system is a group of elements that interact with one another in order to achieve a goal". All living systems are open, so there is continuous exchange of matter, energy or information. In open systems, there are varying degrees interaction with environment from which the system receives input & gives back output in the form of matter, energy & information.

In abovementioned study, system includes development of protocol on care related to maintenance of thermoregulation in preterm neonates by investigator & operationalizing it among the caregivers of preterm neonates for promotion of their skills in providing care related to thermoregulation in preterm neonates. These elements of system are caregivers & protocol on maintaining thermoregulation in preterm neonates.

Input: A matter, energy, information & individual's efforts that enters into a system is called input. In the abovementioned study, the input is reviewing literature on care related to maintenance of thermoregulation in preterm neonates in the form of instructional booklet for the caregivers.

Throughput: It is the process of transferring the information entered in the system into useful terms. It is the process by which information received in the system is utilized & it further leads to formation of product. It may be utilized by system itself or can be transferred to the environment. In this research study, throughput is operationalizing the system. It includes assessment of the skills in caregivers with regard to care related to thermoregulation in preterm neonates & difficulties they may come across with preterm neonates & difficulties they may come across with preterm neonates in relation to maintenance of thermoregulation. It further refers to facilitate the environment for development of skills of caregivers in maintenance of thermoregulation in preterm neonates. It includes communicating & motivating the caregivers of preterm neonates to follow the protocol guidelines for promotion of skills development, in care of preterm neonates for maintaining thermoregulation of preterm neonates are developed demonstration & return demonstration till they are fully skilled.

Output: Output is the end product of the system. In this research study, the output is the success or failure of operationalized system for development of skills of caregivers in providing home care related to maintenance of thermoregulation of preterm neonates.

Feedback: Feedback is the process by which the system continuously monitors itself & the environment for information to guide the operation. In the present study, feedback will be given to input as well as to the throughput of the system. Feedback to the input will be given in the form of recommendations after implementing protocol. Recommendations will include positive/negative results of the development of skills areas that need improvement & modifications if needed in the system.

Table 6.2: Conceptual framework based on General System Theory

Input	Throughput	Output
*Review of literature about preterm neonates thermo-regulatory home care	Investigator system * Facilitate environment	Success or failure of development of skills of caregivers in providing thermo-regulatory home care to preterm neonates
*Development of protocol about preterm thermoregulatory home care	* Involving caregivers	
*Providing instructional Booklet on preterm neonates thermoregulatory home care to caregivers	* Educating caregivers by giving demonstration for promotion of skills in providing thermoregulatory home care to preterm neonates Operationalize the system	

SUMMARY

- A theory is a set of interrelated concepts, definitions & propositions, that present a systematic view of phenomenon by specifying relations among variables with the purpose of explaining & predicting the phenomenon.
- Theory is classified by two ways i.e. abstraction & goal orientation. By abstraction the theories are classified as grand, middle range & practice level or micro nursing theories. By goal orientation theories are classified as prescriptive or descriptive theories.
- The building blocks of theories are concepts, constructs, conceptual definitions, relational statements & conceptual models.

- Theory is an integral part of research, where theory is tested or verified in quantitative research; theory is generated in qualitative research such as grounded theory & used as a lens in other qualitative research studies & mixed methods research studies.
- The main purposes & uses of theories, models & frameworks in research are to clearly identify the variables of the study, provide an overall framework for conducting the research study & help to understand the study concepts & their relationship with each other to provide foundation for theory testing or theory development research.
- Conceptual or theoretical frameworks are developed using the concepts from existing theories, previous research findings & own experiences. The steps of development of conceptual/theoretical models are i) identification of general concepts of the study ii) reviewing literature from existing theories of nursing & related disciplines iii) development of logical construct iv) evaluation & revision of conceptual/theoretical framework v) establishing of congruity in model.

BIBLIOGRAPHY

1. Burns N,. Grover S.K. (2008), Unnderstanding nursing research. Building an evidence based practices, 4th edition, Noida: Reel Elsevier India Pvt Ltd.
2. Gil Wayne, Dec.8,2020. www.nurselabs.com/nursing theories
3. Hage J. (1972), Techniques & problems of theory contraction in society. New York: John Wiley & sons.
4. Murphy F., Williams A., Pridmore J.A. Nursing Models & contemporary nursing: their development, uses & limitations. Nursing Times; 106:23.
5. Polit D.F., Beck CT. Nursing Research: Principles & Methods. Developing a conceptual context. P.114-136.
6. www.nursekey.com/theoretical & conceptual framework
7. Roger M.E., (1970) An introduction to the theoretical basis of Nursing. Philadelphia: F.A.Davis.
8. Roy C. (1976): Introduction to Nursing: An adaptation Model. Engiewood Cliffs, NJ: Prentice Hall.
9. Silvia M.C. (1976). Nursing Research: Testing Nursing Theory: State of the Art. Advances in Nursing Science, 9 (i), 1 – 11.
10. Silvia M.C. & Sorrell, J.M. (1992). Testing of Nursing Theory: Critique & Philosophical expansion. Advances in Nursing Science, 14 (4), 12-23.
11. Sukhpal Kaur, Amarjeet Singh. Simplified Nursing Research & Statistics. (2016) CBS Publishers & Distributors Pvt Ltd. 52-65.
12. Sharma Suresh. (2019) Nursing Research & Statistics. Elsevier, New Delhi.139-159.
13. Steven B. (1979), Nursing Theory: Analysis, Application & Evaluation. Philadelphia,

Lippincott.

14. Stewart D., Klein S. (2016). The use of Theory in Research. International Journal of clinical Pharmacology.
15. Young A. Tylor S.G. & Ren penning K M (2001): Connections: Nursing Research, Theory & Practices. St. Louis: Mosby. P 27-28.

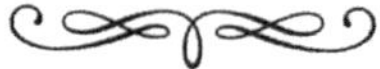

CHAPTER

7 Designing Research

Swati Kambli

Learning Objectives

This chapter helps the reader to –

- Define the concept of research design & approaches.
- Explain the elements of research design & factors influencing the selection of design.
- Enumerate the types of research.
- Describe the types of basic, applied, quantitative, qualitative & mixed method design.
- Discuss the internal & external validity of research designs.
- Develop skills in planning of different types of research designs.
- Explain the process of developing systematic review, meta-analysis & meta-synthesis.

INTRODUCTION

A research design is overall plan, blueprint, guide or framework used for planning, implementation & analysis of a research study. It provides an outline of how a research will be carried out.

- It includes the descriptions of research approaches, types of variables, sampling design & a plan for data collection, analysis, interpretation & presentation of the research study.
- As a single research design may be inadequate to answer all research questions/hypotheses so investigators use a combination of different approaches.

DEFINITION

At the beginning of every meaningful research, a researcher chooses a framework of methods & techniques to be used & applied in the whole research process. This framework is usually referred to as research design. (**Nemanja Jovancic. May21, 2020. Leadquizzes.com/blog/research-design-types**).

TYPES OF RESEARCH DESIGN

Classification or types depends upon the approach of studying the variables i.e. qualitative, quantitative research or purpose of conducting research.

- Based upon **approach** of studying the variables research design is classified as **quantitative, qualitative, mixed methods & other specific methods.**
- Based on **purpose** of conducting the research, the classification is **Basic & Applied research.**

Quantitative Research Design

It is an inquiry into an identified problem, based on testing a theory composed of variables measured with numbers & analysed by descriptive & inferential statistics. It involves **analysis of numerical data.**

Qualitative Research Design

It is based on field of inquiry about in depth understanding of human behaviour & the reasons that govern human behaviour. **Data collected in descriptive form** rather than numerical form & **analysed by descriptive coding & narrations.** Analysis is done with words, pictures & objects.

Mixed Methods

Combination of several methods are commonly termed as **mixed methods or triangulation.** It might be used in four basic ways in a study, i.e. data triangulation, methods triangulation, researcher triangulation & theory triangulation.

Basic Research

Performed for new knowledge generation & expand theories that describe, explain/predict the phenomenon of interest. The findings of basic research may not be immediately applicable to practical problems. But these do provide a foundation of scientific knowledge for building up further research.

Applied Research

The research is conducted for functional purposes & practical use or application of solution to the problems which are directly related to clinical practice. It can contribute for evidence based nursing practice.

Other Types of Research

Other research designs are systematic reviews, methodological, meta-analysis, secondary data analysis, outcome research, evaluation studies, operational research.

PURPOSES OF RESEARCH DESIGN

Kerlinger has described **2 basic purposes.**

1. To provide answers to research questions.
2. To control variance in relation to research study. This is being done to rule out other hypotheses/other variables as causes of the study outcome which may affect validity of the study.
   - **A design** must be **'created'** which requires making decisions about a number of specific issues like research approach, population, study setting, tools & methods of data collection, plan for data analysis etc, It is a creative process of planning an empirical aspects of investigation.
   - It eliminates biases & reduces margin of error.

KEY CHARACTERISICS OF RESEARCH DESIGN (Deepan Pokhrel. Nov. 30; 2015. liteblog.wordpress.com)

- **Objectivity -** The findings obtained by the researcher should be objective. It is possible by allowing more than one person to agree between the final scores/conclusion of the research study.
- **Reliability -** If the similar research is carried out some other time & in a similar setting, it must give similar results. So the researcher must frame the research questions to make it reliable & provide similar outcomes.
- **Validity -** Any measuring device can be said to be valid if it measures what it is expected to measure & nothing else. So accordingly a tool must be developed.
- **Generalization -** The information collected from given sample must be utilized for providing a general application to the large group of which the sample is drawn.

ELEMENTS OF RESEARCH DESIGN

There are six major elements of research design as follow –

- **The Approach -** The approach of research study depends primarily on the nature of phenomenon under study. It involves the decision about the type of approach selection relevant to the phenomenon under study i.e. quantitative, qualitative or combination of methods etc.

- **Population, sample & sampling technique** – Research design also provides the researcher with directions about population, sample & sampling technique which will be relevant for research problem that is under investigation e.g. in one group pre-test, post-test in one of the quantitative research design only one group is selected & there will be no control group to compare the study outcome. A selection of larger sample size can help in the generalization of study findings.
- **The time, study setting & sources of data collection** - As per the availability of time, the research approach may be selected. e.g. comparing to cross-sectional studies, longitudinal studies need more time. Study setting & the sources of requisite data are the other important elements essential for effective planning to conduct a research study.
- **Tools & methods of data collection** - Tools & methods of data collection are selected which is suitable to particular research approach. e.g. Questionnaire can be used in quantitative approach whereas interviews are used in qualitative research approach.
- **Methods of data analysis** - A research design must also include the description of the methods of data analysis that helps the researcher to collect relevant data, which can be analysed as per the research design plan.

SELECTION OF RESEARCH DESIGN

The selection of research design largely depends on the nature of the research problem, sources available (cost, time, expertise of the researcher), accessibility of subjects & ethical considerations. The important factors that affect the selection of research design are as follow –

Factors Affecting Selection of Research Design

- **Nature of the research problem** - Based on research problem/phenomenon under study the researcher can decide, whether quantitative or qualitative research to be followed e.g. a researcher wanted to plan interventions for problems related to patients who have undergone colostomy. The nature of phenomenon in the given example is quantitative type, so a researcher has to choose a most suitable quantitative study design to study this problem.
- **Purpose of the problem** - Research may be conducted for prescription, description, exploration or correlation of the variables, so the purpose of the research study helps the researcher to select the relevant research design. e.g. A researcher wanted to identify the effect of music therapy on

the neurological status of comatose patients admitted in neurology unit. In this situation, a researcher has to choose one of the experimental research designs to study this research problem.

- **Researcher's knowledge & experience** - Mastery of knowledge & enriched experience in a particular area helps the investigator to have enthusiasm & conduct a research study in the person's area of interest, as the researcher has a good confidence in conducting research in that particular area. e.g. enriched experience in neonatal unit helps the researcher to conduct research in that area.
- **Ethical considerations** - Ethical committee approval & time to time guidance is very essential to conduct a research study. All ethical principles like respect for participants & their rights, informed consent, principle of beneficence, non exploitation, risk minimization are to be incorporated in research study. Selection of a research design is significantly influenced by the ethics of the research study.
- **Subjects/participants** - For a quantitative research, large numbers of subjects/participants are required for generalization of the findings. But only few subjects are required to collect in-depth data in a qualitative research design.
- **Availability of resources** - Good resources like funds, equipments & other facilities are required for smoothness in conducting research study & affects outcome positively. Sometimes because of resource constraints, a researcher has to compromise with non-randomized instead of randomized control trials (RCTs) designs.
- **Time** - Time factor is major deciding factor for the selection of research design. e.g. The longitudinal studies need more time. But the cross-sectional studies may be carried out over a shorter period of time.
- **Control of extraneous variables** - An efficient design can maximize results, decrease errors & maximize control. Control is accomplished by ruling out extraneous variables that compete with the independent variable in quantitative research as an explanation for study's outcome. The means of controlling extraneous variables include the following.

  i. Use of homogenous sample.

  ii. Use of consistent data collection procedure.

  iii. Manipulation of independent variable.

  iv. Randomization.

Types of Quantitative Research Design

1. **True Experimental/Randomized Control Trial (RCT)**

i. **Basic True Experimental Designs**

- **ia.** Post-test only control design
- **ib.** Pre-test post-test control group design
- **ic.** Solomon four group design
- **ii.** **Specific True Experimental designs**
- **iia.** Parallel group design
- **iib.** Split body design
- **iic.** Factorial design
- **iid.** Randomized block design
- **iie.** Cross over design
- **iif.** Latin square design

2 **Quasi-Experimental Design/Non RCTs**

- **i.** Non RCT design
- **ii.** Non-equivalent control group design
- **iii.** Time series design
- **iv.** Time series non-equivalent control group design
- **v.** Time series with withdrawn & reinstituted treatment design

3 **Pre-Experimental Research Design**

- **i.** One shot case study
- **ii.** One group pre-test post-test

Non-Experimental/Observational Research Design

1 **Correlational research design**

- **i.** Cohort research design
- **ia.** Prospective cohort design
- **ib.** Retrospective cohort design
- **ic.** Ambispective cohort design
- **ii.** Case control research design

iia. Nested case control design

iii. Analytical cross-sectional design

2 **Descriptive Research Design**

i. Univariate descriptive design

ia. Prevalence studies/cross-sectional descriptive design

ib. Incidence studies/longitudinal descriptive design

ii. Comparative descriptive design

3 **Exploratory Research Design**

4 **Survey Research Design**

5 **Specific Quantitative Research Designs**

i. Clinical trials

ii. Evaluation

iii. Operational

iv Methodological

v. Secondary data analysis

vi. Meta-analysis

vii. Ecological studies Table1

EXPERIMENTAL RESEARCH DESIGNS

Experimental research is a scientific approach to research, where one or more independent variables included to measure their effect on latter. The effect of the independent variables on the on the dependent variables is usually observed & recorded over some time, to help researchers in drawing a responsible reasonable conclusion regarding relationship between these two variable types.

- Types of experimental research designs are determined by the way the researcher assigns subjects to different conditions & groups. They are of three types, namely true experimental, quasi-experimental & pre-experimental research design.
- All the experimental researchers have a common characteristics i.e. manipulation of independent variable, but a true experiment/RCT also consists of the principles of randomization & control. The application of control is difficult when studies are conducted in natural settings on human subjects. Therefore it is not feasible in nursing to conduct RCTs & nurses primarily depend on pre-experimental, quasi-experimental & non-experimental research designs to generate the research evidences.

- According to Riley, experimental research design is a powerful design for testing hypotheses of causal relationships among variables. Experimental research design is further classified into true experimental, quasi-experimental & pre-experimental designs. The experiments which neither have randomization nor control group for comparison are grouped under pre-experimental category.

TRUE EXPERIMENTAL DESIGN

These are also known as Randomized Controlled Trials (RCT) in biomedical research, in which researchers have complete control over the extraneous variables & can prove that the observed effect on dependent variable is only due to manipulation of the independent variable. There is a great need to use experimental research/RCTs in nursing to justify its practices on scientific evidence.

- Several reasons for lacking RCTs in nursing are lack of experience, education, lack of knowledge of RCTs as a method of research.
- Also it could be due to nature of some of the nursing interventions as it is not possible to have total control in natural settings in which research is carried out.
- The process of RCTs & outcome measurement becomes difficult with several confounding variables.

Essential Characteristics of True Experimental Design/RCT

A true experimental research/RCT must consist of three characteristics: manipulation, control & randomization.

- **Manipulation** refers to conscious control of the independent variable by the researcher through treatment/interventions to observe its effect on dependent variable e.g. A study which is conducted to see efficacy of home remedy i.e. use of banana on the control of diarrhea in infants. In this example, use of banana is the independent variable, is manipulated by the researcher & is used as an intervention for the experimental group, while the control group is kept deprived of it to observe its effect on the control of diarrhea amongst the infants.

In another example, use of play therapy as a pain related measure for toddlers receiving intra-muscular injection in experimental group & withholding for other toddlers in control group is considered as manipulation of independent variable.

Control - It refers to the use of control group for comparison.

- The experimental group receives the planned treatment or intervention & comparisons made with control group to observe the effect of treatment or intervention.
- Generally in healthcare & nursing research, it is not practically & ethically feasible to deprive control group of treatment or interventions. Therefore, the control group in experimental nursing research studies may include the following-
- An alternate treatment or intervention - It is also known as positive control, where in subjects in control group receive other treatment/intervention which may be already tested to be effective e.g. a researcher is conducting a study on effectiveness of boiled potato peel dressing versus the dressing commonly used in the burns wound among patients admitted in the burns unit.
- Standard method of care - This is the most commonly used control in nursing studies, where researchers use existing intervention in control group e.g. A researcher wanted to assess effectiveness of continuation of high protein diet in pre-schoolars diagnosed as protein energy malnutrition & having diarrhea where in such condition proteins are excluded from children's diet to control diarrhea which is caused due to protein deficiency.
- A placebo or pseudo intervention presumed to have no therapeutic value. Placebo is commonly used in biomedical studies to assess the efficacy of drugs. But it is not conveniently used in nursing studies as it is very difficult to design a pseudo nursing intervention.
- Different doses or intensities of intervention/treatment in dose response intensive & longer intervention compared to control group to test whether larger doses are associated with larger benefits or smaller doses will serve the purpose.
- Wait-list control group - There is delay in treatment with the participants in control group till the effect of intervention is compared between experimental & wait list group. In these studies every subject receives the treatment.

Randomization

- Randomization is a process of random assignment of subjects in experimental & control groups or two different experimental groups. In random assignment of subject, every subject has an equal chance of being assigned to experimental or control group. Random assignment eliminates the chances of selection bias in a study. It makes experimental & control group homogenous & as balanced as possible. Randomization is used in RCTs to minimize the threat of internal validity of the study & helps to eliminate the effect of extraneous variables on dependent variables. Through randomization, on an average, the characteristics of subjects in experimental & control groups are similar, thus influence of extraneous variables on dependent variables is eliminated by dispersing the variability of the subject characteristics equally in both the groups.

Methods of Randomization - Random assignment of the subjects can be as follow:

- **Simple flipping of a coin** for each subject, coin landing on its head can be included in experimental group & tail can be included in control group.
- **Lottery system -** Name of the group like experimental/control written on slips of a paper & the lots are drawn.
- **A random table** can be used to facilitate the randomization process. In this subjects, closing the eyes, choose a number from a table of numbers from row/columns till a requisite number is reached for both experimental & control groups.
- **Computer generated random numbers** may also be used for the random assignment of the subjects.

TYPES OF TRUE EXPERIMENTAL DESIGNS

The designs commonly used in True Experimental Research or RCTs are as follow –

Basic True Experimental Designs -

- **Post-test only Control group Design -** Two randomly assigned groups included in this research study i.e. experimental & control group, but both the groups are not pretested before implementation of treatment on the experimental group. Post-test observation is carried out on both the groups to examine the effect of manipulation of independent variable on the dependent variable.

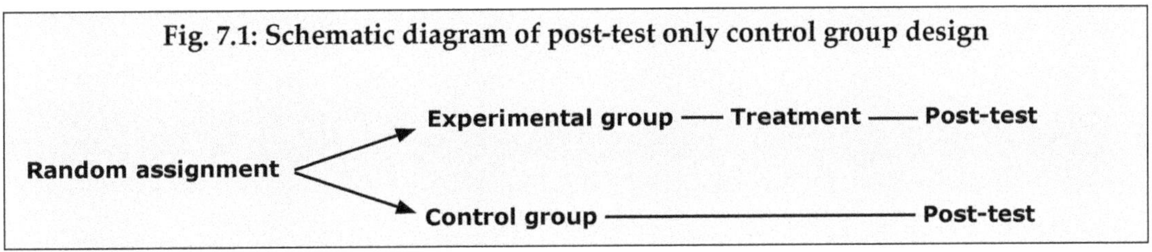

Fig. 7.1: Schematic diagram of post-test only control group design

- **Pre-test, Post-test Only Design** - In this research design, subjects are randomly assigned to either the experimental or the control group. An effect of the dependent variable is made on both the groups. A pre-test is carried out. Later, the treatment is implemented in experimental group only & after treatment observation of dependent variable is made on both groups to examine the effect of the manipulation of independent variable on dependent variable.

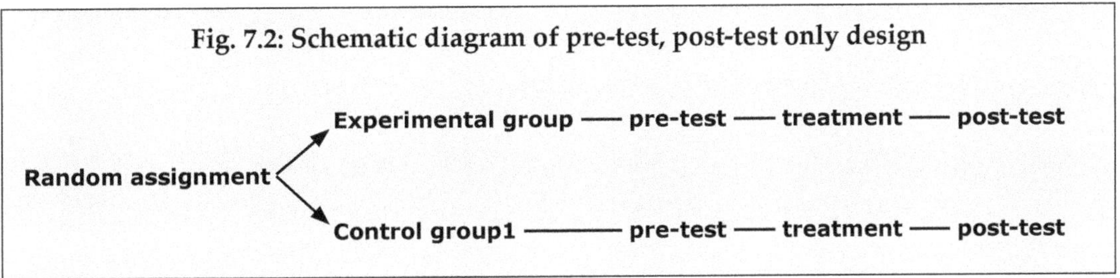

Fig. 7.2: Schematic diagram of pre-test, post-test only design

e.g. such a design could be used for an experimental study to assess effectiveness of cognitive behaviour therapy interventions in reduction of symptoms among patients with obsessive compulsive disorder.

* **Solomon Four Group Design** - In this design, there are two experts (group 1 & group 2) & two control groups. Initially investigator randomly assigns subjects to four groups. Out of the four groups, only experimental group1 & control group1 receive the pre-test, followed by the treatment to experimental group 1 & 2. Finally all four groups receive post-test, where the effects on dependent variables of the study are observed & comparison is made between four groups to assess the effect of independent variable on the dependent variable. To estimate the amount of change in experimental & control group 1 are used as baseline (Fig. 7.3).

The Solomon four group design is believed to be the most prestigious experimental design because it minimizes the threat to internal & external validity. Any difference between the experimental & control groups can be more confidently attributed to the experimental treatment. This design is not commonly used by the nursing & other healthcare researchers as it requires a large sample & statistical analysis related to it.

Fig. 7.3: Schematic diagram of Solomon four group design

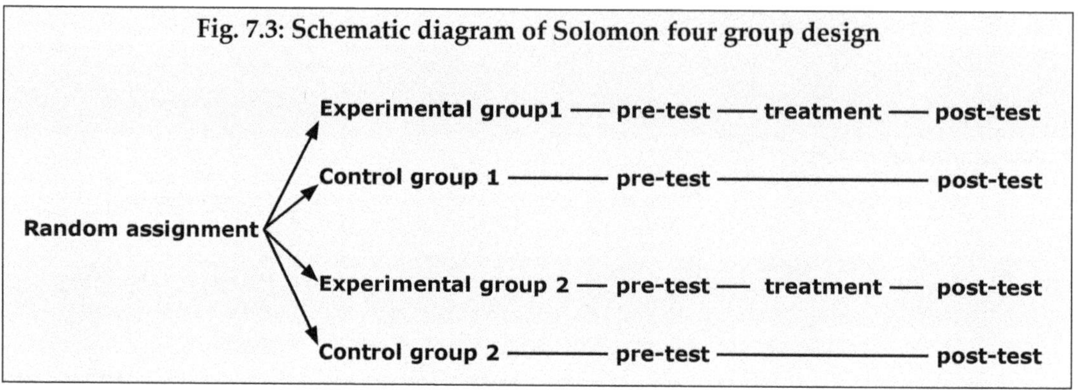

SPECIFIC TRUE EXPERIMENTAL DESIGNs

Parallel group design - There are two or more treatments/interventions are compared, where participants are randomized in different experimental groups & after implementing the different treatments the outcome is assessed & compared in two more experimental groups.

Split body design - In this design, the body is divided into left & right half & one side serves as an experimental arm & another side is used as a control arm. Split body design is considered as the most robust design in clinical trials research as experimental & control groups are truly homogenous in this design.

Factorial design - In this design, a researcher manipulates two or more independent variables. This design is useful where there are more than two independent variables, called factors to be tested e.g. a study to identify an effect of massage with coconut oil versus mustard oil on the thermoregulation of neonates.

Randomized block design - It is used where the researcher wants to bring homogeneity among selected groups. It is a simple method to reduce the variability among the treatment groups by a more homogenous combination of the subjects through randomized block design e.g. a researcher wants to examine effects of two antidiabetic drugs on patients with diabetes. In this example, to ensure homogeneity among subjects under treatment, a researcher randomly places the subjects in homogenous groups (blocks) such as patients with type I, type II diabetic patients with different blood sugar levels. Out of the two factors one is not experimentally manipulated; like there are two factors: type of anti-diabetic drugs & type of patients with diabetes with different blood sugar levels is simply grouped in different blocks with similar characteristics to ensure homogeneity.

Table 7.1: Randomized block design

Type of anti-diabetic drugs	Type I diabetic patients	Type II diabetic patients
A	A1 Blood sugar < 200 mg% A2 Blood sugar > 200 mg%	A1 blood sugar < 200 mg% A2 blood sugar > 200 mg%
B	B1 Blood sugar < 200 mg% B2 Blood sugar > 200 mg%	B1 blood sugar < 200 mg% B2 blood sugar > 200 mg%
C	C1 Blood sugar < 200 mg% C2 Blood sugar > 200 mg%	C1 blood sugar < 200 mg% C2 blood sugar > 200 mg%

Cross over design - In this design, subjects are exposed to more than one treatment, when subjects are randomly assigned to different orders of treatment. It is also known as repeat measures design. This is a group of designs that attempts to achieve control by entering all subjects into all treatments. This design is more efficient in establishing the highest possible similarity among subjects exposed to different conditions when groups are compared, obviously have equal distribution of characteristics. Sometimes this design is not effective, as when subjects are exposed to two different conditions, their responses of the second condition may be influenced by their experience in the first condition. e.g. when we compare the effectiveness. Listerine solution & Saline mouth care protocol, first we administer Listerine mouth care protocol on group 1 & Saline mouth care protocol on the subjects of group 2. Later the treatment is changed for each group where group 1 receives Saline mouth care & group 2 receives Listerine mouth care. In such studies subjects serve their own control.

Latin square design - Latin square design is primarily used in agriculture field. But it can be used in the healthcare sciences field. e.g. a nurse researcher is investigating efficacy of four different skin local applications in treatment of dermatitis. In this design every patient will receive every product. To use this design, the researcher take first four patients as rows of Latin square design & order positions of four skin applications as column of the Latin square design, then next four patients will become part of next Latin square design & thus every patient will receive each product application. A restriction in the assignment of treatments in this design is that each row & column is like a complete block. A requirement of this design is that number of treatments, rows & columns must be equal. The advantages of this design are that it helps in controlling more variations than completely randomized or randomized complete block designs because of its two way stratification results in a smaller mean square of error & the data analysis is simple with this design. It may have some disadvantages such as in this design the number of treatments is limited to the number of replicates, which seldom exceeds 10 & if it has less than 5 treatments, the degrees of freedom (df) for controlling random variation is relatively large & df error is small

Table 7.2: Latin square design

1	2	3	4
1 A	2 B	3 C	4 D
1 B	2 C	3 D	4 A
1 C	2 D	3 A	4 B
1 D	2 A	3 B	4 C

Advantages of an Experimental Design

- These designs are the most powerful methods to establish the causal relationships between variables.
- For the purpose of research as an explanation, causal relationship may be established among the variables by experimentation especially in studies involving physical objects, where the variables are more easily controlled than in human studies.
- There is better extent of purity in observation as the study is conducted under controlled environment.
- Conditions not found in natural setting can be created in an experimental setting in a short period of time that may take years to naturally occur where the independent variable is manipulated by the investigator (therefore very useful in genetic studies).
- Randomized experimental designs completely remove any accusations of conscious or subconscious biases from the researcher & practically guarantee external validity.
- These designs completely remove effect of extraneous variables.

Disadvantages

Sometimes, the result of the laboratory based RCT cannot be replicated in studies conducted on human beings due to danger to physical, psychological health of human subjects & ethical problems.

- Many of the human variables neither have valid measurable criteria nor instruments to measure them. e.g. patient welfare, or level of wellness cannot be measured on any scale or by any instruments. If a modified experimental group design is used, there may be a mismatch of research design & the variable measuring instruments..

- RCTs conducted in natural settings such as hospitals/community it becomes difficult to impose control over extraneous variables.
- One of the main drawbacks in conducting experiments on the effects of nursing care on acutely ill hospitalized patients is that the patients discharged from hospitals in shorter periods of time that there is little opportunity to study the effects as they occur. Only by a difficult & costly procedure, these discharged patients can be followed up in their homes to observe the expected results. So it is not possible due to several constraints.
- Another disadvantage of this design is that it is very difficult to get co-operation from the study participants as it may involve medical or surgical treatment or intervention, which may make the prospective subjects reluctant to participate in research study.
- As the sample size for the experiments involving human beings is often kept small, the study findings cannot be generalized to target population. Representativeness of findings of such study is questionable.
- In research involving human beings, the phenomena are usually very complex & occur due to multiple reasons that the simple experimental approach does not help. A more complex approach is required, which may be possible with great difficulties through experimental approach.

There are many limitations to conduct RCTs with human beings. However, the quasi-experimental designs could be more practical on human subjects especially with nursing intervention trials.

QUASI-EXPERIMENTAL RESEARCH DESIGNS

The quasi-experimental studies lack certain characteristics like true experimental studies. They are also called non-randomized controlled trials. This design involves manipulation of independent variable to observe its effect on dependent variable, but it lack randomization of subjects in experimental groups which is one of the essential characteristics of the RCTs. Sometimes, these designs even lack control groups. Most of the nursing research studies have followed quasi-experimental research designs.

Main characteristics

- There is manipulation of independent variables to observe the effects on the dependent variables.

- This design lacks randomization of participants to experimental groups, which is the important characteristics of the RCTs & sometimes they lack control group also for comparison.
- Independent variables are not manipulated in a completely controlled situation.

Types of Quasi-experimental Research Design

The various types of quasi-experimental designs include as follow-

Non-randomized (non-equivalent) control group design, time series design (interrupted time series, time series with multiple institution of the treatment, time series with intensified treatment & time series with withdrawn & reinstituted treatment).

- **Non-randomized control group design**- It is also known as non-equivalent control group pre-test post-test design. It is identical to the pre-test post-test control group design, except that there is no random assignment of subjects in experimental & control groups. In this design both experimental & control groups are selected without randomization & dependent variables are observed in both groups before the intervention. Later the experimental group receives treatment & after that post-test observation of dependent variables is carried out for both the groups to assess the effect of treatment on experimental group. This design is shown in figure below-

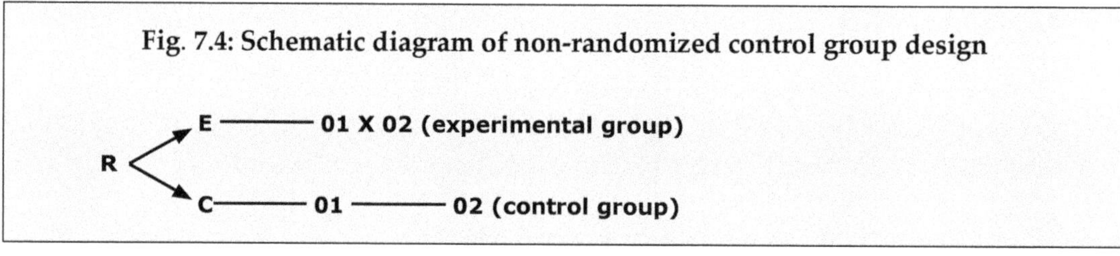

Fig. 7.4: Schematic diagram of non-randomized control group design

- **Non-equivalent control group post-test only design-** This design involves two non-randomized groups, i.e. experimental & control group. It is similar to the non-equivalent control group pre-test, post-test design except that it has only post-test & no pre-test. This design is diagrammed as shown in figure below-

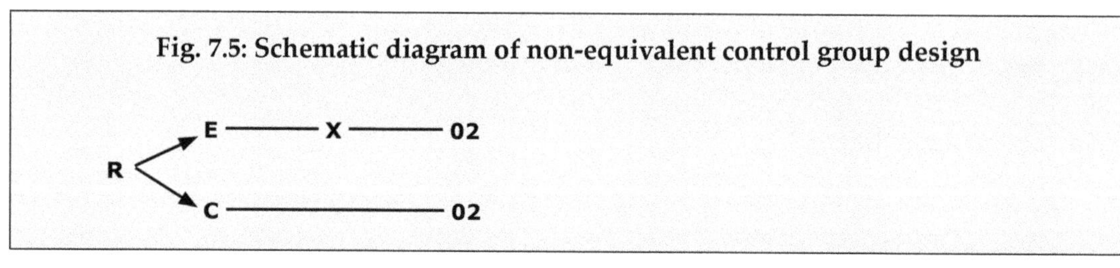

Fig. 7.5: Schematic diagram of non-equivalent control group design

- **Time series -** It involves only one group i.e. experimental group & there is no control group for comparison. In this design, series of observations are made in experimental group before implementation of intervention & again series of observations are made after the implementation of intervention. This design is useful when the investigator wants to measure the effects of treatment over a longer period of time. e.g. a researcher may evaluate muscle power of a group of patients having hemiparesis. After assessing muscle power for as long as three weeks, participants are demonstrated about specific exercises to improve muscle power of affected side. Then weekly muscle power would be evaluated for improvement for next three weeks.
- **Time series non-equivalent control group design -** In this design investigator makes series of observations in an experimental & a control group before implementation of intervention in the experimental group & again series of observations of outcome variables is made in both groups. It is shown in schematic diagram below-

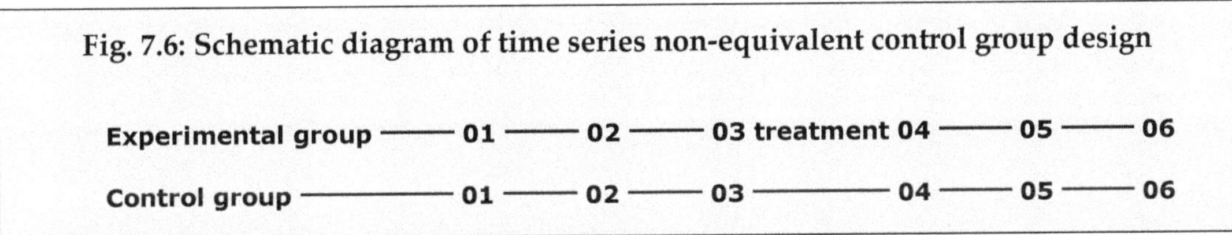
Fig. 7.6: Schematic diagram of time series non-equivalent control group design

e.g. a study carried out to prevent gastrointestinal problems in children with colostomy admitted in pediatric surgical unit of one hospital as an experimental group & control group is selected from another unit of same hospital/another hospital. Before intervention is implemented in experimental group, observations in relation to nutritional status & colostomy drainage are collected monthly in both experimental & control groups for comparison.

* Time series design with withdrawn & reinstitution treatment design

In this design, an investigator would continue to carry out observation of variables & implement short-term intervention & again carry out outcome variable observation & then administer new intervention & then again observe the outcome variables. Then again a new treatment is administered & outcome variable is observed & effect of different interventions are compared e.g. an investigator carries out a study to assess the effectiveness of 3 or 4 types of disinfectants in reducing flora for disinfection of pediatric operation theatre at pediatric hospital. In this example, researcher first carries out culture samples during different shifts & then carry out disinfection of operation theatre with different disinfectants & then collects culture samples during different shifts. After use of each type of disinfectant several culture samples are collected before & after the process of disinfection. In between two interventions, there could be a wash period to eliminate the risk of residual effect of previous interventions, which is a major disadvantage of this design.

Advantages & disadvantages of Quasi-Experimental design

Advantages

- These designs are more practical to conduct research studies in nursing so frequently used. But there is absence of large sample size, randomization &/or absence of control groups.
- It is more suitable for real-world natural setting than true experimental designs.
- The impact of independent variables is observed, evaluated under naturally occurring conditions.
- There are chances that causal relationship is established in this design, wherein some of the hypotheses are practically answered through this design.

Disadvantages

- It is a weaker design, as there is no control over threat to internal validity.
- There are chances for selection bias due to lack of randomization.
- Other than independent variables, extraneous variables influence dependent variables which may cause confusions in study outcomes, so the results of this design are less reliable & weak for the establishment of causal relationship between independent & dependent variables.

Pre-Experimental Research Designs

These designs are very weak in structure & control. They are not considered as rigorous enough for the purpose of research study. There are three types of pre-experimental research designs i.e. One-shot case study, one group pre-test, post-test designs & static group design.

One Shot Case Study

In this design after introduction of independent variables, the post-test is conducted & there is no pre-test. As there is no comparison group, it is impossible to determine whether the outcome scores are really higher than they would have been without the treatment. As post-test scores are not compared with pre-test scores, also it is impossible to identify, if any change within the group itself has taken place.

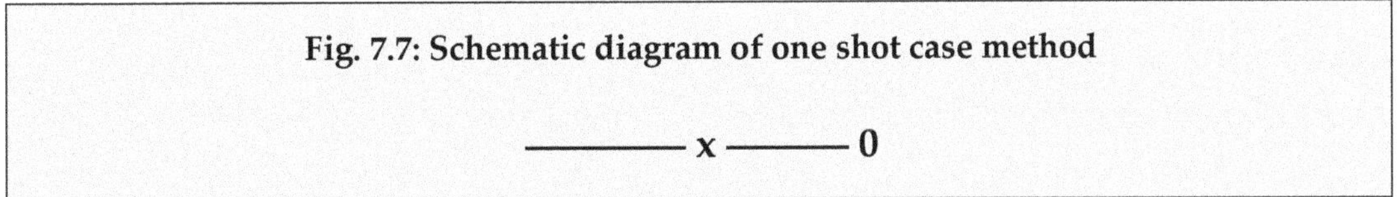

Fig. 7.7: Schematic diagram of one shot case method

One Group Pre-test Post-test Design

It is considered as very weak pre-experimental design as there is no control group & process of randomization in this design. There is pre-test observation of the dependent variables is made before introduction of independent variable in the selected experimental group, then there is implementation of independent variable & a post-test observation of dependent variables is carried out to assess the effect of independent variables on the experimental group. e.g. a study on the effect of virtual soft skills training for nursing students in enhancing transition to workplace. In this study, one group pre-test & post-test design was used to examine nursing students knowledge of soft skills. The data was collected using structured questionnaire using google forms. The questionnaire comprised 25 items on different themes related to soft skills. Pre-test was conducted to assess prior knowledge of students. Virtual training was conducted for consecutive five days using zoom meeting. The post-test was conducted on day 5 using same tool to assess the effectiveness of virtual soft skill training.

Static Group Design

In this design two or more groups are placed under observation, where only one of the groups is subjected to some treatment while the other groups are held static. All the groups are post tested & the observed differences between the groups are assumed to be a result of the treatment.

Advantages & Disadvantages of Pre-Experimental Group Designs

Advantages

- These designs are convenient specially in nursing & other health science disciplines & to conduct studies in natural settings.
- Most suitable for neophyte researchers in the field of experimental research.

Disadvantages

- These designs are considered as a very weak experimental designs to establish causal relationships between independent & dependent variables as there is no control of threat to internal validity. It may have selection bias, which can be a very serious threat in using this particular design.

Campbell & Stanley (1963) have discussed about internal & external validity. Internal and external validity discussed here is in context of experimental designs & not in context of measurement.

Factors Influencing Internal Validity

- **History** - The threat of history occurs when the specific events occur between first & second measurement & this event influences dependent variables e.g. besides the experimental treatment, there is lots of information through mass media which may affect dependent variables so as a researcher; one cannot conclude that change in subject's behaviour is the result of treatment or effect of information of mass media.
- **Maturation** - The processes within subjects which act as a function of the passage of time i.e. if a project lasts after several years, most participants may improve the performance regardless of treatment e.g. improvement of height, weight in children as a process of natural growth in a study in relation to effect of particular nutritional protocol on height & weight of children.
- **Testing** - The effects of taking pre-test on the outcomes of taking a post-test. Generally without treatment the scores in second test are higher.
- **Instrumentation** - The changes in the instrument, observers or scores which may produce changes in outcomes. Instruments like thermometers, blood pressure apparatus, should be checked for their accuracy at regular intervals & the same instruments should be used throughout the study to minimize the errors of measurement. All instruments before using for actual study, should be checked for validity and reliability of the tool.
- **Statistical regression** - It is also known as regression to the mean, caused by selection of subjects on the basis of extreme scores or characteristics e.g. effect of extra classes for slow learners expected to have immediate improvement in their test performances. Can be taken care of with the process of randomization and inclusion criteria in selection of sample.
- **Selection of subjects** - The biases which may result in selection of comparison groups. Randomization is the solution to the problem.

- **Mortality -** It is the loss or dropout of study subjects during the course of study. If the subjects who remain in the study or join later are not similar to those who dropped out, the results could be affected. The longer the period of study, the more are chances of subject mortality.

External Validity

- It refers to the extent to which the study results can be generalized to a large population. It explores the generalization beyond specific experiments to check if the results/findings can be the same with other settings/with other subjects population.
- **Hawthorne effect -** When the subjects are observed, their behaviour changes & this is called Hawthorne effect, that may affect the outcome of the study.
- **Experimental effect -** It is a threat to study results when researcher's characteristics, or behaviour like mannerisms, facial expressions etc. may influence subject's behaviour.
- **Reactive or interaction effect of testing -** A pre-test might increase or decrease a subject's sensitivity or responsiveness to the experimental variable. People might not respond to the treatment in the manner they finally do, if they had not received the pre-test.
- **Novelty effect -** When the treatment is new, subjects & researcher may be interested about new methods of doing the things. Once the treatment becomes more familiar, results might differ.
- **Time, place & person -** A study which is conducted on diarrhea in infants during rainy season, findings of such study cannot be applied during summer season, as incidence & causes may differ of diarrhea in infants during summer season. Health problems/disease pattern in various countries depends upon various factors like culture, lifestyle & prevalence of diseases there, so research conducted in tropical country cannot be generalized in western countries.

NON-EXPERIMENTAL RESEARCH DESIGNS

In non-experimental research designs, the researcher collects the data & describes phenomenon as they exist/occur naturally. There is no manipulation of independent variables as there are no interventions in these designs like an experimental research design. Also there is no random assignment of the subjects to the groups. Data obtained are analysed & the results may lead to the formation of hypothesis that can be tested experimentally. As it is one of the types of research designs of quantitative approach, the observations are represented by numerical data that can be statistically analysed. Questionnaires, interviews & critical incident technique, are used for data collection in non-experimental research designs.

It is also known as observational research design in biomedical research literature, which is one of the broad categories of research designs.

Need for Non-Experimental Research Designs

- This is used by nursing researchers very frequently.
- Following are the situations in which only non-experimental designs can be used.
- In these designs the independent variables cannot be manipulated.
- The studies in which it is unethical to manipulate independent variable, as manipulation may cause physical or psychological harm to subjects.
- Sometimes practically it is not possible to conduct experiments.
- Type of studies like descriptive studies do not require any experimental approach.

Types of Non-Experimental Research Designs

Classification given below is much understandable about the non-experimental research designs. It is given in hierarchical levels of evidence i.e. from higher to lower level of evidence.

Correlational research designs

- Cohort research design
- Prospective cohort design
- Historical/retrospective cohort design
- Ambispective cohort design

Descriptive research designs

- Cross-sectional descriptive design
- Incidence studies/longitudinal descriptive design
- Comparative descriptive design

Exploratory Research Design

Survey Research Design

Correlational Research Designs

It is a research design where researchers study the relationship of two or more variables without manipulation of independent variable or without any intervention. e.g. this design was used for a study on 'effect of alcoholism on the occurrence of liver cirrhosis among people from slum areas of Mumbai city, This design is used to examine the relationship between variables, i.e. naturally occurring between independent & dependent variables.

Main Characteristics of Correlational Research Designs

- In this design, the researchers examine the strength of relationships between variables by determining how change in one variable is correlated with change in the other variable.
- Generally, these studies have independent & dependent variables but there is no manipulation of independent variable.
- The relationship of independent & dependent variables are measured by using the correlation coefficient statistical measure, when results range between -1 & +1, that indicates positive/negative relationship between independent & dependent variables. However, a zero results of correlation coefficient indicates no relationship between independent & dependent variables. Other statistical methods can also be used to find out the statistical relationship between two or more naturally occurring independent & dependent variables.

Types of Correlational Research Design

Three basic correlational research designs are discussed in this chapter i.e. cohort research design, case control research design & analytical cross sectional research design.

Cohort Research Design

A cohort is a group of people who have something common & who remain a part of group over an extended times. To investigate an occurrence of a disease in a cohort group, a longitudinal approach is used. The existing presumed causes are compared with homogenous control group e.g. a researcher longitudinally observes a homogenous cohort of alcoholic & non-alcoholic people for the development of cirrhosis of liver.

- These studies are also called incidence studies which are designed to measure the exposure & outcome in the context of time.

- Also in these studies individual subjects are followed over time to measure the exposure when it happens; then they measure the outcome at a point in time after exposure. As the outcome happens, it is measured exactly or appropriately, then the incidence of new cases can be determined in cohort studies.
- The cohort studies could be prospective, retrospective or ambispective.
- The main disadvantage of cohort studies is that they tend to be very expensive & time consuming.
- Due to high attrition of subjects between measurement the study is substantively weakened.
- This design is inefficient for rare outcome & for those with a very long latency period i.e. time from exposure to outcome.

Prospective Cohort Design

This type of research includes longitudinal observational study design. In this study a group of subjects with similar characteristics, is followed over a time period.

- The prospective cohort studies are helpful in determining the causes of different diseases & disorders. The important characteristics of this study is that the subjects with homogenous characteristics are selected & specific independent variable is observed for longer period of time to assess the effect of independent variable on the causation of particular disease or disorder e.g. a prospective cohort study on predictors of incidence of varicose veins among nurses working in selected hospitals of Mumbai city.

Historical Cohort Design

This design is also known as retrospective cohort design. A researcher collects data from past records & does not follow up with patients. Thus in this design, all the events i.e. exposure, latent period & outcome i.e. development of disease have already occurred in the past. Researcher just collects data & establishes the risk of developing a disease, if exposed to a particular risk factor. e.g. one researcher wanted to assess study outcomes in women with breast cancer treated with different kinds of treatments. He/she plans to evaluate the records to look after the survival & different kinds of treatment details between 2010 and 2016. This approach to a study is possible, if the records on follow up are complete with all necessary details. In these studies, a risk ratio or odd ratio gives an assessment of relative risk of a disease/disorder.

Ambispective Cohort Design

In this design which moves both forward & backward in time, the exposure is measured twice i.e. historical & real time during the study period. The study allows a more precise manner of exposure in term of time e.g. exploring & evaluating causative factors of different kinds of malnutrition among under five children & its effect on risk of developing various kinds of infectious diseases among schoolars & adolescents.

In this design, studies begin with population, where two years, who are exposed & who are not exposed to risk factors, are taken & among them presence or absence of a disease or disorder is assessed & compared at a particular one point in time.

Descriptive Research Designs

The purpose of descriptive research designs is to observe, describe & document the aspects of a situation as it naturally occurs & sometimes to serve as a starting point for hypothesis generation or theory development.

Characteristics of Descriptive Research Designs

- In this design the phenomenon occur in natural setting.
- There is no manipulation of independent variable.
- These designs are mainly information/knowledge acquisition studies.
- These designs can be used to develop theories, assess & justify current practices, or determine other practices in similar situations.
- Bias is prevented through operational definitions of variables, large sample size, random sampling techniques, valid & reliable research tools.

Types of Descriptive Research Designs

Descriptive research designs are: cross sectional design, exploratory design, comparative design, survey & longitudinal design.

Cross Sectional Design - These are also known as prevalence studies or epidemiological studies in which the researcher collects data at a particular point of time. Data analysis is carried out on a group of subjects at one time rather than over a period of time. Important characteristics of cross sectional studies are the exposure & outcome measured at the same point of time. There is minimum risk involved in these studies. Causality cannot be established in this research design. Relatively inefficient for studying rare disease conditions as a large sample is required to analyse the data. Researcher may conduct prevalence studies to estimate the percentage of people with a given disease in the population e.g. a researcher is interested in assessing the awareness on Covid-19 infection among the people. Cross sectional studies could be of the following types:

A) Exploratory design

B) Comparative design

A) **Exploratory design** - It is used to identify, explore & describe existing phenomenon & its related factors. It is not only a simple description or observation of the frequency of occurrence of phenomenon e.g. an exploratory study to assess multifactorial dimensions of dementia & measures to improve cognitive brain functions for elderly people living in selected urban areas of Mumbai.

B) **Comparative design** - It involves comparing & contrasting two or more samples of study subjects on one or more variables, often at a single point of time. Comparison of the groups is being done on the basis of selected attributes e.g. knowledge, perceptions & attitudes; physical/psychological symptoms & so on e.g. a comparative study on growth & development pattern among rural & under five children in district Raigad, Maharashtra.

Survey Research Design - It is used to collect information from different subjects within a given population having same characteristics of interest called sample survey & if the entire population is involved, it is called a population survey, such as census. Information is collected about prevalence, distribution & interrelatedness of phenomenon in a population such as opinion polls, customer survey & health survey. It helps to collect wide range of data from a given population, such as actions, attitudes, opinions, perceptions, behaviours, awareness, practices & so on. Based on the nature of phenomenon under study, surveys are classified as descriptive, exploratory, comparative & correlational surveys.

Longitudinal Research Design - It involves data collection at multiple points of time i.e. data are collected from the same subjects at different point of times, which may vary from few months to many decades. It can be used as longitudinal RCT. Longitudinal studies can be classified as trend, panel & follow up studies. Longitudinal studies can be used in combination with other observational studies e.g. turn over rates or absenteeism rates among the health care workers can be studied during the course of the year.

Advantages & Disadvantages of Non-Experimental Research Design

Advantages

- It can give a direction for conducting experimental studies.
- When ethically not possible to conduct experimental studies, non-experimental studies are better to provide an insight into a real life situations.
- Sometimes there are many constraints like lack of time, shortage of funds, very much inconvenience to conduct experimental studies. In such cases, non-experimental research design is most feasible.

Disadvantages

- The results obtained & relationship between dependent & independent variables can never be absolutely clear & error free, as inferential statistics cannot be used in non-experimental research design.
- In these design groups are selected non-randomly, which may not be homogenous & there is much variation in traits/characteristics which may affect generalizability of the study results.

Other Research Designs

Certain research designs cannot be considered as experimental or non-experimental research designs. Some of these designs are discussed as follow-

- Methodological studies
- Systematic Reviews
- Meta-analysis
- Secondary data analysis
- Outcome research
- Evaluation studies
- Operational research

Methodological studies - Healthcare professionals frequently use tools developed by other disciplines, such as Psychology & Sociology. Standardized tools are always preferred in the research studies, as their validity & reliability is already established. But most of the times standardized tools are not available especially for nursing studies. Methodological studies are conducted to develop, validate, test & evaluate the research instruments & methods. For these studies, relevant, specific & exhaustive literature review is needed to identify the theories & understand the construct. The steps to be followed in methodological research are-

Step 1 - Operationally defining the behaviour/construct to be measured.

Step 2 - Preparation of the draft of the tool based on extensive review of literature.

Step 3 - Testing validity & reliability of the tool.

Step 4 - Try out the tool i.e. checking feasibility,.

Step 5 - Preparation of the final draft of the tool.

For example, a researcher may develop a tool to assess the neurological status of patients with raised intra-cranial pressure admitted in neuro unit.

Systematic Reviews

Systematic reviews are considered the most reliable resources in healthcare professions. They are research studies that make up the top level of the evidence-based information pyramid & as a result, they are the most sought after information for questions about health. There is a difference between systematic review & literature review. Literature review tries to find out, all published material on a particular subject, whereas systematic reviews focus on answering a question comprehensively by considering all aspects of it. Since the systematic reviews are generally associated with health related fields, their main objective is to ensure the results of the review providing evidence that answers relevant questions.

The predefined protocols, the amount of information reviewed, the evaluation process involved & the efforts to eliminate bias are all a part of what makes health professionals consider systematic reviews to be the highest level of evidence based information available. As a part of the process, systematic reviews tend to look at & evaluate all the RCTs, or all the cohort studies, for the specific topic. By evaluating a vast amount of comparable studies, a systematic review is able to provide answers that have a much stronger level of evidence than any other individual study.

Processes involved in systematic reviews are: setting up criteria, searching for information, evaluating information found. The characteristics of systematic review are well defined & internationally accepted. The following are the important features of the systematic review & its conduct –

- Clear objectives & questions to be addressed.
- Inclusion & exclusion criteria
- Comprehensive search to identify relevant studies (published, unpublished)
- Approval of the quality of included studies, assessment of the validity of their results.
- Analysis of data extracted from the included research.
- Presentation & synthesis of findings extracted.
- Transparent reporting of the methodology & methods used to review.

As a scientific enterprise, a systematic reviews will influence healthcare decisions. Ultimately, the quality of a systematic review & recommendations drawn from it, depends on the extent to which methods are followed to minimize the risk of error & bias e.g. having multiple steps in process, reduces the risk of subjective interpretation & also of inaccuracies due to chance error affecting the results of the review. To promote evidence based practice in nursing profession, it is a prime need today to develop systematic reviews specially in India. Various databases to identify systematic reviews are Pub med, CINAHL, TRIP database.

Meta-analysis - In 1976, Glass coined the term meta-analysis, it indicates analysis of analysis. A meta-analysis statistically merges the outcomes of various studies. It follows a quantitative approach. Meta-analysis is considered as the statistical analysis of a large amount of analysed results from individual studies for the purpose of integrating the findings. When the results of several similar studies are analysed together, the findings of such studies start with selecting studies with similar variables & population samples, followed by identifying & coding study characteristics. After statistical analysis the reporting of assessed findings of meta-analysis is done.

Steps followed in meta-analysis

1. Defining hypothesis
2. Review of literature to locate similar studies with a specific theme/topic
3. Input data - Empirical findings of gathered data is entered into statistical database.
4. Effect sizes are calculated - All statistics is converted into a common metric system. Then central tendency & variability is calculated.

5. Analysis of variables - Moderating variables in case of heterogeneity are analysed with mean difference or weighted regression to see if variable is accounted for the difference in the effect size.

Secondary data analysis - In this design to test a new hypothesis, the data collected by one researcher is analysed by another researcher. The collected data in one research which is unused or un analysed is utilized by another researcher. These studies are time saving, convenient & cost-effective. A secondary analysis can be performed with both quantitative & qualitative data.

Outcome research - It involves the evaluation of care practices & systems in place. To develop evidence-based practice & to improve health care services, outcome research is conducted. It is planned to assess or record the results of health care services, with measures such as powerful effect on the provision of health care & the development of health policy. A large number of nursing & multidisciplinary journals focused on outcome research

Evaluation studies - These studies are an applied form of research design, which involves the judgment about how well a special programme, practice, procedure or policy is working. When nursing personnel follow nursing process approach & evidence based practice, evaluation studies become more important in the nursing field. These studies may also be used to assess effectiveness or value of processes, personnel, equipment & the material used in a particular setting. Evaluation studies uses original aims & objectives as a benchmark to assess the effectiveness of particular activity. There are two types of evaluation research i.e. formative & summative evaluation. In formative evaluation, the focus is on the evaluation of a programme rather than outcome. Summative evaluation is conducted after the completion of the programme. In evaluation studies contribution to knowledge & research methodology remains a secondary objective. Example of the evaluation study can be - An evaluation study on the effectiveness of implementation of preventive measures for control of pandemic of Covid-19 infection in the state of Maharashtra.

Operational research - In this design, there is an application of the scientific method of investigation to the study of complex human organizations & services. The main objectives of operational research are to develop new knowledge about institutions, programmes, use of facilities of an organization. It is very useful in the improvement of health care studies. Also can help in 'effectively designing a hospital/ward for efficient flow of man, money, material etc. Example of this research design is - An operational research design on the job satisfaction of nurses working in tertiary care hospital of Mumbai city.

QUALITATIVE RESEARCH DESIGN

Qualitative research design is about understanding the human behaviour & reasons that govern such behaviour. This design is used to describe life experiences of the subjects & understand the meaningfulness of those experiences. In nursing very rarely this approach is followed. An interest of qualitative research design began in nursing profession in 1970s. Like quantitative research design, no numerical data is collected in qualitative research design, but narrations of the subjects are collected & interpreted. The design for qualitative research approach is emergent in nature i.e. a design that emerges as the researcher makes ongoing decisions based on what has been learnt.

Importance of Qualitative Research Design

- For the development of healthcare sciences, this approach is building a knowledge base.
- There is also a contribution towards social sciences by investigating social & cultural phenomena.
- It follows an inductive approach for discovery or expanding knowledge, about an area of interest that has received little research attention.

Characteristics of Qualitative Research Design

There are certain basic characteristics of these designs as follow –

- It emerges as study advances.
- It is dynamic.
- There are multiple strategies of data collection i.e. triangulation.
- It follows holistic approach which strives for an understanding of the whole.
- Researchers act as an instrument & there is intense researcher's involvement in the study.
- Data analysis is an ongoing process which is required for the formation of subsequent strategies & to determine when further field work should be done.

Phases of Qualitative Research Design

Exact form of this research design cannot be known & decided in advance. But the three main broad phases of qualitative research design are as follow –

- **Orientation & overview phase –** Initially, researchers presume the type of knowledge expected to be obtained. Beginning of research design enables them to plan further for the research study.
- **Focused exploration -** In this phase of qualitative research design, the important aspects of the phenomenon are more focused. More information is gathered about the phenomenon from a variety of people so at this phase focus is on exploration of the important aspects of the phenomenon under study.
- **Confirmation & closure -** In this final phase, efforts are undertaken to confirm that the findings gathered are trustworthy by discussing with study participants the authenticity & correctness of findings & then the study is closed finally.

Phenomenological research - It is a study of experiences of human beings. It is a movement in philosophy which attempts to uncover how human awareness is leading to social action, social situation & developing an understanding of social world. The aim of this design is to trace out precisely the live experiences of people & generate theories or models of the phenomena being studied. Phenomenological research involves gathering 'deep' information & perceptions from the people with inductive methods such as interviews, discussions & observations & representing that information from perspective of the individual. Three processes must occur in this research design include that a person must communicate an experience to the researcher; then the researcher must translate the experience; & then researcher communicates his/her understanding in writing, so that the relevant persons can relate their understanding of this information to the past & further experiences.

Ethnographic research - It was developed by anthropologists as a mechanism of studying cultures. It involves the description & interpretation of cultural behavior. The central aim of ethnography research is to provide rich, holistic insights into people's views & actions, as well as the nature of the location they reside in, through the collection of detail observations, record analysis & interviews. In healthcare research, ethnography provides access to health beliefs & healthcare practices in particular cultural or subcultural groups. Therefore, ethnographic inquiry facilitates understanding of cultural behavior & practices affecting health of people.

Characteristics of Ethnographic Research

- It is labour intensive & time consuming endeavor/process.
- Certain level of intimacy by researcher with cultural groups is required to study culture.
- Researchers use themselves as an instrument to collect data through informal interactions & observations than using formal tool.
- Information on three major aspects of cultural life is sought: cultural behavior, cultural artifacts & cultural language/speech.

Grounded theory - This is an inductive technique developed for health related topics by **Glaser & Strauss (1967).** The term grounded theory means the theory development from the research is 'grounded' or has its roots in the data from which it was derived. It is an approach to study of social process & social structures. In this design, there is an ongoing interplay between data collection & data analysis. The focus in this design is the development & evolution of social experiences, the social & psychological stages & phases that characterize a particular event or episode.

In general, grounded theory should be used when little is known about the topic. So this design follows inductive approach. A researcher permits a theory to emerge directly from the data i.e. the theory is grounded in the data. Purposive sampling technique is used to collect the data. Data collection begins with an individual case & simultaneously data analysis goes on. The data may be collected by using questionnaires & from verbal/non-verbal communications with subjects. Each data collection episode builds on the prior collections & the conceptualizations that has been developed up to that point. Collected data is constantly compared with previously collected data. Pertinent concepts are identified & assigned codes. Researcher continues this process until saturation (no new learning) occurs. All records are maintained systematically.

The purpose of grounded theory research design is to go forward from description of experience to generate or discover a theory. In grounded theory the researcher generates a general explanation i.e. a theory of a process, action, or interaction which are shaped by views of large numbers of participants e.g. A study was carried out to explore & describe the nurses' perceptions of the factors affecting their responses to burnout syndrome.

Historical research - In this design, the researcher attempts to examine the past events to identify what exactly happened in the past & its effect on the person. It is seen usually that our action today are rooted in the past. It can help in examining the current events & prevent committing same mistakes made in the past. Steps followed in this design are: identification of research topic & formulation of research question/problem. Data collection or review of literature: & evaluation of materials; data synthesis; & report preparation of the narrative disposition. Data is collected from primary/secondary sources. Always primary sources are better than secondary sources. Information collected from yearbooks, reports, census reports etc. Verbal history can be obtained during interviews of persons who had direct/indirect experience with the knowledge of the chosen topic. Relics are also valuable source of information. They include articles like clothing, buildings, books, maps or any other objects that might provide meaningful information about past.

Action research - Action research focuses on problem solving process. In this research design, group of people identify a problem & actions are taken to solve it & identify success of the efforts taken, if not satisfied, whole process is tried again. It increases an understanding of how change in one's actions/ practices can mutually benefit healthcare professionals within an organization. Taking an action through planning & fact findings brings about future an organizational change.

- Data collection methods used in this design are: interview, observation, story telling, sociodrama, drawing & painting, plays & skits.

Importance of Action research in health science -

- It can improve health care practice & healthcare research.
- The habit of thinking, the ability to work harmoniously with others & professional spirit will improve.
- Healthcare knowledge, actions & consciousness will benefit from action research, as it will help to recognize strengths & areas need improvement.

Case study - H. Odum defines case study method as a technique by which individual factor whether it is an institution or just an episode in the life of an individual or a group is analysed in its relationship to any other in the group. Case study is often used when the selected case might offer insight into a unique situation or more information to be collected about a particular phenomenon within a real life context. On the basis of the purpose of carrying out case studies, they are classified into three major categories i.e. descriptive, exploratory & explanatory case studies. In health care sciences, this methodology has been used since a long time for in depth study of a single patient or a group of patients to generate a knowledge for solving patients' problems with specific diagnosis. In case study data are collected by observation or by personal interview method. In case studies, the stress is more on the qualitative analysis of the collected data.

Meta-synthesis - Qualitative meta-synthesis is an interpretation of qualitative research findings that are themselves interpretative synthesis of data including phenomenologies, ethnographies, grounded theories & other integrated & coherent descriptions or explanations of phenomena, events as cases that are hallmarks of qualitative research. This is done to move toward evidence based practice. Also it allows for a collective way of viewing specific research within a discipline & integrating the findings into a form that is readily accessible & understandable. It helps to build new theories. It primarily generates theories such as programme theory, implementation theory, or an explanation theory of the working of particular interventions.

Sandelowski & Barroso (2007) have described six steps of meta-synthesis as follows–

- Formulation of research question
- Conducting a systematic literature search
- Screening & selecting appropriate research articles
- Analysing & synthesizing qualitative findings
- Maintaining quality control
- Presenting findings

Triangulation (Mixed Methods)

Combination of several methods are commonly termed as mixed methods, multiple methods, methodology pluralism & triangulation. Triangulation is one form of combining more than one method. In the same study i.e. primarily have qualitative or quantitative approach. Combination of methods used in research study can include increased confidence in study data & better understanding of a phenomenon & integration of theories. This process can decrease the chances for biases within the research process & the analysis of the data while validating the results obtained. Triangulation might be used in four basic ways in a research study: a) data triangulation; b) methods triangulation; c) researcher triangulation; d) theory triangulation. The most commonly used triangulation is the methods triangulation in recent studies.

Data triangulation - The multiple data sources are used in this method, so the conclusion is validated. There are three types of data triangulation i.e. time, space & person triangulation.

Time triangulation - In this type of triangulation data collection is done on the same phenomenon or same informant at different times. There can be interval of data collection of hours or months.

Space triangulation - In this method, data collection is done at different sites, so that consistency of data is assessed.

Person triangulation - Different types of people or informants collect data. Different people have different perspectives of the same phenomenon, so data collection by different persons widens the perspectives on the phenomenon of interest.

Methods triangulation - To have comprehensive understanding of phenomenon, both quantitative & qualitative data collection techniques are combined e.g. a researcher is interested to assess problem of absenteeism among the healthcare professionals working in various units of J.J. Hospital Mumbai city. So in this out-structured qualitative data measurement tools, that breadth & depth of information may be obtained. There are two types of methods triangulation i.e. concurrent & sequential types. In concurrent type both quantitative & qualitative methods are equally used at the same time. In sequential type, both the methods are followed by one another & one type of the methods dominates while using sequential type of triangulation method.

Researcher triangulation - For the purpose of data collection, analysis & interpretation of data is carried out by more than one researcher. To minimize the occurrence of researcher biases & enhance the quality of data analysis researcher triangulation method is used.

Theory triangulation - During analysis & interpretation of data more than one theory/hypothesis is used. In this method conceptualization of phenomenon occurs.

Combining methods & approaches should be well thought process & supported by strong rational discussion, the purpose & benefits of such decision & the choice of methods. It is believed that mixed method research is adapted by a new generation of researchers but still there are controversial issues about use of mixed methods.

SUMMARY

- A research design is the overall plan, blueprint, a framework or guide used for planning, implementation & analysis of a study.
- Classification of research design is based on approach & purpose of conducting research. Based on approach, research design is classified as quantitative, qualitative methods. Based on purpose, it is categorized into basic & applied research designs. Other types of research designs are mixed methods. Specific types of quantitative methods are evaluation, outcome, operational, methodological, secondary data analysis, meta-analysis & systematic reviews research designs.
- Quantitative research designs are classified as experimental, true experimental, quasi-experimental, non-experimental, correlational, descriptive, exploratory & survey research design.
- The true experimental research design is also called as Randomized Controlled Trials (RCTs), has three important characteristics i.e. manipulation, randomization & control.
- Categorization of qualitative research designs is: phenomenological, ethnographic, grounded theory, historical, action research & case study & meta-synthsis.
- Mixed methods research design includes combination of quantitative & qualitative research designs for the purpose of data collection, analysis & interpretation of data to facilitate comprehensive understanding of phenomenon & provide a complete answer to research question than use of one method alone.

BIBLIOGRAPHY

- Burns N,. Grove S.K. (2005) Understanding nursing research: building an evidence based practices. (4th edition) Noida: Elsevier.
- Bryman, A. (2006) Social research methods. (3rd edition). Oxford University. Press.
- Creswell, J.W., Planno Clarke V,L., (2003) Designing & conducting mixed method research. Thousand Oaks, CA:Sage.
- Cresswell,J.W., (2015). A concise introduction to mixed methods research. Thousand Oakes,CA: Sage.
- Donalck,j.g. (2004) Demystefying nursing research: Phenomenology as a qualitative research method. Urology nursing, 24,516-517.
- Finfgeld,D.L. (2003). Metasynthesis: the state of the art so far. Qualitative Health Research.13 (7),893-904.
- Haidich,A.B. (2010) Meta-analysis in medical research. Hippocratia,14 (suppl.I) 29-37.
- Jacelon,C.S., O'Dell,K.K. (2005) Case & group theory as qualitative methods. Urology nursing,25,49-52.

- Macnee C.L. (2004) Understanding nursing research: reading & using research in practice. (1st edition). Philadelphia, PA: Lippincott
- Monc J.M., Niehans,, L. (2009). Mixed method design: Principles & procedures. Wanut Creek.C.A.: Left cost press.
- Morse J.M., Niehans,L (2011): Mixed method design: Principles & procedures. Forum: Quantitative social research.12 (I), 130-141.
- Paterson,B.L., Thorne,S.E.,Canan,C. & Jillings C. (2001) Meta study of qualitative health research. Thousands Oakes CA:Sage.
- Polit F.D., Beck C.T. (2008) Nursing research: generating & assessing evidence for nursing practices. (8th edition) Philadelphia,PA:Lippincott.
- Thorne S., Jenson L,.Kearney, M.H.. Noblit,G. & Sandelowsky, M.,. (2004) Qualitative metasynthesis:Reflections on methodological orientation & ideological agenda. Qualitative health research., 14, 1342-1365.

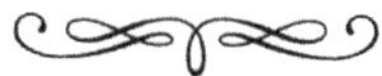

CHAPTER

8 Sampling and Nursing Research

Swati Kambli

Learning Objectives

This chapter helps the reader to –

- Explain the purposes & process of sampling.
- Identify various factors influencing the sampling process.
- Discuss the probability & non-probability types of sampling techniques.
- Understand the sampling techniques used in qualitative research.
- Develop skills in selection & calculation of sample size.
- Identify problems related to sampling process i.e. sampling errors & bias.

Sampling is critical part of research design specially in quantitative research approach. Also it is most important factors which determines the accuracy of research results. It is a process of selecting representative units from an entire population of the study. Sampling is an old concept. In 1786, Pierre Simon Laplace estimated the population of France by using a sample technique, along with a ratio estimator. He also computed probabilistic estimates of the error. Alexander Ivanovich Chuprov introduced sample surveys to Imperial Russia in the 1870s (Cochran 1963 & Robert et al. 2004).

Sampling is a part of daily life e.g. when we prepare meals, we check a portion of it to confirm whether it is cooked or not & about taste, flavours of the items. Similar concept is applied in research as it is not possible for the researcher to study an entire population, therefore the representative sample is selected from the population to conduct the research & make the inferences about the population. It is a process of acquiring knowledge/information regarding a phenomenon about entire population by carrying out a research on part of it.

Population

Population is the collection of the elements which has some or the other characteristics in common. Also it is the entire aggregation of cases in which researcher is interested. Populations are not restricted only to human subjects but consist of everything like records, blood samples, schools/colleges etc.

Target & Accessible Population

Target population - It is the aggregate of cases about which the researcher would like to generalize e.g. All diabetes mellitus cases all over Mumbai city.

Accessible/source population - An aggregate of cases that conform to designated criteria & that are accessible as subjects for a study, e.g. All patients diagnosed as diabetes mellitus admitted in J.J. group of hospitals. Researchers usually sample from an accessible population & hope to generalize to a target population.

Criteria

The criteria which specify population characteristics are referred to as **eligibility/inclusion criteria.**

- Sometimes, a population is defined in terms of characteristics that people must not possess i.e. **Exclusion criteria.**
- It is important that sample should be a good match with population construct. Construct validity is enhanced when there is good match between eligibility criteria of sample & population construct.

Samples & sampling -

- **Sampling** - It is a process of selecting a portion of the population to represent the entire population so that inferences about population can be made.
- A sample is a subset of population elements.
- An element is a most basic unit about which information is collected. Usually in nursing research the elements are humans.

Purposes of sampling -

- **Economical** - The researchers can have economy of time, money & resources with the help of the sampling as it is not always possible & economical for the researcher to study the entire population.
- **Quality of data** - Success/outcome of the research study depends upon quality of data, & good quality of data will be generated by handling fewer number of people, which would not be possible in case the entire population was involved. Also it is possible to generate the study results faster.

- **Precision & accuracy of data -** With a small number of sample, it is possible to accurately follow all scientific steps of research study, where there are less bias, errors, so that the data collected from small sample will be more precise & accurate.

Characteristics of a good sample - In order to apply the study findings for an entire population, a good sample for the research study must have following characteristics -

- **Representativeness** - It is the important characteristics of sample that it should be closely related to those of the population. A representative sample is one whose key characteristics are closely approximate those of entire population.
  - If sample is not representative of the population, external validity (& the construct validity) of study is at risk.
- **Free from bias & errors -** A sample is good when it is not selected deliberately for study. Sample should be free from sampling errors & bias.
- **Approximate Sample Size -** In quantitative research designs, as the sample size is larger, findings of the study can be generalized to the population. But in qualitative research designs smaller sample size is helpful till the data saturation occurs.

Sampling Process

Selecting a part of the required population which represents entire population is termed as sampling process. It should be very systematically carried out. Sampling process is based on specific selection criteria. As per the specific selection criteria, sample selection is done. **The sampling process includes following criteria –**

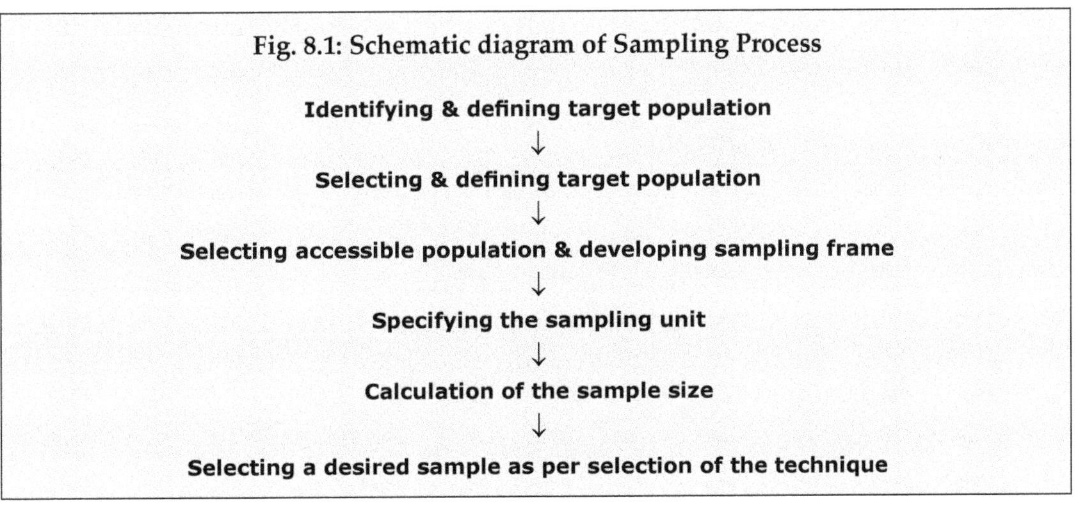
Fig. 8.1: Schematic diagram of Sampling Process

- **Identifying & defining target population -** Depending upon the phenomenon under study & set criteria of population for which study findings will be generalized, target population will be identified & defined.
- **Selecting accessible population & developing sampling frame -** Accessible population is readily available for the purpose of conducting a research. After complete description of accessible population, researcher must develop a sampling frame to select a sample from accessible population.
- **Specifying the sampling unit -** Sampling unit selection should be based on the specific inclusion & exclusion criteria, so that confusion in selection of sampling unit is prevented.
- **Selection of sampling technique -** Selection of sampling technique i.e. probability or non-probability is one of the important stages of sampling process. Several factors can influence in selection of technique are: types of population, type of phenomenon under study, availability of resources & researcher's knowledge.
- **Calculation of sample size -** Sample size calculation should be done in such a way that study findings can be generalized. Details are discussed under the subtitle of sample size calculation.
- **Selecting a desired sample as per the selection of technique -**

  Whatever plan for sampling process is prepared, should be implemented to ultimately select a representative part of population, which is used for the process of data collection by the researcher.

CLASSIFICATION OF SAMPLING DESIGNS

Overall sampling design is classified as Probability & Non-Probability sampling Designs. Researchers can specify probability that an element of the population will be included in the sample. Most respected as greater confidence can be placed in representativeness of probability samples.

Probability Sampling Design

This technique is based on the theory of probability & it involves random selection of elements of population. In this design every population element has equal chance to be selected as the subject.

- In this technique sampling units are selected randomly (by chance) & neither investigator, nor the population elements have any conscious influence on what is included in sample.
- Sample is representative of population so findings of the study can be generalized.

- Through the process of randomization, the danger of unknown sampling bias can be minimized. Hence probability sample is preferable & a greater degree of accuracy of estimation of population parameters is achieved.
- A further advantage is that probability sampling allows researchers to estimate the magnitude of sampling error which is discussed further in this chapter.
- This technique is further classified in five subtypes: **Simple Random Sampling, Stratified Random Sampling, Systematic Random Sampling, Cluster or Multi-Stage Random Sampling & Sequential Random Sampling.**

  Simple Random Sampling - It is a most basic probability sampling design. In this design, every population element has equal chance of being selected as the subject & each subject is being selected independently of the other members of the population.
- There are two essential prerequisites to implement simple random technique i.e. population must be homogenous & the researcher must have list/sampling frame of the elements/members of the accessible population. A sampling frame is the technical name for the list of the elements/members of the accessible population.
- There are three basic procedures followed to draw sample as follow-
  - **Lottery method -** This method is the simplest, oldest of all methods used to draw a sample & it is a most familiar procedure in simple random sampling. If a sample of 10 students is drawn out of a list of 50 students from a particular class then 50 slips of paper are prepared, numbering from 1–50. Then we need to shuffle/mix them properly in a container & closing the eyes pick up 10 slips randomly. All the subjects bearing the number are selected by the researcher, become the subjects for the study.
  - When a number is replaced & has a chance to be selected again is known as sampling with replacement, referred to as unrestricted random sampling.
  - When number is set aside, does not get a chance of being selected again, known as sampling without replacement/restricted sampling.
  - Lottery method is useful for drawing a small sample of a population. It is time consuming & tedious, if population is very large.
  - **Use of table of random numbers -** Tables are developed by **Kendall & Smith (1939). Fisher & Yates (1963) & Tippett (1927).**

- To select a random sample out of a given frame, one should simply start to read numbers from a Table of Random Numbers at any randomly selected point & pick out numbers within the range of the frame.
- Easy to use & readily accessible. Ideal for obtaining a random sample from relatively small populations. Not very useful for large populations.
- **Use of Computer -** If population is very large then computer can be used to draw random sample. Computer can be programmed to print out a series of random numbers as the researcher desires.

Advantages of Simple Random Sample

- All elements have equal chance to be selected.
- Easiest, most simple.
- Requires minimum knowledge of population in advance.
- It is free from classification errors.
- Sampling errors are easily computed. Accuracy of the estimate is easily assessed.

Disadvantages

- It does not make use of the knowledge about population which researcher may have.
- The size required for this design is usually large.
- If the sample is Widely dispersed geographically then it requires lots of time & cost will be very high.
- It is difficult to researcher to have up-to-date lists of all elements of the population.

Stratified Random Sampling

It is an improved type of random/probability sampling. In this design, the population is subdivided into homogenous groups/strata & from each stratum, random sample is drawn. e.g. University students are selected course wise & from each course they are selected year wise. Stratification is needed for -

- Increasing a sample's statistical efficiency.
- Providing adequate data for analysing the various sub-populations &
- Applying different methods of analysis to different strata.

According to the weightage of the sample & proportions, stratified random sampling is further divided into two categories: proportionate & disproportionate stratified random sampling.

- **Proportionate Stratified Random Sampling -** As per the size of the total population, the sample is selected from each stratum. The sample size of each stratum seems to be proportionate to the population size of the stratum. The important thing in this technique is to select the same sampling fraction for each stratum irrespective of the differences in the strata's population size.
- **Disproportionate Stratified Random Sampling -** In this technique the sample size need not to be proportionate to the population size of the stratum, so two or more strata will have different fractions. Thus the difference between proportionate & disproportionate stratified random sampling is their sampling fractions only. Sampling fraction is the ratio of the sample size to the size of the stratum. e.g. a researcher would like to conduct a study on nursing staff of three different hospitals from Mumbai city, which includes 150 nurses from government hospital, 200 nurses from Municipal Corporation hospital & 250 nurses from private hospital. As per the following table, researcher has selected sampling fraction i.e. ½ for proportionate stratified random sampling & as per the table 8.1 and 8.2 researcher has selected different sampling fractions.

Table 8.1: Example of Proportionate stratified random sampling

Stratum	A	B	C
Population size	150	200	250
Final sample size	½	½	½

Table 8.2: Example of Disproportionate stratified random sampling

Stratum	A	B	C
Population size	150	200	250
Sampling fraction	⅓	¼	⅕
Final sample size	50	50	50

The accuracy of this design is mostly dependent on the sampling fraction allocation by the researcher. If there are any errors in alotting sampling fractions, a stratum may be under-represented or over-represented, resulting in skewed results.

Merits

- This technique is superior than simple random sampling technique, as it ensures representation of all groups & is more representative of the population which is being sampled.

- It can be kept small in size without losing its accuracy & it saves time, money & efforts of the researchers. With this technique, the most inaccessible subgroups can be sampled.
- Characteristics of each stratum can be estimated & existing relationships between two or more stratum can be observed & hence comparison can be made between subgroups.
- As variability within subgroups is less, so there is higher statistical precision.

Demerits

- It requires accurate information on proportion of population with stratum.
- It becomes a costly affair to prepare stratified lists of all members.
- There is always a possibility of faulty classification & hence leading to increase in variability.

Systematic random sampling - In this sampling technique a list/sampling frame is prepared from target population. Then the first subject is randomly selected. Later on systematic sample is formed by selecting every nth item from target population where 'n' is referred as sampling interval. Sampling interval is determined by dividing the size of the universe by size of the sample to be chosen. e.g. 320 traveling expense vouchers selected from a universe of 32,000 vouchers. Sampling interval would be 100.

Merits

- It is simple to follow.
- This technique distributes sample more evenly over the entire listed population
- It is less cumbersome, saves time, cheaper than simple random sampling technique.
- It is statistically more efficient & provides a better representative sample when population elements are randomly distributed.

Demerits

- It is not truly random & may not be appropriate to select a representative sample. All items selected for the sample are determined by constant interval.
- May result into a badly biased sample.

Cluster/multi Stage Random Sampling

In this technique the population elements are scattered over a wider area & a list of population elements is not readily available. As the use of other methods are too expensive & time consuming, cluster sampling is adopted for a research study.

- A sampling unit is drawn from cluster of population elements by simple random selection/stratified random selection procedure.
- This technique is most often used in large scale studies when population is geographically spread out.
- It consists of groups rather than individuals.

Types of Cluster Samples

- **One stage cluster sample -** e.g. A research study on job satisfaction of group of nurses who are selected randomly is conducted from a particular hospital.
- **Two-stage cluster sample -** In this technique, the list of clusters is prepared from the population. Then the units/elements are selected by simple random sampling/systematic random sampling technique in the second stage. E.g. Various hospitals list is prepared & then nursing supervisors are selected by simple random/systematic random sampling for research study on identification of conflicts & various strategies of conflict resolution.
- **Multi-stage cluster sample -** Sampling is being done for more than two levels. e.g. Various hospitals having neuro speciality from a particular state are selected first. Then various patients with diagnosis of cerebrovascular accident will be selected as a cluster by simple random sampling/systematic sampling technique & later on convalescent patients are selected as elements by simple random sampling/systematic random sampling technique as per the inclusion criteria of the study.
    - **Steps involved in cluster sampling –**
        1. Identify clusters. e.g. schools, colleges, factories, sections of school/ departments of factory.
        2. Examine the nature of clusters. Clusters should not be homogenous as internal characteristics will not represent overall population. e.g. city blocks contain different income/social groups combined as one cluster.
        3. Determine the number of stages i.e. single stage/multistage clusters. It depends upon geographical area of the study, the scale of the study, the size of the population & the consideration of the costs.

Merits

- This technique is economical in terms of time, money etc.
- Easy for a large population & require only a list of numbers.
- Same cluster/population can be used again for study.

Demerits

- This technique is the least representative of the population, as limited clusters included in the sample, leaving of a significant proportion of the population unsampled, giving rise to high possibility of high sampling error.
- There are chances of having overrepresented or underrepresented cluster which can skew the study results.

Sequential Sampling

In this technique, initially a small sample size is selected & inferences are drawn. If not possible to draw the results, then more subjects are added until clear cut results are drawn. e.g. A researcher is studying association between alcoholism & liver cirrhosis. Initially smallest sample is selected & inferences are drawn. If not possible, then sample is added till meaningful inferences are drawn.

Table 8.3: Sequential sampling

No of subjects Alcoholics (A)		Non-alcoholics (B)	Having cirrhosis of liver	
			A	B
20	7	12	2	1
30	18	22	5	3
50	28	22	10	4

The above Table shows addition of subjects until results are drawn. It is observed in the above values, out of 50 subjects, 28 alcoholics had almost double incidence of cirrhosis of liver as compared to 22 non-alcoholics.

Characteristics

- This technique is used in problems involving alternatives (to accept/reject/ continue analysis)
- Total size of sample is not decided in the beginning of the study.

Merits

- A study can be conducted on best possible smallest representative sample.

- With the help of this technique the inferences can be drawn.

Demerits

- Not possible to study a phenomenon at one point of time.
- To collect the sample, repeated entries are needed.

NON-PROBABILITY SAMPLING

In this technique, the individuals in the population do not have equal chances of being selected in the sample. So there are chances that methods of sampling are likely to result in a biased sample than random methods. In this technique generalization of study findings to entire population is not possible. In spite of all limitations of non-probability sampling, it is still used in nursing & other disciplines. The drawback of this technique is that an unknown proportion of the entire population is not sampled.

Uses of Non-Probability Sampling

- Less likely than probability sampling to produce accurate & representative samples
- It is used to show that a particular characteristic is existing in the population.
- In qualitative research approach, pilot & exploratory study, this technique is used.
- When population is limitless it is used.
- With this technique, study findings cannot be generalized to entire population.
- When there are limited resources like man, money & materials.

Types of Non-Probability Sampling

Classification of non-probability sampling is: purposive, convenience, volunteer, quota, snowball & genealogy.

Purposive Sampling

This technique is based on the belief that researcher's knowledge about the population can be used to handpick sample members. Researchers might decide purposely to select subjects who are judged to be typical of the population/particularly knowledgeable about the issues under study. Also this is an objective method for assessing typicalness of selected subjects. Newly developed instruments can be effectively pretested & evaluated with diverse. This technique is frequently used by qualitative researchers.

Merits

- Simple to draw the sample.
- Useful in exploratory, pilot & qualitative research study.
- Economical in terms of resources, less field work is required.

Demerits

- Considerable knowledge is required about population under study.
- Not reliable, there are chances of conscious bias.
- Members of population do not have equal chances to be selected.

Convenience Sampling

It is probably the most common of all sampling techniques. It uses most conveniently available people as study participants. Also called as accidental sample. e.g. distribution of questionnaire to particular class of students/or people on the streets.

Subjects are readily accessible for the researcher & may help save time, money & other resources.

Uses of Convenience Sampling

- It is used in pilot studies, so that basic data is obtained without problems of using random sample selection methods.
- Useful in recording a particular quality of a substance/phenomena that occurs within a given sample.
- It is very useful for detecting relationships among different phenomena.

Merits

- Easiest, cheapest type of technique, least time consuming & saving resources.

Demerits

- The sample selected is not representative of entire population & there is sampling bias.
- Findings of the study with this type of samples cannot be generalized to the population.

Volunteer Sampling

Through a published advertisement researcher requests target population to participate in the study & interested participants may voluntarily participate in the study. e.g. a nurse researcher is interested to assess the effect of gluten free diet on prevention of coeliac disease. The features of volunteer sampling technique is as follows -

1. Researcher only disseminates the information about the research activity to the target population.
2. The interested participants volunteer to participate in the study.

Merits

- It is economical, in terms of efforts, money & time to locate participants.
- Large amount of data can be collected in limited time period.

Demerits

- Sample is not representative of population.
- As persons who come across the advertisement only participate in the study so it encounters systematic errors/bias.
- Study results lack generalizability.

Quota Sampling

It is the technique in which the researcher identifies population strata, determines how many participants needed in each stratum. In this technique information about population characteristics, researcher can ensure that diverse segments are represented in the sample, preferably in proportion as they occur in population. e.g. correct number of men/women.

- Stratification should be based on one/more variables that would reflect important differences in the dependent variable under study. Such variables as gender, ethnicity, education & medical diagnosis are often good stratifying variables.
- Quota sampling is procedurally like convenient sampling so it shares many of the same weaknesses as convenience sampling.
- Despite its problems, quota sampling represents important improvement over convenience sampling & should be considered by quantitative researchers.

Snowball Sampling

This technique is used by the researchers to identify potential subjects in studies where subjects in studies are hard to locate e.g. a researcher wants to conduct a study on the prevalence of HIV/AIDS among commercial sex workers, truck drivers & persons with substance abuse disorders. In this situation snowball sampling is the best choice to select a sample.

Types of Snowball Sampling

- **Linear Snowball Sampling -** In this technique a linear chain is created as each selected sample is asked to provide reference of only one similar subject.

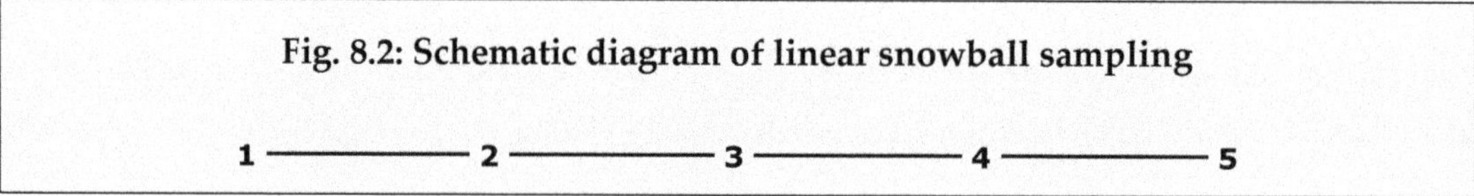

Fig. 8.2: Schematic diagram of linear snowball sampling

- **Exponential Non-discriminative Snowball Sampling -** In this technique, each sample is asked to provide a reference of at least two similar subjects due to which sample size grows exponentially & a large size is achieved

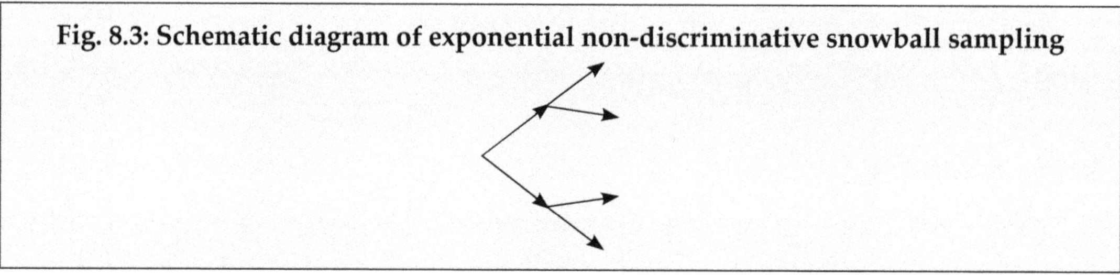
Fig. 8.3: Schematic diagram of exponential non-discriminative snowball sampling

- **Exponential Discriminative Snowball Sampling -** In this technique in the beginning one sample is selected who provides two references of similar subjects. Out of which, one subject should be active to provide further references & another could be nonactive in providing references & same process is repeated further.

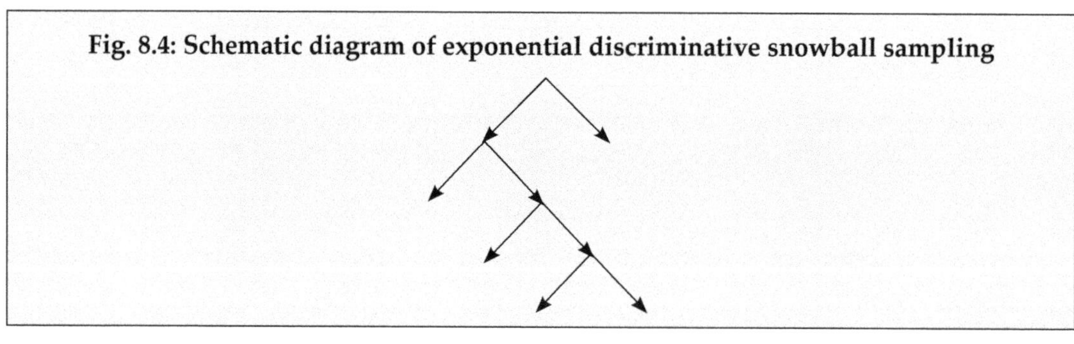
Fig. 8.4: Schematic diagram of exponential discriminative snowball sampling

Merits of Snowball Sampling

- The chain referral process permits the researcher to reach populations that are difficult to sample.
- This technique is simple, economical in terms of man, money, material etc.

Genealogy Sampling

In this technique all the members of entire related families are selected. It begins with identifying first participant who is willing to participate in the study & then further he/she is asked to refer to close relatives of the same family, who may be living in other areas of village or other villages. This is mainly used for rural population which are socio-culturally & economically homogenous & it is also used for genetic studies, to identify patterns of genes in traditional families.

Merits

- It is useful for drawing a representative sample from traditional rural community.
- Economical in time & efforts as sample is identified through reference from family members.

Demerits

- There are problems of systematic errors/bias.
- It has limited usefulness as subjects are selected from a family so it lacks diversity of sample characteristics.

Sampling in Qualitative Research

The aim of most qualitative research is to discover meaning & to uncover multiple realities, so generalizability is not a guiding consideration. In qualitative research studies, there are no definite rules to determine sample size. It is largely a function of the purpose of inquiry, the quality of the informants & the type of sampling strategy used. It also depends upon the variety of characteristics needed for research. The more the variety, the bigger is the sample size needed. If less number of characteristics needed for research then the sample size can be small or kept at a level till data saturation occurs. Data saturation depends upon the number of factors/scope of research question. The broader the scope, the sample size should be larger. Mostly non-probability sampling technique is used, as sample size remains small. Usually in qualitative research, subjects have information richness, so in-depth information about phenomena under study is collected. Thus in qualitative research emergent sampling technique is used. As study advances, new sampling technique is added. Some of the commonly used sampling techniques are as follow-

- Convenience sampling technique, snowball sampling & purposive sampling techniques which are already discussed in this chapter.
- Sample size usually needed in different kinds of qualitative research is as follow-
    - Ethnography – 25–50.
    - Phenomenology – 10 or less than that.
    - Grounded theory – generally 20–30 informants selected who can best contribute the information to develop a theory.

Sample Size Basics in Quantitative Research Approach

- A largest sample size should be used if possible as sampling error is inversely proportional to sample size.
- The larger the sample, the sample is more representative of the population likely to be as compared to a smaller sample.
- Smaller samples tend to produce less accurate estimates than larger ones. In other words, the larger the sample, the smaller the sampling error.
- When samples are too small, there are chances that quantitative researchers run the risk of gathering data that will not support their hypotheses, even when their hypotheses are correct, therby undermining statistical conclusion validity.
- The results drawn by sample should stand closest to the true population values.

Sample Size Determination

A sample is selected out of target population. Sample drawn should have similar traits like target population. Sample size should be adequate to represent the population. In conduct of research & evaluation of research process, sample size has been considered one of the major aspects. This chapter presents some of the simplest ways to calculate sample size for a research study to draw conclusions & generalization of the study findings. The methods followed as in **quantitative research studies** to determine the sample size are sample size determination nomogram table, power analysis with statistical formulae & sample size determination software. So an accurate sample size can be estimated.

- Thumb rules for estimating sample size lack scientific basis & not appreciated by various scientists. In case of lack of resources like computation of sample size, the following thumb rules can be used.
  - A large sized health science trial should include nearly 300 subjects, in each group; a midsized trial nearly 100 subjects in each group & small sized trial at least 50 subjects in each group.

Factors Affecting Sample Size Requirements in Quantitative Research-

- **Homogeneity of the population -** If the reason to believe that the population is homogenous, a small sample may be adequate.
  - For clinical studies that deal with bio-physiologic processes in which variation is limited, a small sample may adequately represent the population.
- **Design effect -** This includes the type of study & the number of variables under study & the sampling strategy. Quantitative studies require a larger sample size than qualitative studies.
- **Resources available -** A larger sample size, even though effective, may be costly, so researchers need to decide, if sufficient resources are available.
- **Sampling method used -** Efficiently selected smaller samples are better than badly selected larger samples. Comparing to non-probability sampling, probability sampling is more effective & meaningful for study outcomes.
- **Co-operation & attrition -** In most of the studies, not necessary that everyone invited to participate in the study agrees to do so. So in developing a sampling plan good to begin with a realistic estimate of percentage of people likely to co-operate. Researchers should expect a certain amount of subjects loss & recruit accordingly. To enhance co-operation of subjects, recruitment method can be face to face. Also courtesy towards subjects can be shown by pleasant non-threatening approach. Persistence is needed for success of the study. Acknowledgement & incentives like expression of gratitude towards subjects can enhance their participation. Assurances provided regarding anonymity/confidentiality of their participation in the study.
- **Subgroup analysis -** Researchers are sometimes interested in testing hypotheses not only for an entire population but also for subgroups. When a sample is divided to test for subgroup effects, the sample must be large enough to support these divisions of the sample.
- **Sensitivity of the measures/measurement factors -** Instruments vary in their ability to measure variables/key concepts of the study precisely.

Bio-physiologic measures are very sensitive & measure phenomena accurately. Psychosocial values contain some errors & lack precision. So larger samples needed to test hypotheses adequately.

- **Generalizing from samples -** Ideally, the sample is representatives of accessible population & accessible population is representative of the target population. Inferences about generalizability of study findings can be enhanced by comparing sample characteristics with population characteristics, when this is possible.

Sample Size Determination by Using Table

It is not very easy to calculate sample size by using various formulae which are available & recommended. Therefore a Table is given by experts (2006) based on sample size calculation formula by Krejcie & Morgan (1970). In nursing research studies, generally 95% confidence level & 5% margin of error is considered ideal.

- **Power Analysis -** A procedure known as power analysis (Cohen, 1988) can be used to determine sample size. To estimate sample size with power analysis is a gold standard. It helps to decide on how 'large a sample' is required for quantitative research study. The main components of the power analysis are as follow-
  - **Power -** A researcher specifies the power to be achieved. Thus for that level of power, required sample size can be estimated e.g. to find a popularity of a television serial amongst the viewers, researcher feels 75% of people like to view this serial so the power here is 75%. Then data is collected from 100 viewers, it will yield result 75% of the times & a non-significant result only 25% of the times.
  - **Effect size -** Power analysis builds on the concept of an effect size, which expresses the strength of relationships among research variables.
- If there is a reason to expect that the independent & dependent variables will be strongly related, then a relatively small sample should be adequate to demonstrate the relationship statistically. When there is no prior reason to believe that relationship will be strong, then small samples are risky.
- **Sample size calculation using computer -** The neophyte researcher may use the user friendly, a preformatted software to determine the sample size. The clinical researchers may use the sample size calculator (http://www.sample-size.net/about-this-site) of UCSF clinical & Translational Science Institute for sample size calculations in advanced level clinical research studies.

- **Confidence levels -** The confidence level remains expressed as a percentage & represents how often the true percentage of the population pick an answer lies within confidence interval. The 95% confidence level means one can be 95% certain; the 99% confidence level means one can be 99% certain. Nursing & most of the other researchers use 95% confidence level. Higher confidence level requires a larger size of population.

Probability & sampling errors -

Sample is expected to be representative of population it is derived from. But it is not necessary that each sample will be representative of the population it is derived from. A sampling error is the difference in sample & population from which it is derived from in terms of characteristics, behaviour, qualities or figures of entire population. Sampling error occurs as a result of calculating estimate (mean, total, proportion etc) based on a sample rather than the entire population. This is due to the fact that the estimated figures obtained from the sample may not be exactly equal to the true value of the population. Salant & Dilman describe that statistics based on samples drawn from the same population always vary from each other (& from true population values) simply because of chance. This variation in sampling error & the measure used to estimate the sampling error is the standard error.

- Following formula can be used to estimate standard error of the proportion-
- Se (p) = [(pq) /m] where Se (p) is the standard error of a proportion, p & q is the proportion of the sample that do (p) & do not (q) have a particular characteristic & n = the number of units in the sample. (cs.fit.edu/.../CSE5800/sampling techniques.pdf).

Reasons for sampling errors -

- When sample is drawn from different subjects from same population but subjects have individual differences.
- Frequent cause of error is biased sampling procedure.
- Most common error is **systematic error** wherein the results from the sample differ significantly from the results from entire population.
- There are **two basic reasons** for sampling error.
    - **Chance error** - Error occurs by chance e.g. a study conducted on diarrhea among infants from two cities & where the second city had a large number of slum dwellers, wherein hygienic conditions are poor, so it comprised of large number of infants with diarrhea, thus the results are skewed.

- **Sampling bias** - It occurs when sample is selected that possesses particular characteristics e.g. a study is conducted to identify the effect of virtual teaching on learning of 5th standard students. This study will be biased towards those children who have facilities of computer, laptop or android mobile phones, but the ones who do not have these facilities are excluded.

Types of sampling bias -

- **Self selection bias -** This types of bias occurs when participants in the study have preference over the study to participate or not. e.g. volunteer sampling.
- **Exclusion bias -** This happens when some people of the group are eliminated from the study as the situation of children with electronic gadgets discussed above.
- **Healthy user bias -** When sample selected is more healthier compared to general population.
- Ben Shlomo Y, Brookes S, Hickman M, 2013 have included following reasons for sampling bias –
  - Any pre agreed sampling rules are deviated from.
  - People in hard-to-reach groups are omitted.
  - Selected individuals are replaced with others e.g. if they are difficult to contact.
  - There are low response rates.
  - An outdated list is used as the sample e.g. it excludes people who have recently moved to an area.

Minimizing sampling errors/bias -

This can be achieved by a proper & unbiased probability sampling & by using a large sample size. The following things can help to minimize sampling errors/ bias.

- Avoiding convenience/judgment sampling.
- Sample frame should match target population which is well defined.
- The sample selected should be representative of entire population, matching overall traits of target population.
- If sample is large then there are less sampling errors.

SUMMARY

- Population is the aggregate of people/entities in which the researcher is interested & to which the results are to be generalized.
- Sampling is a process of selecting representative units from an entire population.
- A good sample must be representative of the target population under study & free from bias/errors & of an adequate size to generalize the findings.
- A sampling process involves the steps as: identifying & defining the target population, selecting accessible population & developing sampling frame, specifying the sampling unit, selecting sampling technique & calculation of sample size, selecting a designed sample as per the selection of technique.
- The sampling techniques are mainly classified as probability sampling technique & non-probability sampling technique.
- The types of different probability sampling techniques are: simple random sampling, stratified random sampling, systematic random sampling, multi-stage cluster sampling & sequential random sampling technique.
- The types of different non-probability sampling techniques are: purposive, convenience, volunteer, quota, snowball & genealogy sampling techniques.
- The factors affecting sample size are: design effect, resources available, nature of the study, sampling methods used, level of homogeneity of population, effect size, degree of accuracy desired from the estimates & degree of confidence.
- Sample size calculation is done by: using table, power analysis & by computer a pre-formatted soft wares.
- A sampling error is the difference in sample & population from which it is derived in terms of characteristics, behaviours, qualities or figures of entire population. There are various reasons responsible for sampling bias & sampling errors & can be minimized by: by selecting a proper & unbiased probability sampling, by using a larger sample size, avoiding purposive/convenient sampling, matching sample frame with population from which it is derived & selecting sample which is representative of entire population.

BIBLIOGRAPHY

- Burns, N., Groove S.K., (2005) The practice of nursing research: conduct, critique & utilization (5th edition) St. Louis, MO: Elsevier
- Chavan J., Biswas T., (2013) How to calculate sample size for different study designs in medical research? Indian J Psychology Med., 35 (2): 121-126.

- Dempsey PA, Dempsey A.D., (2000) Using nursing research: Process, critical evaluation.& utilization. 5th edn., Philadelphia: Lippincott Williams & Wilkins.
- Goodman, L.A. (1961) Snowball sampling. Annals of Mathmatical Statistics,32,148-170.
- Heckathorn D.D. (1997) Respondent driven sampling: a new approach to the study of hidden population. Social problems, 44, 174-199.
- Heckathorn D.D., (2002) Respondent driven sampling: deriving valid estimates from chain referral samples of hidden populations. Social problem. 49, 11-34.
- Kerlinger F.N. & Lee, H.B. (2000) Foundations of behavioural research. New York. NY: Harcourt Brace.
- Nursing Research society of India. (2013) Nursing Research & Statistics. 1st edition. New Delhi.: Dorling Kindersley.
- More J.M., (2000) Determining sample size. Qualitative Health Research. 10 (1), 3–5.
- Pattop, M.Q., (2002) Qualitative evaluation & research methods. (3rd edn) Thousand Oaks, CA: Sage.
- Sagalnik, M.J., Heckathorn, D.D. (2004) Sampling & estimation in hidden populations using respondent driven sampling. Sociological Methodology, 34, 193-239.
- Tabo,L.A. (1995) Principles & practices of nursing research. Boston, M.A.: Mosby.
- Ukande U. (2001) Population, sampling & data collection in Proceedings of workshop of Nursing Research Society of India.
- Thompson S.K. (2002) Sampling. 2nd edition New York: Jossy Bass.

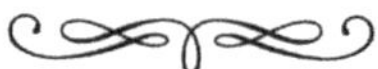

CHAPTER

9 Instruments and Method used for Data Collection

Nancy Fernandes Pereira

Learning Objectives

This chapter helps the reader to –

- Understand the use of different instrument for collecting data.
- Choose the appropriate instrument for their research project for collecting data.
- Design instruments for their research study.
- Understand strength and weakness of every instrument.

Introduction

Data collection instruments are means to collect information to answer all the questions that have been posed. It follows a methodological process of collecting information, then analysing to provide solution to the questions posed by researcher. It enables to provide all the required information on a particular research question or subject matter of interest. The collected information can be contributed to hypothesis testing which would enable to explain the phenomena under study. The collected data provides a vantage position to researcher while making prediction based on the findings of the expected trends.

To acquire the relevant and appropriate data it is important to use an appropriate instrument. Researcher from different field use number of instruments namely; Questionnaires, opinionnaire, inventories, checklist, rating scales and methods like observation, interview. Depending on the nature of the research question/study the research, setting may use any one or more than one instrument to collect the required information. The instrument chosen depends upon the objective of the study, design, time, money and subject or sample of the study. It also depends on purpose of collecting data whether it is empirical or qualitative in nature. Every researcher needs to develop the required skill in developing the instrument and effectively using it.

Data collection methods vary along following important dimensions

1. *Structured*: Research data often collected according to a highly structured plan which indicates what information is to be gathered and exactly how to gather it. Sometimes it's appropriate to impose minimum of structure and provide them opportunities to reveal information in natural way like in field studies.
2. *Quantifiable*: If statistical analysis is to be done, data should be quantifiable. For qualitative analysis data may be collected in a narrative form.
3. *Researcher's obtrusiveness*: Methods of data collection differs in terms of the degree to which clients are aware of their role i.e. client status. If they are fully aware of their role their responses may not be normal and if data is collected unobtrusively ethical problem may arise.
4. *Objectivity*: The method adopted should be as objective as possible, though in certain researches especially phenomenological based research the subjective judgment of the investigator is considered valuable.

Instruments are divided into two categories

1. **Mechanical devices**: It includes almost all instruments used in physical sciences i.e. telescopes, monitors, thermometers, microscopes etc. The social and behavioral sciences use tape recorders, cameras, films, video tapes, computers etc. Mechanical devices allow precise measurement that can be replicated with accuracy.
2. **Clerical methods**: They are useful when researcher studies people; their feelings, emotions, attitudes, judgment. Instruments used here are filed records, histories, case studies, questionnaires, interview schedules etc.

Clerical devices are less reliable, less accurate and less precise. Therefore two challenges are faced by researchers are:

1. To develop clerical instruments that is precise.
2. To define concepts that is amenable to mechanical devices.

It's often more time consuming and valuable to use a tested instrument than to design a new one. Instruments are developed to gather many kinds of information. It's the researchers prerogative to decide by which method these data are to be compiled, compared and analyzed for a particular study. Rather than use a available data the investigator may want to develop a new data gathering instruments appropriate for a particular study. The kind of data to be gathered from individual or inanimate objects may require the use of the same or different type of instrument, depending on the format and appropriateness of the tools.

Data is collected by measuring a variable i.e. 'Measurement', observing a phenomena using 'observation' –check list or inventory, by asking questions directly that is 'interviewing' using an interview schedule, or collected as responses to a 'questionnaire' in a written format where it would be 'self-reporting'.

Sources to develop instruments

a. Review of Literature (ROL) – other studies, books for description of various tools/instrument.

b. Discussion with experts, researchers, faculty.

c. Combination of different instruments available.

d. Formation of new instruments to collect data – for this exercise, concept realization of entire process is very important.

Researcher may try to find out

1. **Facts**: The purpose of a specific research study may be to gather data based on historical recollections alone. The investigator might want to include facts on the activities and personal background of the respondent, their likes/dislikes, information they can supply about other individuals, observations or perceptions, statements about life style, plans, motivations etc. made by them.
2. **Attitude and feelings**: The respondent may be asked to answer direct questions about their thoughts on the items or the researcher may choose to develop an instrument that may provide insight into the sample's attitude and feelings. Since human beings tend to be biased 50% of the times, we should design our instruments keeping this in mind.
3. **Judgment**: The instrument should be so designed that it provides sufficient information for the subjects to make a decision. Judgments related to quality and quantity might be set up on five point scale from strongly agree to strongly disagree. The sample must have a sufficient knowledge of the topic to make a valid judgment.
4. **Psychomotor skills**: An instrument is so designed, so that the observer simply checks off whether the psychomotor skill is used or not. The

researcher determines the specific levels to be attained and tests the length of time necessary to attain the skills. The learning of such skills is mandatory and often expected to be mastered within a specific time.

Bio Physiological Methods used to study physical and physiological parameters:

Bio-physiological Methods they seek to measure in vivo and vitro parameters in individuals. In vivo measurements are done directly in or on living organism, whereas, in vitro measurements are performed outside the body as in case of checking the blood sugar level. The measures often involve the use of highly complex instrumentation and technological system as seen in the Table 9.1.

In vivo Bio Physiological Methods: **In vivo** is Latin for "within the living." It refers to tests, experiments, and procedures that researchers perform in or on a whole living organism, such as a person, laboratory animal, or plant. The measurements are directly performed over the organism or study subject by using specialized instruments or equipment's. e.g.: BP, ECG

In vitro Bio Physiological Methods: In vitro is Latin for "in glass." It describes medical procedures, tests, and experiments that researchers perform outside of a living organism. An in vitro study occurs in a controlled environment, such as a test tube or petri dish. They are the measurements carried out outside the organism or study subject by using specialized instruments or equipments. e.g.: Radiological Measurements, Biochemical Measurements, Microbiological measurements.

Advantages

1. They are relatively more accurate and error less.
2. They are more objective in nature.
3. Provide valid for targeted variables Ex: thermometer for temperature.
4. Easily available in hospital settings.

Disadvantages

1. Some of instruments are very costly.
2. It requires significant amount of training, knowledge and experience.
3. The results produced by these instruments may be affected by environment.
4. The use may cause fear and anxiety among participants.
5. Use of some method may have harmful effect.

Table 9.1: Different types of instruments

Body function	Variable to be assessed	Instruments
Circulatory	BP, Blood volume	BP apparatus, stethoscope, Doppler, ECG. Respiratory readings.
Respiratory	Respiratory volume, O_2 saturation	Spirometer, pulse oximeter.
Neurological	Systemic body temperature	Thermometer, EEG.
Muscular-skeletal	Muscle contraction, Muscle tremors/strength, range of motion, motor response	EMG, accelerometer, monometer.
Gastrointestinal	Gastric motility, Gastro-intestinal activity.	EGG
Gentiourinary	Renal obstruction, prostatic obstruction, urine flow.	Renal arteriography

In-vitro measures gather data from respondent or participant by extracting some physiological material and subjecting to laboratory investigation. Whereas Bio-Chemical measures are performed in laboratory using chemical to study potassium level, electrolyte level, hormonal level, haemoglobin level etc. while microbiological studies are studied by withdrawing blood sample from the respondent and identifying the bacteria. Cytological or Histological studies are conducted by collecting tissue from the individual and/or other obtained through tissue biopsy, or understanding what's happening to the human body through X-ray, CAT scan.

Today many nurses researchers conduct nursing studies that included physiological measures to assess the outcomes of nursing care and nurse researchers use different kinds of bio-physiologic measures in research. e.g., to study the effect of walking versus yoga exercise on the heart rate, blood pressure in adult with respiratory condition.

1. PHYSICAL MEASUREMENTS

Studies linking physiological and psychological variables require physiological measurements. The data may be collected through different methods where a respondent may report the manifestations or discomfort, researcher may observe through direct participant or indirectly, laboratory test finding may be used as data, parameters may be assessed using electronic monitoring devices like ECG monitor, etc. Most common physical measurements including taking temperature, blood pressure, weight, etc.

Physiological measures which are measured directly or indirectly. Among COPD patient's tolerance of exercises can be directly observed through PFT, O_2 saturation. Others are anxiety and depression scales. Monitoring of room temperature in ICU/OT. Thereby assess body temperature through rectal mode for accuracy.

Physiological variables can be measured through laboratory test where information can be obtained e.g. Hemoglobin (Hb) level/activated partial thromboplastin time (APTT). Consider the following points while selecting the physiological measure for a study:

- Physiological measure which is relevant to the study.
- Does continuous or particular point in time measurement is required.
- How often is it needed to measure i.e. its frequency.
- What are the limitations?
- How was a physiological variable measured in previous studies?
- Use of structured and unstructured observation to enrich measurements of variable.

Points to be remembered while considering selection of bio-physiological measures

Is the equipment or lab analysis readily available?, can it be easily acquired or affordable.

Can the equipment be operated and interpret the results or is the training required for the same.

Can permission be obtained to use the necessary equipment? Does the measure need to be direct or indirect, e.g. To check the BP one may need to use arterial line or use BP apparatus. Does the monitoring need to be continues or periodical and is it adequate. Can data be simultaneously recorded? Will single measure of dependent variable be sufficient? Can research variable be measured using non-invasive procedures? Is the measure used sufficiently accurate and sensitive to variant? Care should be taken while selecting appropriate instruments or laboratory findings to practical, ethical, medical and technical considerations.

The bio physiological measures are very objective, relatively precise and sensitive. Selection is difficult: review of literature of similar studies, manufacturer's catalogue and exhibits at the conference.

2. QUESTIONNAIRE

It is the most commonly used instrument when information gathering is desired from widely dispersed population. It can be used to study any research problem. The researcher has to have/develop skill in framing questions. It has a wide scope for using in research. Whether a research is framing interview schedule or observation check list one requires forming question. Which maybe structured, unstructured open ended or close ended? When question is asked to the study sample by the researcher it's referred to as interview but the same question written and given to the respondent is called questionnaire using paper and pencil. Where in the method becomes questioning used to collect data.

Meaning of a Questionnaire is a systematic compilation of questions put in written format to the study population with the objective to elicit information desired for research study. The instrument is in printed form designed to elicit response in written form or oral as in interview.

Sample may not be able to elaborate or ask for clarifications. The questionnaires are simple method of exploring new areas/topics.

Types of a Questionnaire: structured, unstructured.

Structured questionnaire: the question requires definite answer which are more objective. There is no freedom in the responses made. They are easy to compute and analyse. Whereas questions used in check list or multiple choice questions limits the response.

Unstructured questionnaire: the questions provide opportunity to respond freely. It encourages participant to answer. Unstructured questionnaire is often used in qualitative research when designing a question guide or interview guide.

Types of questions: Open ended questions, closed ended questions.

Open ended questions: allow free flow of response from participant of the study. The participant can express in their own words, no clues are provided. These types of questions provide opportunity for depth of information. e.g. what is the role of nurse in disaster management? Data from open ended questions are difficult to interpret; one would need to do content analysis to find the meaning. Open ended question cannot be used to obtain data from large samples as in survey study hence need to be avoided but can be used in qualitative studies. In open ended questions responses can be open and flexible. The open ended question allows respondents to complete the questionnaire with an appropriate response. The questions may be broad or narrow, like why, what, how, what do you think?, How do you feel about…? **Narrow questions** allow only limited flexibility. **Broad questions** like, "What are some of the advantages of attending training in government institutions?", "What are the problems nurse's face when using PPE kit?"

Narrow question would be; "What has been the most important academic advantage for enrolling in government institution for training?", "What is/was your greatest problem wearing PPE Kit?" Open ended questions have the advantage of permitting respondents to express their feelings. Their responses may trigger new insight for the researcher though the disadvantage is difficulty to tabulate.

Closed ended questions: restrict the response from the participant the Yes/No type. The answer could be forced choice, where multiple options are given to choose one best response. Best to use closed ended questions when research wants to cover a large population in exploratory/survey method. e.g. Does nurse play a role in disaster management? Yes/No/Unsure. Data obtained through close ended questions are easy to tabulate. Closed ended questions can have a set of specific list of alternatives. Respondent's answers are limited to the offered choices; there is no opportunity to express their opinion. They may take the form of "forced choice questions" it may include ascending or descending scales, yes/no check offs…

Developing questionnaire: Should know the information to be sought. The researcher has to prepare a blue print of the questions to ensure all domains/content have been covered. It should be framed at the educational level of respondent i.e. Language used should be simple and clear. Researcher should review literature to identify any instruments or questionnaire published and is available covering similar area so that permission can be taken to use.

If questionnaires are picked from published researches permission needs to be taken from the author. While using an existing questionnaire need to add or delete items

Characteristics of a good questionnaire:

1. Questionnaire covers the topic for which it is designed and encourages the respondent to answer.
2. It clearly states the purpose of data collection and is accompanied by covering letter introducing researcher and consent of participant.

3. Information is collected which is not available in literature/library.
4. Simple, clear and not too long instrument i.e numbers of questions are adequate to obtain all essential information.
5. The question deals with one concept, no duplication, should be logically arranged and ambiguous or vague terms are avoided e.g. how heavy the emergency was last night." to enhance tool validity and reliability.
6. Questions are placed keeping in mind the psychology of the respondent from simple questions to very personal or sensitive questions.
7. Questions are grouped based on the sub topics, and clues or leading questions are avoided.
8. If multiple choice questions are used same number of alternatives should be used throughout the questionnaire.
9. Double negative questions in one question should be avoided. e.g. "Do you believe nurses should not administer medication without doctor's order? Yes or No."
10. Ensure questions are grammatically framed correct.
11. Ensure that threatening or sensitive questions are not placed in the beginning of the instrument but at the end.
12. Include important questions in the beginning and less important items later.
13. Leading or influencing questions should be carefully placed in appropriate place in the instrument, so that it does not lead or interfere with the other.

If the questionnaire is well prepared it's easy to tabulate the data and enter the responses for analysis in pre-tabulated sheet, it is also able to give the researcher sense of the information they are getting generated at a glance. Questionnaire should be accompanied by a covering letter explaining the purpose of the study, researchers name and approximate time required to complete the questionnaire and if supported by organization or institution. To ensure questionnaire is posted/returned by the respondent in a self-addressed stamped envelope should be included. Questionnaire should be checked for its clarity and effectiveness through the implementation of pilot study. The instructions should be clearly stated in the beginning of the questionnaire.

Advantages of a questionnaire:

1. Relatively simple

2. Rapid and efficient
3. Can be distributed to widely scattered population through mail. Today with Google forms available via computer can reach samples in remote places too.
4. Easy to tabulate the data
5. Anonymity can be maintained.
6. Respondent has time to contemplate on their responses.
7. Can be easily tested for its validity & reliability.
8. Measurement is enhanced as all samples respond to same questions.
9. In written format of questionnaire absence of the researcher/interviewer also reduces the bias.

Limitations of a questionnaire:

1. May become lengthy if we probe in depth.
2. Respondents may omit certain areas in between, if unable to clarify.
3. Amount of information gathered can be limited.
4. Respondent may omit responding to some questions.
5. Data is limited to voluntarily supplied responses by the sample.
6. All samples may not compile to the request to participate.
7. If questionnaire is to be posted response may be poor.
8. For some statements the respondent may be forced to make a choice.
9. Cost of printing, postage, return envelopes etc.
10. Items may be misunderstood.
11. Only the literate can answer, literate and differently abled sample will be lost.
12. Nonverbal cues cannot be observed.
13. Researcher has no opportunity to interact.
14. Constructing a good questionnaire requires considerable effort.

When respondents are promised anonymity, the researcher is then unaware who have returned questionnaire as a result difficult to follow up. The researcher has no control as to which respondents have answered or not if respondents have to post the questionnaire.

3. SCALE

Scales are a form of self-report, which are precise means of measuring phenomena. Scales is a device designed to assign a numerical score to individuals to place them along a continuum with respect to the attitude being measured. Scales are constructed to discriminate among people with different attitude, fears, motives, perceptions, personality traits and needs. Scales are used to measure psychological variables, and physiological variables like pain, nausea, or functioning capacity of individual.

Types of a scale: Rating scale, Visual analogue scale, Likert scale.

Meaning of a Rating Scale: Rating is a term used to place value to opinion or assess situation on a scale. It's used to quantify variables understudy which otherwise does not carry a numerical value. They are the crudest form of measure involving scaling technique. Rating scale indicates the degree to which an attribute is present or absent on a continuum from low to high or least to maximum.

Requirements of a good rating scale: measure what it is supposed to measure. An ordered series of categories of a valuable that are assumed to be based on a underlying continuum. A numerical value is assigned to each category and the fine distinction between categories value with the scale.

1. Avoid statements which are so extreme that no sample or respondent would select them.
2. Clearly state the behavior or trait to be placed on the scale.
3. Divisions on the scale should be adequate, not too many nor too few, best to have five, maximum ten based on the attribute being assessed.
4. Respondent rating should be provided with clear instructions, to avoid generosity or error due to halo effect or logic.
5. The items should be rated by more individuals for better understanding, and feedback compiled.
6. The statement/items should be organized in descending or ascending order.
7. Appropriate respondents should be selected to respond to the items.

Rating scale should be used where in the respondents are in a position to rate and if needed can provide quotes to support their responses. There are different types of rating scales used by researchers like *Numerical scale* where in the respondent tick the appropriate number to indicate the presence or absence of the attribute. *Descriptive rating scale* is where descriptive phrases are used and the response is placed on the scale. Mostly used to describe behavior of an individual or how they are like hence may also be called behavioral scale. *Ranking scale* is where in the respondent merely places the variable understudy/ item in order of possessing the attribute.

Advantages of a rating scale

a. Simple form of scoring variables.
b. Number of attributes can be numerically scored.
c. Helpful to measure variables/objectives which need paper-pencil method. e.g. Personality, various competitions, for appraisal of performance/ practical skill.

Limitations of a rating scale

1. Emotions may affect rating of attributes.
2. As its self-rating respondents may over rate or underrate on traits/behavior or performance.
3. Respondents are unable to justify scoring and may give absurd response.
4. There could be error of generosity in rating or halo effect in rating if respondents are asked to rate their colleagues. Therefore the rating may have central tendency effect where midpoint score may be awarded.
5. Respondents may be cautious and hesitant that they have a tendency to rate all individuals low or high, it's called as stringency error.

4. ATTITUDE SCALE

Uses a list of statements containing adjectives to describe how an individual would respond/react to the situation/feeling. The purpose of psychosocial scale is to quantitatively distinguish among people in terms of the degree to which they can be characterized by some personal traits. The respondent is expected to score on the scale their point of view to the statement. Just as thermometer permits a quantitative differentiation between two different temperatures, so also the scales that measures attitudes attempts to distinguish between individuals who are more or less favourable towards some concept or situation.

Define an Attitude scale: It is an individual disposition/reaction or response to situation, phrases, slogans, opinion, and people where in every individual from their own psychology can differ in their response as being favourable, neutral or unfavourable

Types of attitude scale: Likert scale (LS), Sematic Differential, Q-sort, Thurstone technique.

Characteristics of a good attitude scale

1. Extremely positive and negatively worded statements can be placed on a continuum.
2. Abstract variables can be measured quantitatively by giving numerical value.
3. Statements can be disguised to avoid directly asking the respondent to indicate their attitude to the topic.
4. The author works out the norms and tries to standardize the scale before implementation.
5. Researcher works out the norms and tries to standardize to get sum score.
6. The number of items/statements should not exceed 25 to 30 maximum.
7. Should have a four point scale.

Advantage of an attitude scale: Help to identify the attitude of individual or group to certain phenomena. Helps to identify attitude towards sensitive topics or identify attitude and score it.

Limitations of an attitude scale:

1. Respondent may not necessarily express their true response which could result in hiding their true attitude.
2. Respondent may not be clear to express or not able to evaluate their true attitude.
3. The respondent may not have encountered the situation, as a result may not be able to express and response could be hypothetical.
4. The scoring on the continuum scale may not be equally spaced to reveal true attitude.
5. Similar score obtained by several respondents indicates favourable position is uncertain.

Likert scale (LS): The most common method of attitude measurement named after social psychologist, Rensis Likert. These scales consist of several declarative statements expressing a view point on a subject. Respondents are asked to indicate the degrees to which they agree or disagree with the opinion expressed in the statement on a scale. Likert scale comprises of equal number of negative and positive statements to elicit attitude related to a topic to avoid bias. Each response category is assigned a value wherein value of 1 given to the most negative/unfavourable and value of 5 given to most positive or favourable response. Scale value of negatively expressed items must be reversed before analysis.

To use Likert scale one needs to develop a large pool of items/statements that clearly state favourable or unfavourable attitude towards the issue/topic understudy.

Neutral statements or extreme statements that virtually every one would agree or disagree with them should be avoided. It's important to select items that focus on one concept about 10-20 statements to suffice for Likert scale. The aim is to spread out people with various attitudes along a continuum of favourability.

Response choices commonly address agreement, evaluation or frequency. **Agreement** response are strongly agree (SA), agree (A), uncertain (UNC), disagree (DA) and strongly disagree (SDA). **Evaluation** responses are rated as good or bad, positive or negative, excellent or terrible. **Frequency** responses are rarely, seldom, sometimes, frequently, usually. They provide a 5 point scale but some may add two or more points such as slightly agree or slightly disagree. Uncertain or undecided terms cause the respondent to sit on the fence. Statements which are positively worded tend to get a higher score than statements negatively worded.

SDA	DA	UNC	A	SA

e.g. –

1. People with blood cancer have a short life span.
2. Elderly women give birth to preterm babies.

The responses to statements should reflect variability, if variability is lacking the statements is not making a contribution to discriminate among individuals on the basis of their attitudes.

Advantage of Likert scale: It is extremely efficient way to measure characteristics of individuals in a way that permits a researcher to quantify different gradation, strength of possessing those characteristics. It's easy to construct. They are used for comparisons in both directions and intensity of attitude. Can be used for large group of individuals also can be administered verbally and written.

Disadvantage of Likert scale: Actual opinion may not be marked on the scale by respondent.

To understand the actual state of mind or opinion the instrument should be administered number of times which may not be feasible in a study undertaken. The respondent may feel imposed or forced to respond to the limited option; which can be taken care by reducing the 'Yes' and 'No' type by including adequate number of positive and negative statements.

Sematic Differential (SD): This technique is often used to measure attitudes. It was developed by Osgood, Suci and Tannenbann (1957). It's a graphic rating scale, respondents have to give a judgment of something along an ordered dimension. These scales are bipolar in nature as they specify the two opposite ends of a continuum; such as good—Bad, Important –unimportant, strong – weak, beautiful—ugly and so forth.

The adjectives which can be used are as follows: **Evaluative**: valuable-worthless, good-bad, Fair-unfair..., **Potency** adjective like strong-weak, large-small.., and **Activity** adjective like active-passive, fast-slow. Scoring is same as in Likert scale where in positively worded adjective are scored higher. It may be scored on a seven point bipolar scale.

Advantage of Sematic Differential: It's highly feasible and easy to construct. Virtually anything can be rated like person, situation, abstract concepts etc. it provides opportunity to include several concepts in the same form. This permits comparison if same bipolar scales are used. As a result it's difficult for the respondent to disguise their true feelings and can arouse the interest of the respondent to the most difficult subject or situation, as it provides indirect approach.

Disadvantage of Sematic Differential: Difficult to test its validity and reliability as response may change with time or mood of respondent. Researcher needs to be well trained to interpret as it covers the psychological domain.

Thurston technique: This technique was developed by L. L. Thurston in 1920; it's more or less same as Likert scale and measures aptitude. It's a method of equal appearing interval. Attitude is a one-dimensional linear continuum where equally scaled interval is applied to statements. Researcher collects a great number of potential items that relate to the topic of interest. The statements cover full range of possible attitude towards the object from strongly negative to strongly positive with adequate coverage of intermediate and neutral positions. It requires the respondent to agree or disagree with a large no of statements related to the topic or object understudy. Large no of judges are required to classify independently the statements in to equal categories of favourability. The judges only rate each statement in terms of favourability which they believe is expressed by the statement without reacting to it. e.g.: To measure attitude towards suicide. "Individuals who attempt suicide are weaklings and no better than losers" It may be assigned positive or negative in terms of unfavourability. Researcher averages the category rating for each statement, across all the judges. Statements of considerable disagreements are deleted and final drafts of statements are selected about 20 to 30 statements in such a way that they are well distributed. To which the selected respondent will tick/agree or disagree.

Administration of the instrument: The respondent checks the statement to which he/she agree or check 2–3 statements which best indicates their viewpoint. Scale value does not appear on the instrument and statements appear in random order. The average of the scale value that the individual endorses would be considered that respondents scope. Hence if a statement of low value gets a high score, it is possible that the statement is ambiguous or poorly worded and therefore is not considered.

Advantage: Statements are valued.

Disadvantage: Difficult to construct than Likert scale. Time consuming and elaborate work is required. Statements given to the judges may end up expressing their own attitude in the rating. If the judges are biased they may end up influencing or distorting.

There are number of standardized scales like quality patient care having 68 items, Slater scale having 84 items, etc....

Guttman Scale: includes a set of statements which relate to a individual's attitude towards a single topic or aspect. The statements are arranged from low to high according to the difficulty, and the respondent selected what applied to them best; e.g. self-efficacy scale. When respondents agree or disagree to a statement they would probably also agree/disagree to the previous statement. This type of scale does not provide adequate variation of perception of situation or feelings of individual. It's difficult to construct but has better reproducibility.

Q-sort: was devised by William Stephenson. It's similar to questionnaire and is effective in ranking attitude and judgments. Statements are typed on cards, slips of paper and given to the respondent and they are asked to pile them in piles of 9 to 11 ranging from most to least important on a relative scale. It's effective specially when there are at least 50 statements. Here the number going in each pile is predetermined; it helps the rater to distribute the statements evenly over the whole scale. Thus a respondent is forced to make a choice.

Advantage: It has a provision for completeness, as it forces the respondent to complete the entire exercise/activity. It's inexpensive and adaptable to many situations or theory. Attitude, beliefs of an individual and variables can be measured precisely. Powerful for in-depth research into human, their attitude and behavior. Data being objective is simple to analyse in Q-sort.

Disadvantage: It's time consuming, especially when administering to a large number of respondent or participants. It cannot be mailed like questionnaire. It's difficult to develop valid statements. Respondents or participants may make choice mechanically to complete the task; as a result the importance of the statement may differ on different days in the mind of the respondent. Hence it's difficult to establish its reliability. It is difficult to correlate the data with the hypothesis. On the part of the researcher it requires a lot of forethought while analysing the data e.g.: Approval—disapproval, Most like me—least like me, Highest priority –lowest priority.

Delphi technique: is used to measure the judgment of a group of experts for the purpose of making decisions, assessing priorities or making forecast. First a panel of experts on a particular subject are invited to participate in a research study. They may include nursing practitioners, scholars, specialist, educators or other stake holders are asked to give their opinion on the statements in the instrument. The instrument may gather opinion, estimates or future predictions on some special topic. The responses are collected and results are summarized and returned to the experts to get again their opinion and feedback. Using combined information of all the experts a new instrument is developed. Each individual responds to the new instrument. This process is usually repeated at least four times until the resulting data are in consensus of the opinion, predictions or belief of all experts. This is useful for planning course of action, finding consensus of opinion or for predicting future conditions or situations. **Advantage**: expert opinions are obtained with great demand on time. Each expert can review the other judge's responses and can compare and evaluate their own opinions with the other respondent. Members of the expert panel may remain anonymous. Their response rate is reasonably consistent. Results are extremely useful because they represent a form of accumulated knowledge which would be difficult to obtain otherwise.

Disadvantage: It's costly and time consuming. The complete activity is dependent on the cooperation and speed of responses of the experts participating. There is high possibility of biases being introduced therefore only certain type of individuals who are disciplined may be invited to participate. Results are opinion which may or may not represent reality.

Vignettes: brief descriptions of an event or situation to which respondents are asked to respond. Description may be fictions or based on fact, but are always structured to elicit information about the respondent's perception, opinion or knowledge about some phenomena under study. Vignettes are often written, narrative descriptions; videotaped vignettes are also used now. The questions posed to the respondents after presentation of the vignette may be either open ended e.g. "How would you handle this emergency situation" or a closed ended e.g. "on a ten point rating scale score how well do you think the nurse handled the situation". To collect adequate information approximately well-constructed 4 to 10 vignette in a study are normally enough. Hence vignettes are economical means of eliciting information about how individuals might behave in situations that are difficult to observe.

Advantage: easy to construct and economical. It's possible to manipulate experimentally the stimuli by randomly assigning vignettes to small groups.

Disadvantage: They can be mailed like questionnaire therefore expensive. The respondent may not describe or state their true feeling or behavior as a result response may get biased. E.g.: if the statement is: "How patient would react related to nurses with different types of personalities and different personal style of interaction." If the response would affect the respondent then they may not reveal their true response/behavior.

Visual analogue scale: are also called as magnitude scales. They are useful in scaling stimuli. It is beneficial in measuring variables like pain, mood, anxiety, alertness, craving for cigarettes, quality of sleep etc. a clear stimuli has to be stated with one cue appearing for each scale. A vertical or horizontal line is drawn of approximate 100mm with right angles at each end and anchors are placed at both ends which are bipolar. These anchors include the entire range of sensations possible in a phenomena being measured. The respondents are asked to place a tick mark on the line to indicate the intensity e.g. of pain/ stimuli. A ruler is then used to measure the distance between the left end of the line and mark placed by the respondent. The measure obtained is the value of the stimuli. No Pain ——————— Worst Pain

4. CHECK LIST

It's a list of statements indicating action carried out or a behavior taken place in a particular span of time, to which the respondents either places a tick (√) or cross (×)/yes or no. The purpose of this list is to draw attention to various aspects of an object or situation to ensure that an important aspect is not missed out. In nursing check list is used often to ensure no steps of a procedure is left or if the participant has performed all the steps of the procedure. It can be compared to a shopping list type consisting of prepared statements. It merely records the presence or absence of the event/activity or task done in a study undertaken. In nursing it helps prevent errors or to ensure evidence based practice is carried out. It helps to gauge the extent to which skill is achieved or the progress made. It's calculated based on the sum number or yes indicating the steps or behavior occurred and sum number of no Scores are obtained for every individual participant and then calculated for the group i.e. are all nurses performing the procedure correctly or not.

Meaning of a Check List: It includes enumerated statements to which the respondent has to respond.

Types of check list: there are mainly three types or styles.

i) Procedural check list,

ii) Communication checklist and

iii) Task check list.

Where to the statement the respondent, in the space provided indicates (yes/ no) indicating the activity performed or not (P/A) indicating participation or absence from the activity.

From the list of alternatives the respondent selects the most appropriate action/statement by encircling or underlining it. Procedural checklist help to assess if a procedure is carried out as per plan and all steps are performed, while communication checklist helps to assess the clarity of disseminated information; a well communicated information builds trust, helps in problem solving and facilitates creativity. Task check list ensures the list of assigned task are completed.

To make a good check list be clear of the purpose, plan the type of checklist; is it to confirm task done or read and respond. Keep it simple and clear preferably to keep the sentences short. Keep few or group the activity in to subgroup for easy analysis. They should be in logical flow, complete, comprehensive and terms used should be at the level of the respondent. Care should be taken that it discriminates the quality of information collected.

Advantage of a check list: can be used in survey design study to understand the number of activities performed by the participants. Hence convenient and efficient to get a range of areas covered. It shows the productivity and motivation of participant using checklist.

Limitations of a check list: The respondent without paying much attention may simply tick as an activity in a rush to get done. If care is not taken important observation checked out using a checklist may be missed out. As researcher may give lot of focus to get it right while constructing it may consume time.

5. STANDARDIZED TEST OR STANDARDIZED INSTRUMENTS

These are tests that have stood the test of time and can be used in any setting or geographical location. Majority of the Psychological test are standardized. They are published and accompanied with a manual, which gives information about its usage. e.g. Personality test, Aptitude test, Test for Intelligence, Attitudinal scale etc. When using standardized test the permission has to be obtained and credit has to be given to the author of the instrument.

METHOD OF UTILIZING THE INSTRUMENTS

There are major methods i.e. measuring a variable like *measurements*, observing a phenomenon i.e. *observation*, asking questions directly i.e. *interviewing* and responding to a question in a written format i.e. *Self- reporting*.

1. Interviewing

Interview involves verbal communication between researcher and the study subject/sample during which information is provided to the researcher.

An interview is one of the most important methods for collecting data used in qualitative researchers. Interview method allows researcher to collect information from individuals from real life situations and roles they perform. Interviewing requires proper planning and details need to be worked out before the interview. Questions for the interview should be correctly developed. Interview based on the type of study may be conducted face to face or via a telephone. Good interview helps to focus on the study samples world. It's the second most common method to gather information. The interview schedule/ interview guides are similar. Interview schedule are set of questions readout to the respondents while interview guide provides ideas but allows interviewer the freedom to pursue relevant question or topic in depth to support the study. It's an effective tool especially in exploratory studies. Both Interview schedule and guide can be structured and unstructured these are used in conjunction with the interview especially in qualitative studies.

Meaning of Interview technique: Interview is a two-way method where information and views are exchanged. When used in research the conversation is conducted with a definite purpose to obtain information on the topic of researcher's interest.

Purpose of interview: Information gathering, ordering, evaluation or appraisal of situation behavior description, providing the basis for inferences or predictions. All this requires factual recall or presentation of opinion.

Types of interview: Structured, Semi-Structured, Non/Unstructured, Focused. *Structured interviews*: uses questions formulated before the collection of data, the flow of questions is regulated with regard to the order of the questions, and based on available time. It provides the researcher increased amount of control over the content of the interview where in the interviewer is not supposed to change the specific wording. The questioner used during an interview is called as interview schedule, which contain the question in a desired flow to maintain smooth flow as well as not to intimidate the respondent. This method provides the research an opportunity to explain the meaning of the question or modify the way in which the subject can understand it better without changing the essence of the question. Each interview has to be conducted in precisely the same manner.

The researcher needs to ask the precise question as it has been designed. If the respondent does not understand the question can be repeated. If the responses are lengthy, they can be printed and given to the person for selection of a response. Range of responses can be decided by the researcher.

Semi-structured interviews: Few questions are formulated but the researcher goes by the flow of response and new questions might emerge as the interview progresses. The researcher is free to probe as they choose to acquire information. This type of interview is also refereed to semi standardized interview.

Non/Unstructured interviews: Few introductory questions may be formulated to get the interview started. The researcher has free rein to put questions as the interview progresses based on objective of the study. Often there is no time limit as information is sought from the respondent until no new information is provided by the study subject/sample. In this method researcher has complete freedom too. It's also referred to as Non-standardized interview.

Focused interview: Interview for collecting data in qualitative research is mostly individual interview but sometimes group interviews can help in drawing out information which is difficult to elicit during individual interview. The objective of a focus group interview is to get collective views on a certain defined topic of interest from a group of individuals who might have undergone an experience which researcher is interested to study. Focus groups interview help researcher to elicit opinions, attitudes and beliefs held by individual from the community. In focus group the number of members in a group should be 8 to 12 individual maximum 15. Interviewer should not insist on response if the individual is unwilling to make a response. Interviewer has to give suitable clues and more chance to the subject to speak and explain his/her point of view.

Steps of interview: It has mainly three steps-*First step* is prepare for the interview i.e. is preparing the questions to be asked, clear cut sequences of how it's going to flow, purpose of interview. *Second step* is actual execution of interview where in client is made comfortable, consent taken, recorder placed appropriately. *Third step* is Recording and interpretation of response where in documenting simultaneously/immediately or after interview. It is best to use recorder so that actual wording can be transcribed.

i) Designing interview questions: developing questions and maintaining the sequence, and progressing from broad and general to specific and narrow. Questions should be grouped based on the area, sensitive aspects reserved for last and general or safe topics covered first to enable build trust and confidents like less interesting data like age, education, income and demographic data are collected last as they can be collected from clients records too. The questions framed for the interview is dependent on the educational level of the sample; after developing the interview schedule, it should be given to experts for feedback and for validating the content.

The researcher should pretest the interview schedule before commencing for pilot study so that it's error free before final study. It's preferable to test on subjects similar to the samples of final study. This will enable the researcher to identify problems in design of questions, sequencing of questions or procedure of recording the responses. Pre-testing of the interview schedule allows confirmation of the reliability and validity of the interview schedule.

ii) Interviewer's preparation: If the researcher is going to have assistance for the interview, this interviewer should be trained so that they develop the skill of interviewing, it's important that they practice. The interviewer should be familiar with the content of the interview. Interviewers must anticipate situations that might occur during subject and thus facilitate an effective response to a particular situation. Role playing can give an insight to the interviewer into the way of a subject and thus would help facilitate an effective response to a situation. The interviewer has to learn to create a permissive atmosphere in which the sample will be made comfortable and encouraged to respond to any sensitive area. The interviewer has to practice to maintain unbiased verbal and nonverbal attitude and manner to be able to get cooperation from the respondent. The interviewer has to practice posing the questions, phrasing of wording of questions, tone of voice when put the question. The interviewer has to be careful of nonverbal body language like raising of eyebrow, change of body posture, shifting in the seat etc. which could communicate a negative or positive reaction to the samples response from the researcher interviewing, which could alter the response from the sample. The interviewer has to be dressed appropriately when going to interview the study sample. Take prior appointment to avoid waste of time for both researcher and study sample specially if the interview would take too much time or is lengthy. Provide correct information to the sample before taking consent for participating in the study. The interviewer has to choose an appropriate place where it's quiet and no disturbance, privacy is ensured so that the sample/subject is comfortable in the environment. This will facilitate the respondent providing correct information related to the area of study.

Use of Probing questions in the interview: Used by the researcher to gather more data in a specific area of interest. While probing the researcher my repeat the question, may explain or reframe the question or ask the sample to explain the statement made, or press for correct response. The interviewer may pick on the response and dig deeper for information and meaning. The interviewer while probing must take care not to bias the responses and not to probe in such a way that the subject/sample feels they are being grilled or cross examined.

iii) Documentation of the interview: To avoid forgetting or distorting the information the interviewer may document the data during the process of interview or immediately after the interview. Documentation may be done using video tape/audio-recorder or handwritten notes may be maintained. If recorder is used should ensure the sample is not distracted or becomes guarded when responding. Researcher should remember to take permission to record/ write script of the interview to avoid breach of trust.

Advantages of interview Schedule

1. Data from every interview are useable, whereas this may not be true of questionnaire.
2. Depth of responses assured, since researcher can pursue questions of special interest.
3. Can be combined with other tools.
4. If subject fails to understand it can be repeated or simplified.
5. No item is likely to be missed/overlooked, plus gives researcher opportunity to ask questions previously not asked or included in interview schedule.
6. Verbal or non-verbal cues can be picked up.
7. Can be administered to illiterate/those critically ill samples.Respondents do not get influenced in answering the current question by looking ahead at the other questions.
8. Face to face or telephonic interview can be conducted.
9. Classification of responses is possible.
10. Higher response rate than written questionnaire, therefore more representative sample can be obtained as drop out is less as compared to questionnaire.
11. Interpersonal skills may be used to facilitate co-operation of sample to extract information.
12. Complex situations & sensitive issues can be probed by the interviewer after establishing rapport and atmosphere of confidence and trust.

Limitations of interview

1. Time consuming for an interviewer specially if there is lack of time also preparation of the schedule is expensive.
2. May require research assistant if it's a big project which can add to the cost of the research project; at times suitable assistant may be difficult to find.
3. Cost depends on the place, number and length of interviews this may limit the sample size.
4. Interviewee may not have a choice in relation to place and time of interview.
5. Artificiality of the interview
6. Lack of trust
7. Level of entry
8. Elite bias, there is threat to subject bias to validity of the findings.
9. Hawthorne effects
10. Constructing knowledge
11. Ambiguity of language
12. Interviews can go wrong.
13. Presence of a researcher can influence responses of respondents
14. Reports of events may be less complete or inaccurate than information gained through observation.

How to ensure success of using interview method for data collection?

One needs to develop **questioning skill to** eliciting – try to use open ended questions for interviews. Open questions uses 'who', 'what', 'why', 'where', 'when', 'how', they elicit responses that are open-ended and more descriptive or narrative in nature.

The other skill required is **Listening skills**

An interviewer needs to follow the content of what is being said, listen to the meaning underneath the words, and then gently bring this into the conversation. He or she offers or reflects back what they have heard, so that the respondent can confirm, deny, or elaborate. This way of working creates empathy, deepens the conversation and ensures the meaning has been understood.

Problems one may encounter related to interview method: Interview is effective for obtaining opinion, attitude, values and perceived behavior, but ineffective for obtaining actual behavior patterns. Sample may consciously give response that seems to be what the interviewer wants. Every subject/sample may not be available for interview. In some situation of the study the presence of the interviewer may alter the response of the sample; they may become conscious or nervous as their responses are being recorded or written down which may add to a degree of biasness in their response. Since the interviewer has to immediately note down it can become mechanical and errors may occur; also time is lost when trying to document response. Interviewee may lose their chain of thoughts, while their responses are documented.

Tips for success when using interview method:

1. Try to interview a variety of people representing diverse views to gather range of information and get depth of information.
2. Prepare beforehand, be familiar with the structure of the interview.
3. Interviewer should be aware who they are going to interview.
4. Use the mirroring technique
5. Be flexible and open to new lines of enquiry
6. As a general rule, tape your interviews

2. Observation technique

Meaning of Observation technique is recording down information as seen how individual act behave in situations. It is conducted in natural setting, often helps to get true picture of what's happening, feelings, how individual think.

Types of observation: Structured and Unstructured, participatory and non-participatory.

Structured observation: used to collect data of the physiological parameters. Constructive as well as destructive behaviors etc. can be observed observation is more ridged and less flexible. An observation check list would be used to document.

- Define carefully what is required to be observed.
- Need to determine how observation is to be made, recorded and coded.
- Require to develop a category for organizing and sorting observed behavior or event.

- To ensure all aspects observed are properly documented; 15 to 20 categories are preferably to be developed.

Unstructured observation: used mostly for qualitative research.

- Spontaneously observing and recording what is seen with a minimum of prior planning.
- Gives freedom to the observer, lacks objectivity, cannot remember all details of the observed event, notes can be made.
- Observation can be photographed or videotaped for extensive examination later on.
- It provides a detailed description of an individual's behavior in a natural environment.

Method of observation is intense, needs more than one observer to avoid missing an important event. As individual researcher can observe a person for maximum 30 minutes

Participatory observation: The researcher becomes part of the study group members who are being studied. The researcher as a member of the group is noted by the study group as they perform activity alongside them, the degree of participation will vary based on what the researcher desires to observe. The researcher may adopt role of learner, visiting member of health team, or a listener, the best being an active participant observer.

Non participatory observation: Where in the researcher stays away from the study group under his/her observation, tries to be unnoticed especially when observing behaviors or performance of activity which may get altered by their presence like dealing with children or especially abled individuals etc.

Steps of observation: step one *plan for observation,* according to the objective of the study what, when, where and how the observation will be carried out, how documentation will be done, duration of observation, the frequency of activity to be observed. Will assistance be required for observation; if yes, they should be trained so that there is no difference or any aspect missed? Design the instrument for documentation, get it validated from experts and check its reliability. Step two execution of the observation focus on what is to be observed, keep at hand material in which to document i.e. the instrument. Follow the plan for observation. In Third step it is documentation and interpretation of the observation. Which can be done simultaneously as the observation is being done or immediately after the activity or event is observed so as not to miss out i.e. when the observation is still fresh in mind.

Advantages of observation

1. Observations make important contribution to data gathering as important aspects of activity, event or behaviors can be noted for descriptive studies.
2. Observation is direct rather than indirect through the use of questioner, interview or elicited through situational scenario.
3. Observation can be compared to set standards of practice/protocol and accordingly scored.
4. It's carried out in natural setting like in clinical area, class room during practice session etc.
5. Helps to understand the cause of certain behavior, help in bring about change in performance, skill/competency during procedures

Limitations of observation

1. High level of subjectivity as individual may see what they want or know.
2. May focus on those aspects during observation which has less importance.
3. Difficult to validate as response or behavior may differ as situation changes.
4. Difficult to precisely state the items in the Observation sheet.
5. Risk of distortion of the event being observed especially if non participatory observation is made.
6. It is time consuming and lot of hard work to ensure adequate data is gathered through observation.
7. Lack of familiarity to the setting where observation is carried out may interfere with the observation made.
8. Event being observed if rare may end with inadequate data for drawing out inference. e.g. CPR given to patient in arrest by nurse after BLS training.
9. Researcher may have to travel and stay at the venue to make observation and gather adequate data making the research project expensive.
10. Study sample may be uncomfortable or become conscious when they find they are being watched.
11. The researcher should be skilled to make observation else the gathered data may become invalid.

12. If multiple observers are used, discrepancy may arise in the gathered data if they are not trained.

3. Self-Report

Useful when participants are not able to be closely monitored in setting such as a hospital or in critical care units. In all human science this method is used. Direct questioning and asking the people to report. If a researcher wants to know what individual think, feel or believe the most direct means of gathering this information is to ask them about it. For certain practices when it's not possible for the researcher to personally or directly observe or collect data participants are asked to report using a checklist or self-reporting questionnaire. For certain practices like child abuse, contraceptive practices, drug usage the information can be gathered with self-reporting method, as it may be impossible for a researcher to observe these things. Self-reporting technique can be used for phenomenon's that one can experience by person but cannot be observed by another individual. e.g. pain, nausea, hot flushes, restlessness etc. Self-reporting technique facilitates collect of retrospective data about the past occurrences. Actions always do not indicate state of mind of a sample/participant. This is the most common research instrument used. The term self-reporting may be used in conjunction with other instruments or techniques like observation check list. Self-reporting instrument can be distributed to the respondents directly at any place or it can be mailed to them.

The respondents have great amount of information but unless the statements/questions/items in the instrument elicit this information; the knowledge goes untapped. One of the secrets of meaningful research is asking good questions. The information provided by the participant may not be always trusted especially when questions potentially require them to reveal an unpopular position on a controversial issue, or to admit to socially unacceptable behavior. Once the study design and the type of instrument are selected, the researcher decides the specific information that is needed and then develops a research instrument.

The self-reporting instrument may use open ended questions or close ended questions as discussed earlier in the chapter. Should be accompanied by clear instructions, if the technique for the instrument is self-reporting then the individual/respondent scoring or ticking off the alternative should be explained the method of documenting in the instrument e.g. Frequency of performing deep breathing activity at home or compliance to drug regime at home reporting may be done by the participant or the caregiver. They should be able to record as accurately as if the researcher them selves were recording the data. It's therefore important that the instrument is well organized.

Advantage of self-reporting: Relatively simple method. Items can be constructed rather easily by beginner's rapid and efficient method of collecting information. Data can be gathered from a widely scattered respondent or participant. It is inexpensive as can be distributed or mailed and anonymity can be maintained. It offers a simple procedure for exploring new topic. It can be flexible depending on the type of items, its order and the topic covered. Instrument can be easily tested for reliability and validity. Respondent has time to contemplate their response. Measurement is enhanced as all respondents respond to the same questions. Easy to tabulate as mostly questions are close ended hence analysis and interpretation can be easily accomplished.

Disadvantage of self-reporting: It can become a lengthy instrument, if in-depth probing is used. Respondent may omit certain items/statements in between without giving any explanation. At times some items may force the respondent to select response at random which may not be the actual response, only literates can report. Respondent may find it easy to express orally.

Criteria for selection of a good instrument for data collection

It should be reliable and valid. It should fulfil the objective of the purpose for which it is chosen. The instrument should be adequate for data collection. It should be usable and easy to be administered that it should be accompanied by clear instructions. Should be easy to score and mathematical calculation should be simple. The selected instrument should be easy to interpret; this is the most important task. If the instrument is administered but researcher is unable to interpret, the instrument can fail. It should be economical in terms of time and money. If an apt instrument is available to the researcher but costly the researcher may not purchase the instrument. Equivalent form of the instrument should be available to measure the same variable/attribute/behavior etc.

Guidelines for developing an instrument

1. It must be *suitable for its function*. That is it should be constructed to contain components that get to the heart of the problem than tap the vital elements of the questions being studied.

2. It must be *based on the theoretical frame work* selected for the study. The researcher may need to read extensively to identify which aspects of the theory are appropriate for investigation.
3. It *should be valid,* to the extent that it does not influence the sample's answers or performance and good instrument elicits the data that it was intended to elicit with a minimum of influence. "Will the instrument test what we want to test?"
4. It must *be reliable,* that is if the respondent answers the questions twice within time to remember the items or gain greater proficiency through practice of the skill, he/she would provide a similar response both times.
5. It must be *free of bias.* Instrument should be prepared in such a way that the respondent has no idea of the researcher's attitude towards the topic under study.
6. It must not have built in clues that is it should be *free of clues* as unintentional clues may invalidate a portion of the data and lead to erroneous findings.
7. It must have *proper direction for its use* in simple format for the respondent as well as for whoever would be administering the instrument to gather data.
8. It should be as *easy as possible to administer* the instrument.
9. The instrument should include items that directly *answer the hypothesis.*
10. It should *not permit cheating.* The research instrument should be designed and constructed in such a way that minimizes the chance of cheating. The responses given by each respondent should be solely his/her own.

While designing an instrument the researcher should gather a group of items from sources from such a person with experience from the field who is knowledgeable, accepted theories or hypothesis. Personal experience or material from study reports in books/professional journals. Care should be taken to ensure appropriateness of the items, their clarity, continuity and level of reading difficulty.

Devices used to while collecting information are: Tape records,Video records.

Reliability and validity of research instruments indicate the goodness of the instrument used for collecting data.

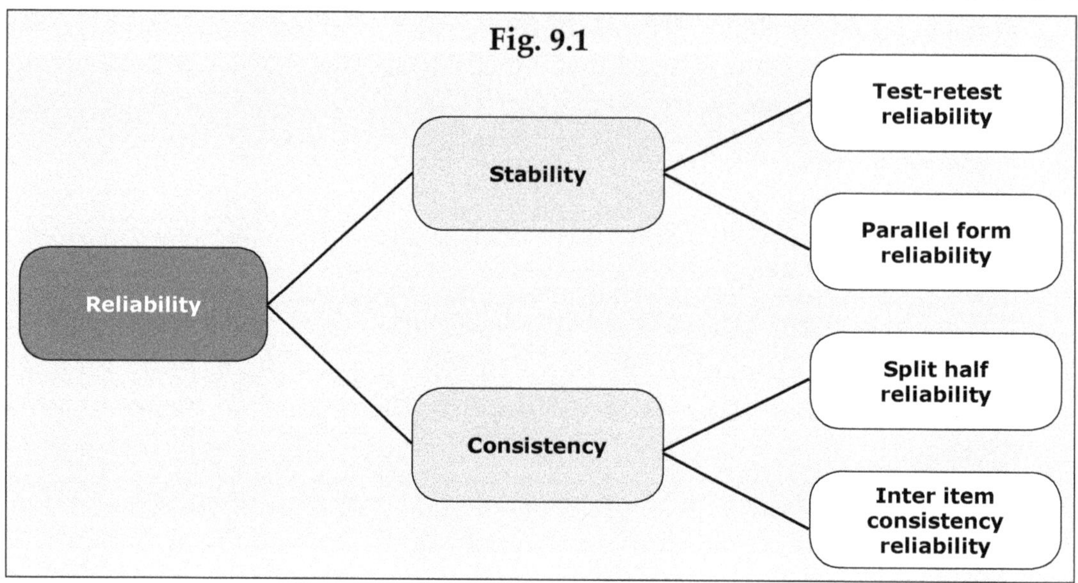

Reliability: It's the ability of the data gathering devices to obtain consistent results. It is the degree of consistency or dependability with which instruments measure the attribute it is designed to measure. Reliability of measure indicates extent to which it is without bias and hence ensures consistency measurement across time (stability) and across the various items/concepts of interest in the instrument (internal consistency) which means 'repeatability' or 'consistency'. A measure is considered to be reliable if it would give the same result over and over (provided the variable understudy has not undergone change). A reliable instrument maximizes true score and minimises the error. e.g. Intelligence test- it does not vary from day to day. Therefore similar results are obtained time after time.

Reliability refers to the accuracy of measuring instrument. e.g. Weighing scale if used to check weight will provide the same reading irrespective of the number of times an individual steps on and off it; if the weighing scale does not show the same reading when the individual steps on and off each time, then the weighing scale is unreliable. Major problem with this approach is that you have to be able to generate lots of items that reflect the same construct. The test should be administered in suitable condition to the group as it uses a statistical approach.

Two basic sources of inaccuracy:

1) Error in the instrument itself.

2) Inconsistency between individuals who are taking readings from the instrument.

Usually reliability is discussed in terms of a reliability coefficient i.e. correlation between two measurements that are obtained in the same manner.

Reliability Testing

1) **Test- Retest -Method**: This mainly tests the stability of a measure i.e. the extent to which the same scores are obtained when the instrument is used with the same respondents twice with an interval of several weeks to may be six months. Then the correlation between the scores obtained is called test retest coefficient. Higher the coefficients better the reliability and consequently the stability of the measure across time.

   Steps:

   - A test is administered to the subjects & after a period of time it is administered again
   - If the test is reliable & the trait being measured is stable the results will be consistent both the times
   - Since over a long period of time the things may change so inconsistent results may be obtained, especially if there has been a long time period between testing or change has occurred in the construct being measured the time between the measures is also critical. Shorter the time gap, higher the correlation; longer the time gap lower the correlation.
   - Test retest reliability should be high for stable traits e.g.: intelligence or knowledge test.
   - Unstable traits e.g. Joy, boredom, depression may produce low reliability, but it is because of the nature of the trait rather than the inaccuracy of the test.
   - Reliability coefficient (r) ranges from 0.00 to 1.00 the higher the value the more reliable (stable) the measuring instrument r >.7 is considered satisfactory

   This approach has certain disadvantages; many traits do change over time. Secondly subjects responses on the 2nd testing may be influenced by their memory about the 1st testing, thus we may get spuriously high value of '**r**'.

Test – Retest:

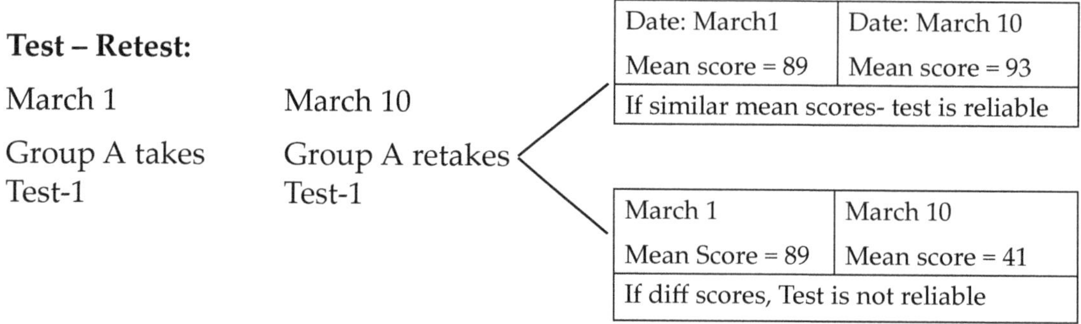

2) **Parallel form reliability**: Consistency of performance on different forms of a test.

Two forms of the test are developed using same specifications i.e. both tests contain the same types of items based on the similar material but are framed/worded differently or arranged question sequencing is changed but have the same response format. When responses on the two comparable sets of measures tapping the same construct are highly correlated (say 8 and above) one can be fairly certain the measure is reasonably reliable, with minimum error variance caused by wording, order or other factors; we have parallel form reliability. Cronbach's alpha is calculated 0.0-1.00.

Step

- Same subjects are given the 1st test, followed immediately by the 2nd test
- Some time may be spaced in between
- These parallel forms of the test supposedly reveal a high correlation
- When the tests are reliable.
- It is difficult to develop sufficient items to construct two tests/scales of the desired length for the same domain. Constructing a large pool of questions and randomly dividing them in to two sets to administer to the same group can be time consuming

Parallel form reliability:

March 1
Group A- Test- 1

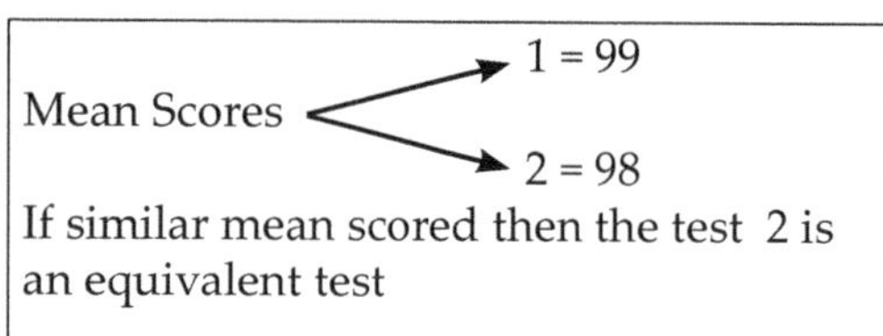

March 1
Group A- Test-2

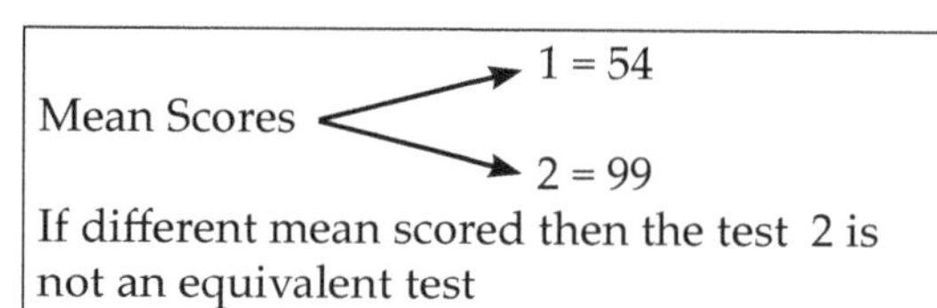

3) **Split half method**: Assess the internal consistency of the instrument. The strategy here is to assess with administering the test twice like in test retest or parallel form. The instrument items are split into two half where separate scores are given to the even and odd numbered items.

The results from each half of the test are compared to determine the internal consistency of the test. If the two halves of the test produce approximately equal scores, then the test is considered to be reliable. Spearman Brown formula is used to obtain coefficient for the entire test.

Advantage: In this method only single test is administered unlike in the earlier 2 methods. It indicates the instrument is reliably consistent, accurate precise stable and equivalent and homogenous.

Three aspects of reliability are focused on Stability, Consistency and Equivalence.

Stability extent to which similar results are obtained on separate occasions it is assessed through test retest approach; where same instrument is administered twice to the same group and scores are compared. Though the scores may not be identical neither largely different. Computing reliability coefficient (**r**) which objectively determine how small the difference is (> .70 = satisfactory > .80 is preferred.)

Consistency is assessed by the parallel form reliability where same construct in two instruments yield same results. Since scales/instruments are composed of one unitary attribute.

Equivalence concerned with the degree to which two or more independent observers agree about the scoring on an instrument. The degree of error can be evaluated through inter-rater reliability. Index of equivalence or agreement is then calculated with these data to evaluate the strength of relationship between the two ratings.

Item Analysis: A test is developed by the investigator to ensure that every item is both reliable and valid. Every item discriminates between a high and low achiever. If every item discriminates highly then it's a good test. Item difficulty is also considered here. Knowledgeable will be able to answer the most difficult question whereas the least will be unable to answer the most difficult question. Least difficult question will be answered by all. Items with difficulty index of about 80 and < 20 should be probably deleted. Tests whose total discrimination index is approximately 50 are preferred, as they provide maximum discrimination. It also ensures that the item/statements belong there or not. The mean difference between the high scores and low score group are tested to detect the significant difference through t-test. The item with a high value are then included in the instrument after which the instrument is checked for its reliability and validity.

Item analysis is based on:

1. Total score rank, from higher to lowest.
2. Select top & bottom 27% for analysis.
3. Tally the response made to each item by the subjects.
4. Compute % of each group that answers the item correctly
5. Average 2% from step 4 to obtain difficulty index of each item.
6. Subtract the % from the two extreme groups to obtain discrimination index

Table 9.2

Items	% correct	Difficulty Index	Discrimination Index
Item A upper 27% lower 27%	100 70	85	30
Item B upper 27% lower 27%	60 40	50	20
Item C upper 27% lower 27%	88 30	59	58

Reliability is concerned with consistency, accuracy, precision, stability, equivalence & Homogeneity.

Homogeneity can be assessed by either of the four methods i.e.

1. Item total correlations.
2. Split half reliability
3. Kuder Richardson's (KR- 20) coefficient.
4. Cronbachs Alpha

Reliable Measure- increases True scores- reduces error component. Increase in error- results in increased unreliability

- A test may be reliable even though it may not be valid
- A valid test is always reliable.

VALIDITY

Fig. 9.2: Validity

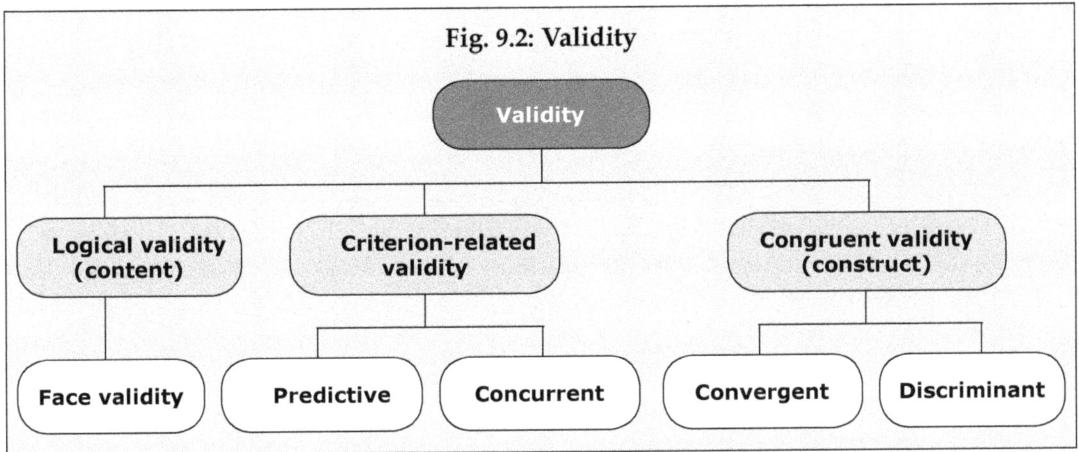

Validity refers to an instruments ability to actually test what it is supposed to test. If the study has to be meaningful and worthwhile instrument must have validity. Validity test show how well an instrument that is developed measured the particular concept it is intended to measure. Validity is concerned with whether we measure the right concept and degree to which an instrument measures what it is supposed to measure.

Valid instrument can be used for prediction. An instrument valid for one purpose may not be valid for another. No instrument should be used in 'research' until its validity is ascertained.

Several types of validity tests are used to test the goodness of a measure.Validity can be checked for its **content** validity, **construction** validity, and **concurrent** or predictive validity, criterion related validity

Content Validity

It's the extent to which the instrument includes the factors or situations under study or an adequate and representative set of items tap the content. More the scale items represent the domain of the concept being measured, greater the content validity. In other words, content validity is a function of how well all the dimensions and elements of a concept have been delineated. Experts or research mentors must judge that the content of the instrument is appropriate. Researchers calculate content validity index (CVI) that indicates the extent of expert agreement which should be 0.9.

- Individuals who are expert in the field under study are the best people to do content validity.
- Jury is better than the single individual opinion.

- Numbers of experts are selected to act as a jury by the researcher.
- Content validity is important characteristics of inventories check lists, evaluation instrument, and Questionnaire and interview schedule.
- Every item must be related to the hypothesis and to the focus of the study.

Criterion related validity is established when the measure differentiates individuals on a criterion it is expected to predict. This can be done by establishing what is called concurrent validity or predictive Validity. Researchers seek to establish the relationship between scores on an instrument and some external criterion. Instrument is said to be valid if its scores correspond strongly with scores on the criterion. Concurrent validity that is degree of correlation of two measures of the same concepts administered at the same time. A high correlation coefficient indicates agreement between two measures. It seeks to establish that measure correlates another criterion. A validity coefficient is calculated, magnitude of co-efficient is estimate of validity (r=.00-1.00) (.70 desirable).

Concurrent Validity

Concurrent validity is established when the scale discriminates individuals who are known to be different; that is they should score differently on the instrument.

Various aspects of the study are broken down for in depth investigation. There is always association with the present behavior of an individual. The research test has concurrent validity, if data resulting from its use are related to behavior in the current situation. e.g. If the students' performance in the clinical area is similar to that in the practical test, the practical test has concurrent validity to that degree.

Predictive Validity

Where the instrument's ability to differentiate between individual's performance and behavior on a future criterion. The difference between predictive and concurrent is the difference in timing of obtained measurements on a criterion.

Degree of correlation between the measures of the concept and some future measure of the same concept because of the passage of time coefficient correlation are likely to be somewhat lower for predictive validation studies e.g.: Can the result of the test be used for predicting the performance of a student in another domain in another situation on some other day.

Construct Validity

It's the interplay between theory & the measurement of the construct that make up theory. Term construct frequently refers to the phenomena of concepts that are not directly observable. The human characteristics that can be observed in human behavior must be clearly defined so that inferences can be verified. If an instrument is developed to identify certain constructs then it must be tested for construct validity. Construct validity testifies how well the results obtained from the use of the measure fit the theories around which the test is designed. The extent to which a test measures a theoretical construct or trait is assessed through different methods **convergent** and **divergent** and **discriminant** validity.

a) Convergent validity is established when the scores obtained with two different instruments measuring the same concept are highly correlated. Researcher search for other measure of consistence where two or more tests theoretically measure the same. The construct are identified after both are administered correlational analysis is done and if its positively correlated convergent validity.

b) Divergent: ability to differentiate the construct from others if it's positively related to other measures 'validity' of the measure is strengthened.

c) Discriminant validity: is established when, based on theory, two variables are predicted to be uncorrelated, and the scores obtained by measuring them are indeed empirically found to be so.

e.g.: When validating a measure of fear related to labour experience. Assessing primigravid and multipara., women's labour experience, it is expected that primi would experience more fear than multipara and if the result obtained are in contrast to this then the validity of an instrument is questioned though some group differences would be reflected in the scores. Logical and empirical procedures are both employed in construct validity. e.g. insecure patients change physicians more frequently is expected to find similar score in all individuals but there would be slight variation in score owing to personality difference.

Face validity: also called ***logical validity***. Refers to whether the instrument looks as though it is measuring the appropriate construct. It is an analysis to see whether the instrument appears to be a valid scale. It has high degree of subjectivity it's a criterion that's questionable when testing validity though, it's least time consuming. It is good for an instrument to have face validity.

Face validity states if item/statement/questions are very 'valid 'moderately 'valid' or not very valid and is specific for a particular subject. It gives the appearance of measuring concepts. Colleagues give their opinion about the instrument. Will this test measure or has it measured the matter and the behavior that it is intended to measure.

Internal and External Validity: It's done in the experimental situation. *Internal validity* refers to interpretation of findings within the study related to data. *External validity* is concerned with generalization beyond the study related to the use of the findings. Researcher attempts to find out whether the studied variable is the causal factor or there are extraneous variables unaccounted for in the study setting. The degree to which researcher is able to accomplish this is called internal validity. The extent to which researcher can make a generalization about the relationship identified in the experimental setting is a measure of the external validity.

Methods used to test validity are:

1. To correlate results from the instruments with that researcher believes to measure the same construct.
2. To utilize a group of independent judges, who observe & record evidence of the participants behavior in situations that spell out concepts in operational terms.
3. Logical analysis & the testing of relationship predicted on the basis of theoretical consideration

Once the instrument is developed its reliability & validity is established. 'Reliability' proportion of accuracy to inaccuracy in measurement in observed scores derived from a set of items consists of *true scores and error*. **Error** may be either *chance error* or *random* or *systematic*; 'Validity' is concerned with **systematic error** & 'reliability' is concerned with random error. **Random errors** are unsystematic in nature and are a result of transient state in the respondent, or in the administration of the instrument. e.g.: When measuring Temperature - ***random error*** introduces distortions caused by temperature fluctuation of an individual, thermometer placement site may be moist or not placed properly, person's attempt to talk while taking temperature. ***Systematic error***/*construct error* measurement error attributed to relatively stable characteristics of the study population that may bias that behavior and/or cause incorrect instrument calibration.

PILOT STUDY

Pilot study is a preliminary small scale study that is conducted before main research to decide how best to conduct a large scale research study. Research problem or question refinement can occur after pilot study. Best methods can be identified for conducting actual study. Pilot studies should be conducted for both quantitative & qualitative research studies.

Fig. 9.3: What should be done to construct an instrument/tool for data collection?

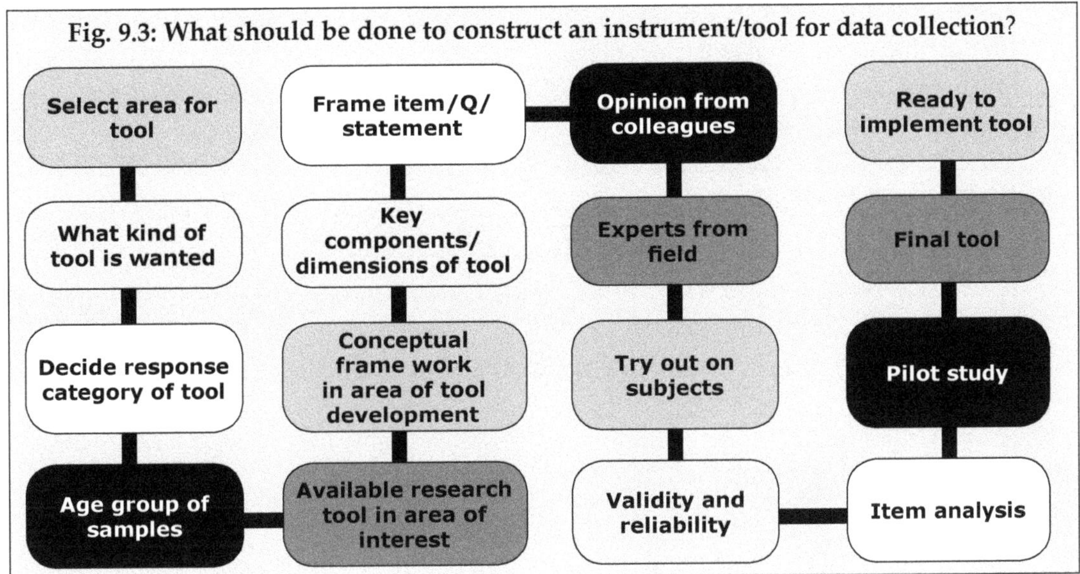

Meaning of Pilot Study

- A pilot study is a small feasibility study designed to test various aspects of the methods planned for a larger, more rigorous, or confirmatory investigation. (Arain, Campbell, Cooper & Lancaster, 2010)
- A pilot study is conducted to prevent the occurrence of a fatal flaw in a study that is costly in time & money. (Polit & Beck, 2017)

Following are Advantages of Pilot Study

- It helps in refinement of problem statement/question
- Helps in identifying potential confounding variables that were not previously known & evaluate the strength of relationships among important variables.
- Helps in refinement of hypothesis/set of hypotheses
- Evaluating sample, study setting/data requirement for research study
- Helps in testing research tool/instruments
- Finalizing research methods
- Assessing & taking care of as many potential problems/issues as possible
- Time, cost & other resources can be estimated
- Assessing whether research goals & design is realistic
- Result of pilot study can help secure funding & other forms of institutional investment

Points to be Considered while Conducting the Pilot Study

- Whatever steps are to be followed for main study, need to be followed for pilot study.

- Same instrument & method planned for main study, need to be followed for pilot study.
- Sample size for pilot study should be 10% of the size calculated for main study.

Limitations of Pilot Study

- Sometimes the result of pilot & main study may differ.
- If sample used for pilot study is included in main study contamination of main study results can occur.
- It can provide only limited information about subjects' responses as sample size is small.

Recording of Pilot Study

Specific record of pilot study to be included in research report. As there will be much more clarity in relation to study design/data collection plan/instrument which can help to conduct the main study smoothly.

CONCLUSION

In this chapter we have discussed various instruments that can be used to gather the required data/information from the participants for a research study. The meaning of the instruments, how they can be developed, its advantage and disadvantage. Every instrument has its own limitation; it's always beneficial to use multiple instruments to gather data and negate any biases originating in the instrument. It's fruitful if the researcher gets familiarized with the different instruments so as to be able to select the most appropriate instrument for obtaining adequate data for the selected research design. It's also important that once a instrument for collecting is designed it's checked for reliability and validity before using for collecting data for a research project.

BIBLIOGRAPHY

- Polit Denis F, Cheryl Tatano Beck, Nursing Research 8th edition, Philadelphia; Lippincott William and Wilkims, A Wolters Kluwer company, 2007.
- Nancy Burns and Susan Grove K. The practice of nursing research: conduct, critique and urilzation, 5th edition, Philadelphia saunders, 2005.
- Keeves, John. P. (ed.) (1998): *Educational Research. Methodology and Measurement, An International Handbook.* London: Pergarnon Press.
- Borg, Walter R. (1989): *Applying Educational Research, A Practical Guide for Teachers.* 2nd edition, New York: Longman.
- Thrustone, L.L. & E.J. Chave (1929): *The Measurement of Attitude.* Chicago: The University of Chicago Press.

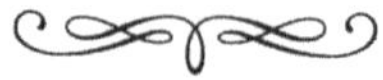

CHAPTER

10 Data Analysis

Nancy Fernandes Pereira

Learning Objectives

This chapter helps the reader to –

- Understand concept and importance of data analysis.
- Analyze data gathered for both qualitative and quantitative method.
- Analyze data using the appropriate method for different types of research design.
- Interpret the data analyzed and present it using the appropriate means to make it meaningful.

Introduction

Data Analysis

It is a process, where the gathered information is organized classified to make sense of the collected information with a view to contribute in discovering new knowledge. Data analysis may also be referred to as ordering of data in order to obtain answers to the research questions. Data analysis is the way by which date is put into order, categorized, manipulated, and summarized so that answers are obtained to research question posed. It is usually the first step taken towards data interpretation. The collected data from a study may be analysed quantitatively or qualitatively.

Interpretation of data is a method using predetermined processes by which the analysed data is assigned, meaning and conclusion is drawn with intention to drawn inference related to the relationship between variables under study.

Data analysis uses many ways and techniques, based on the research design the researcher may use the method found to be most appropriate that is analysing using descriptive or inferential statistics. Data analysis provides an opportunity to make decisions which are more scientific and effective. Before proceeding to collect data a researcher should know what are the statistical measures that can be used so as to choose the correct method for computation and for reporting the findings. Data analysis helps the researcher to organize the *quantitative data* from becoming chaotic, so that it can be evaluated summarized, interpreted and communicated to those interested in the findings. Mere data analysis does not provide answers to research question but interpretation of data is important as it helps to make inferences and draw conclusions.

Quantitative data may use descriptive or inferential statistics. Descriptive statistics used most often are frequency and percentage. Details of statistics will be presented in the next chapter.

This chapter focus on putting the data gathered together to analyse and draw inference. The data has to be organized according to the objectives and the variables being studied with a view to infer from the data. The gathered data has to be classified and displayed in a fashion that helps researcher to understand. It's important to group facts together as grouping scores gives clearer and concise picture. Raw data is difficult to be interpreted by layman or a novice researcher; the data can be interpreted in two ways one can interpret relationship within the study and second the results of the study and inferences drawn, can be compared to theoretical frame work and other research findings, wherein the researcher seeks meaning within his/her own study and concludes in comparison to other researchers with the expectations of theoretical framework.

Descriptive statistics used in complex descriptive studies where data is grouped in nominal, ordinal, interval data. The most basic step is grouping data and presenting them in frequency and percentage calculating mean, median, mode and standard deviations. Standard deviation is frequently used statistics that shows how scores will vary about the mean. Which is basically using nominal measurement where the demographic data gathered about a population is organized based on their attributes like age, gender, education, marital status. Other data may be especially collected based on the topic being studied. When numerically the characteristics of the population is discussed it's referred to as parameter; it's easy to remember as both words start with letter '**p**', while the numerical characteristic of the study sample is referred to as statistics and which can be remembered to avoid confusion as both words start with letter 's', whereas 'SD' is used to indicate standard deviation. Some of the publication may use the symbols instead of writing the words. e.g. mean may be denoted as 'M' or X but later may be more common. Inferential statistic is often used when difference between two groups are required to be studied like in experimental and control group to identify the difference in the score was a true difference or by chance or was it due to over representation or under representation.

The analysis proceeds into four stages where the collected data is first '*categorised*' according to the problem and objectives, '*frequency distribution*' is done according to the number of cases falling in to the formed categories i.e. basically it gives the number of cases in each category and then a comparison is done between frequency and percentage to find the relationship like comparing the score of female samples with the men, *measurement* is use of basic mathematical understanding to describe the data using descriptive analysis which includes calculating mean median, mode and statistical averaging where mean is the arithmetic average of the scores median is the midpoint of the scores analysis and then interpretation is where data is interpreted statistically or analytically; it's difficult of participants break down.

For example day of study, vital sign readings, blood group, type of activity or type of medication the individual is on. The reason for organizing data is to make manifestations possible, relationships, proposition, trends or tendencies to be revealed from the gathered information.

Preparing Master Sheet

The gathered data is firstly tabulated and then presented in Tables. As the data is gathered a spread sheet or a master sheet is prepared based on the skill of researcher manually or computerized. Every item for which information is collected a code can be used and it can be scores using tally. Tally is placing 4 vertical lines and a line across them to indicate bundle of five, the lines are placed every time a score is indicated or a variable appears or behavior has been noted.

Example: Data has been gathered from 30 individuals suffering from the dengue with the help of questionnaire. This has 30 questions with 4 options and demographic data to identify the age, gender, education level, income group, marital status and type of employment.

As seen in the Table below master sheet can be prepared for all items/question then a Table can be prepared.

Table: 10.1

(N=30)

Item	Count of response	Total
Age:		
20-30 yrs	~~1111~~ ~~1111~~	10
31-40 yrs	111	03
41-50 yrs	~~1111~~ 11	07
51 yrs & above	~~1111~~ ~~1111~~	10
Gender:		
Male	~~1111~~ ~~1111~~ ~~1111~~ II	17
Female	~~1111~~ ~~1111~~ ~~1111~~ 111	13

Preparing Tables for Interpretation

Table: 10.2: Distribution of samples according to their demographic variable

(N=30)

Particulars	Frequency	Percentage
Age		
21-30 yrs	10	33.33
31-40 yrs	3	10
41-50 yrs	7	23.3
51 yrs & above	10	33.33
Gender		
Male	17	56.6
Female	13	43.3

The above Table can then be interpreted as "It is observed from the above Table 1 that majority (33.33%) of the samples were in the age group of 21 to 30yrs and 51 yrs and above who suffered from dengue. Only three (10%) and seven (23.3%) suffered from dengue in the age group of 31 to 40 yrs and 41 to 50 yrs respectively. The Table also highlights, of the 50 sample seventeen (56.6%) were males and thirteen (43.3%) were females. It's concluded that more male suffered from dengue as compared to female though the difference in number is small." The age groups in this Table have been arranged in interval of 10 units. One can arrange based on the quantum of data in interval of 3, 5, and so forth. If score for each attribute was scored it would not make much sense for example weight or respiratory rate of a person as shown in the Table below.

Table: 10.3

(N=30)

S. No	Weight in kg	Tally	F	Resp. rate	Tally	F
1.	35 kg	~~IIII~~ ~~IIII~~ ~~IIII~~	15	14	~~IIII~~ ~~IIII~~ 11	12
2.	36 kg	~~IIII~~ ~~IIII~~ 11	12	15	1111	04
3.	37 kg	II	02	18	1111	04
4.	38 kg	I	1	20	1111 1111	10

If each attribute as seen in the above Table is scored on tally sheet or master sheet, it's difficult to understand and the master sheet would be exhausting, hence best to arrange them in class intervals as seen in Table 10.2.

Data when organized becomes easy to interpret and is understandable at a glance. Data gathered for questions stating Yes/No can be code as 1 for 'Yes' and 2 for 'No' the number of 1 or 2 can be counted; else just as indicated in the table above tally marks can be placed (Table 10.4). Once the data collected is transferred on to the master sheet one has to check for mistake and get it corrected. The data after entering should be checked for accuracy, completeness so that no aspect is missed out nor any question response is marked on the master sheet. When questionnaires are returned they should be checked to see if any question has not been attempted. Check to ensure uniformly the same pattern of entering the response is done. Check the response if it is written legibly, and completely, check for responses made like "don't know", "not sure", if it for dietary recall response such as "cannot remember" or incorrect spelling which cannot be comprehended; can be separately listed and accordingly interpreted as incomplete response or minus those response and according write the 'N' for that question. In case information has been collected using interview schedule, the chances of missing a question is less as compared to questionnaire, if the researcher has appointed a research assistant to collect data, then data should be checked out, if not understood what is documented with the research assistant or checked out in the field or content validated before entering in the master sheet to ensure no omission is there. The data once organized in a homogenous group according to the characteristics.

Table: 10.4: Master sheet

N=20

Sam-ple no	Q.1				Q.2				Q.3				Q.4				Q.5		Q.6	
	a	b	c	d	a	b	c	d	a	b	c	d	a	b	c	d	Y	N	Y	N
1		1			1							1			1		1		1	
2	1				1						1				1		1		1	
3	1					1						1			1			1	1	
4		1			1						1			1			1		1	
5-20	1				1				-	-	-	-			1			1		1
Total	**3**	**2**	**-**	**-**	**4**	**1**	**-**	**-**	**-**	**-**	**2**	**2**	**-**	**1**	**4**	**-**	**3**	**2**	**4**	**1**

The Table indicates the response scored for each option for a given question. The correct option is bolded, from which a Table of frequency and percentage for the questions asked can be drawn. As seen in the Table Q.1 two samples (%) chose the correct option while three (%) chose incorrect option. Similarly the remaining items can be analyzed. In the above Table it may be noted that sample no 5 had not responded to Q. no 3. Tabulating the data provides opportunity to place the data in a Table arranged in rows and columns the data arrangement may be simple or complex, care should be taken when tabulating data to avoid mistakes. Complex data may be seen especially when tabulating like a demographic data which highlights religion economic strata level of education or pretest and more than one post-test as in experimental study. Refer example in Table 10.5.

Table 10.5: Distribution of the score related to .....

(N=30)

S. No	Particulars	Pretest		Post-test	
		Frequency (F)	Percentage (%)	Frequency (F)	Percentage (%)
1	Q.1	15	50%	28	93.3
2	Q.2	18	60	30	100%
3	Q.3	15	50%	26	86.6
4-30	Q.4	22	73.3	30	100%

The above Table 2 indicates the frequency before and after intervention as in an experimental study for the frequency percentage is calculated. Which can facilitate clear interpretation "to the Q.1 in the pretest fifteen (50%) responded correctly and the response improved in the post test to twenty-eight (93.3%) which indicate effect of the intervention (could be knowledge/practice/ intervention used).

One could have a prevalence Table e.g. if the researcher intends to study age group having premature deliveries and are the incidences more in rural or urban. The Table would reflect the two variable age and place of residence of the mother.

Table 10.6: Distribution of mothers delivering premature babies with regards to their age and place of residence.

Age at delivery (Years)	Urban Mothers delivering premature babies (N=70)		Rural Mothers delivering premature babies. (N=80)		Total no of Mothers delivering premature babies. (N=150)	
	F	%	F	%	F	%
14-16	23	33	30	37.5	53	35.3
17-19	36	51	23	28.75	59	39.3
20-22	3	4	10	12.5	13	8.6
23-25	2	3	12	15	14	9.3
26-28	6	9	5	6.25	11	7.3
Total	70	100	80	100	150	99.8
Prevalence	**70/500 = 14%**		**80/500 = 16%**		**150/1000 = 15%**	

The Table can be interpreted as "in the age group of 14 to 16 yrs. Twenty three (33%) from urban and thirty (37.5%) from rural gave birth to premature babies. It is observed from the data the incidence of premature birth is slightly higher in rural as compared to urban the overall incidences of premature delivery in this age group is fifty three (35.3%)." In this way the rest can be interpreted. When it comes to prevalence on can state of the over 15% deliveries which are premature 14% are seen in urban and 16% are seen in rural area which indicates the prevalence is not much different in both these sections of the society.

The data since classified/tabulated and presented for better interpretation it's important to ensure the Table is well prepared following the guidelines. One needs experience to prepare Table and a novice researcher may take guidance from expert in preparing a perfect Table.

Tables are important aspects in presenting analyzed data in tabular form which is adequately and properly labeled. Every row and column should be labeled appropriately to describe its content. They should be set up correctly, identified fully and reflect the appropriate information. The Table heading should be clear to enable it to stand independently without additional explanation in text.

If 'Tables' cannot be understood without reading the text, means it's poorly constructed and poorly labeled, though they aid, they are not an end in themselves. Tables show relationships those are easily seen but may be difficult to explain in words. The format used to prepare a Table should be simple containing not more than two variables at a time. If readers find difficult to comprehend the Table they may skip reading the report too.

The research document may have two type of Tables used one General and other for specific purpose. *General* Table used in the document could be ***'reference Table'*** could be both simple and complex providing information like conversion, index Table, Table of figs etc. *Special* Tables would include ***'relationship Table'*** showing relationship between two variables could be event, qualities etc., and comparison Table reflects one or more variable where one is held constant or running in series and another variable is compared with it, e.g. demographic data Table. The other being ***'Continuity Table'*** where it reflects increase or decrease from one cell to another e.g. a Table showing physiological parameter in which for example blood pressure is monitored daily and recorded for 15days or temperature recorded for 5 days thrice. It reflects improvement or deterioration in a parameter.

Title of Table: should be brief yet reflect the essence of the content. Title should not be too long and should be inverted 'V'.[☰]

The columns and rows should be appropriately labeled; the rows should be numbered for clear referencing when comparison is done.

Numbering: Table should be numbered and numbers should run in sequence. e.g. Table: I, Table: II. Tables in appendix should be numbered separately than from the main body of the text.

Placement of Table: It should be within the body of the research report. It should be well balance in one page, Table should not be narrow neither too broad; that is it should have good proportion. If it's a broad Table it can be presented with the page in landscape. It should fit on one page, if the content of the Table runs into the next page or more, every page the Table, columns and row should be labeled. The Table can be broken down in to two or more but the same heading should reflect in the following Tables they may be labeled as

Table 10.1 (A), Table 10.1 (B) since the contents are similar it can be done e.g. if many attributes are included in demographic Table.

Content of the Table: contains numerical data for the readers to understand at a glance. The Table should have lines only if necessary e.g. to separate age and gender/religion, one question from another. In the Table the numerical should be rounded but avoid unnecessary rounding as when percentage is total it may excessed 100%. Numericals should be centered in all columns to appear neat. If there is no score in any column it should not be left vacant/empty place a zero or dash avoid dittos if number is same; figs should be aligned with the decimal point. In case four or more digits it should be separated by a comma e.g. 7, 456 never write 7456 it's incorrect recording. Totals may be placed at the end of column or row as required. Similar content then Table should have the same format.

Tables should not be consecutively in the report or chapter, every Table should be followed by the textual explanation and interpretation, it depends on the institutional/publication house guidelines if the discussion should follow the interpretation or a separate section should be dedicated.

Table is a popular illustrative device to present the data in an effective manner. A well prepared Table is simple, clear and worth thousand words. Other than Table, data can be **diagrammatically** presented in the form of graphs, concept maps, flow charts; it adds visual clarity

Visual Presentation of Data

A graphic presentation offers a visual appeal of the study findings making it apparent. It could be in the form of bar graph, pie chart, line graph. Graphic presentation is referred to as a "Figure."

Bar Graph helps in depicting relationship between two or more variables using rectangular bars. The bars can be presented horizontally or vertically though most preferred is vertically. The 'X' axis represents independent variable while the 'Y' represents the dependent variable. The bar graphs are named according to how the bars are represented as follows: Grouped Bar Graph, Stacked Bar graph, segmented bar graph, Histogram.

Grouped Bar Graph is used to highlight sub grouped of the same group of variables where in the bars are placed side by side like a histogram e.g. response to play therapy in two different age groups toddlers and

pre-schoolers with attention deficit attending child guidance clinic as shown in Fig. 10.1.

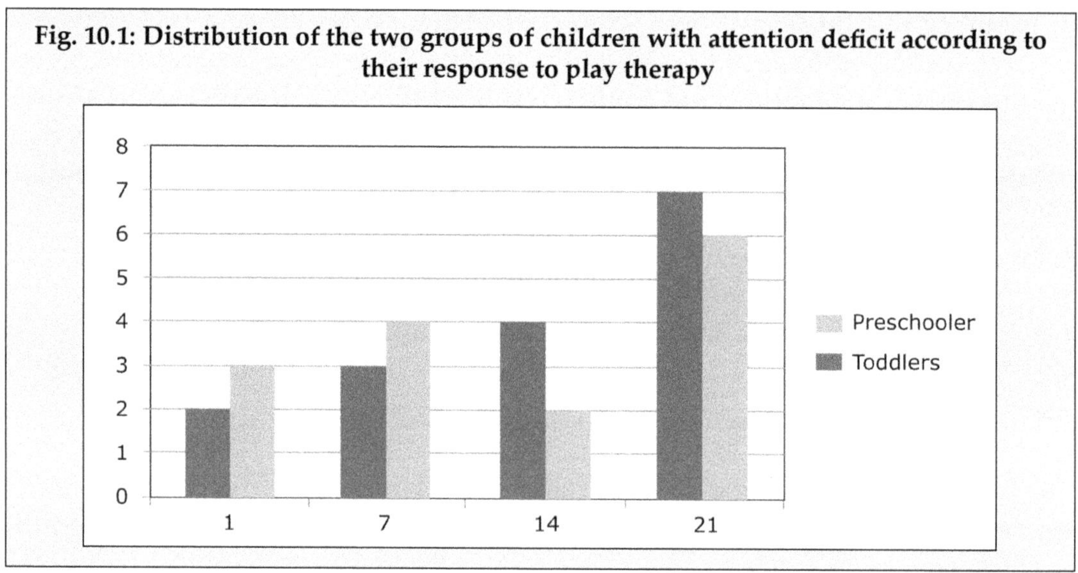

Fig. 10.1: Distribution of the two groups of children with attention deficit according to their response to play therapy

Stacked Bar graph: In this the bars are stacked on top of each other rather than being placed next to each other. The above Figure is presented using stacked bar graph.

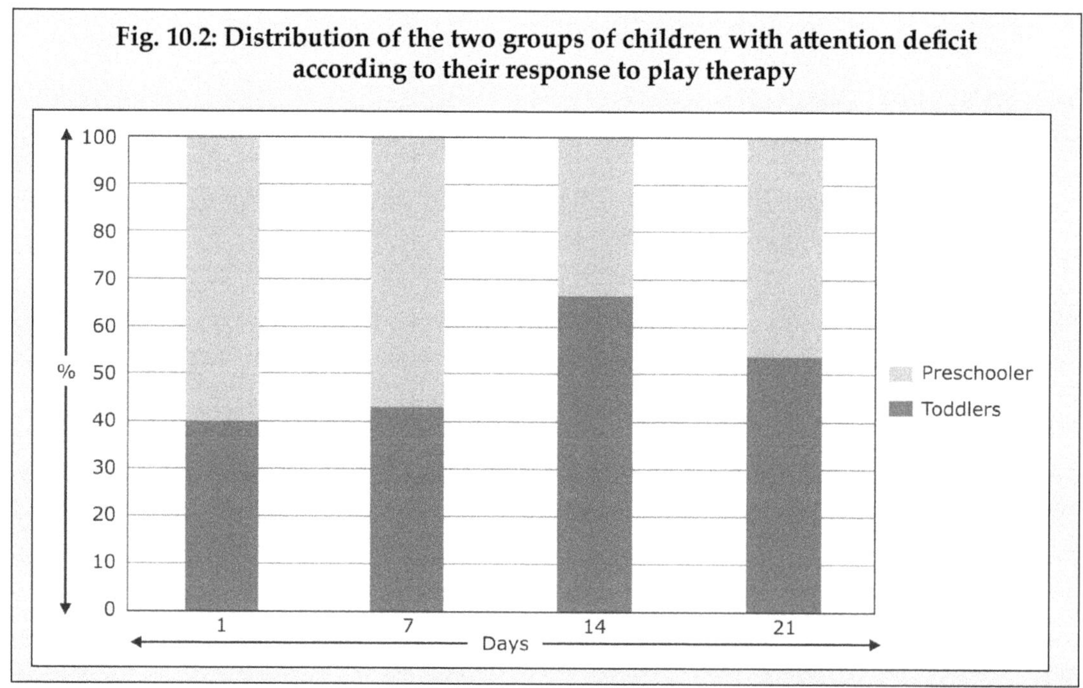

Fig. 10.2: Distribution of the two groups of children with attention deficit according to their response to play therapy

Segmented Bar Graphs: are just like the stacked bar graphs depicting 100% of the dependent variable in the stacked rectangular bar. It's often used in studies having intersection between the variable.

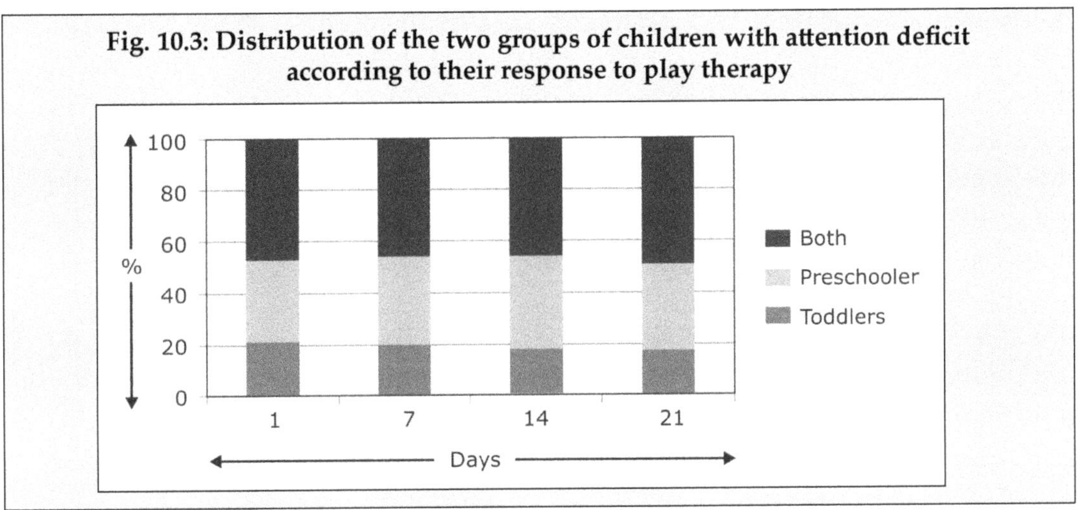

Fig. 10.3: Distribution of the two groups of children with attention deficit according to their response to play therapy

Histogram: Depict numerical data in a continuum and summarize discrete data, used to present variables measured in ordinal, interval or ratio level. Only one variable is presented in a histogram as it shows number of responses that fall in a specific range. The bars are of equal with and touch each other to indicate data is in continuum. Whereas the width of the bar represents the class interval and height of the bar represents the frequency of occurrence of each class interval. It's similar to vertical graph, e.g. number of times candidates appeared for interview and number of sets of applications submitted.

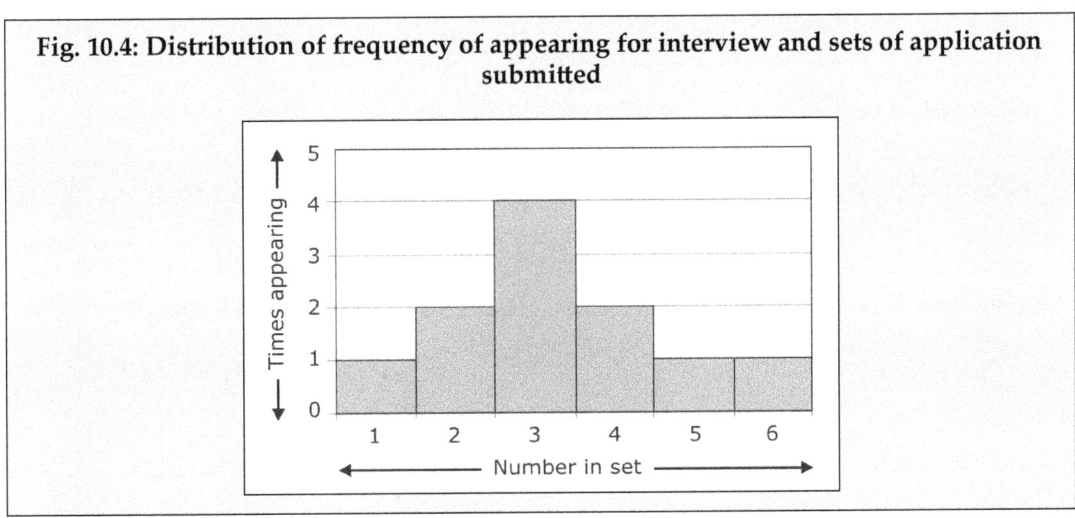

Fig. 10.4: Distribution of frequency of appearing for interview and sets of application submitted

Advantage of Bar graphs: They help to easily understand, simplify and present large data, give information at a glance of key score.

Disadvantage: May not properly be able to describe data, cannot be used without text, and can be manipulated to show the impact.

Pie diagram is a circular diagram depicting 360 degree circle useful to present small data like demographic aspect but not useful for large data. They allow for variation in presentation in research reports. There are different *types* of pie chart like simple pie chart, doughnut pie chart and 3 D chart. Most of the pie diagrams can be easily prepared in the computer.

Simple Pie diagram: depicts the distribution of the frequency or percentage in relation to the characteristic of the population under study wherein only one attribute is presented as seen in Fig. 10.5.

Fig. 10.5: Distribution of samples according to their level of education

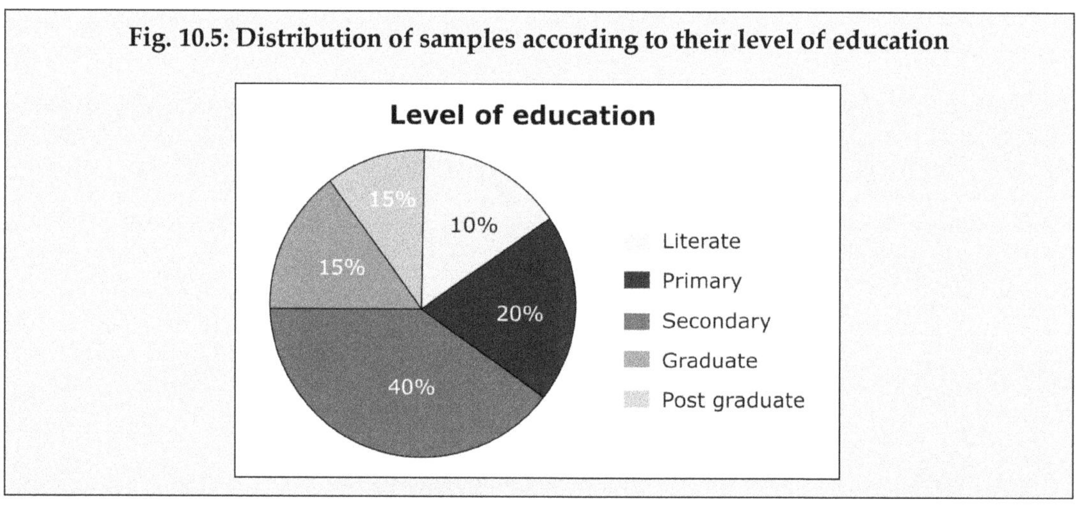

Doughnut chart is a type of pie chart. Below figure shows distribution of educational level of the population under study. Similarly it can be presented in modified doughnut which shows percentage in a split doughnut in Fig.10.6 and Figs. 10.6 & 10.7.

The pie and the doughnut can be presented in the form of 3 D also as it allows variation in presentation and visual appeal.

3D Chart: pie or split pie chart can be presentation of percentage of attributes of the samples understudy in three dimensional image as seen in Figs. 10.8 and 10.9.

Fig. 10.6 distribution of samples according to their level of education

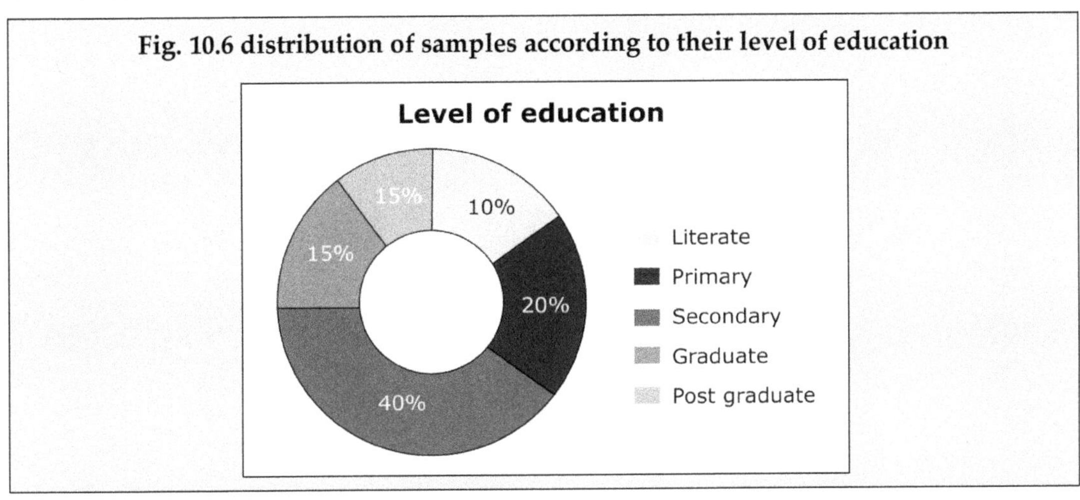

Fig. 10.7: Distribution of samples according to their gender

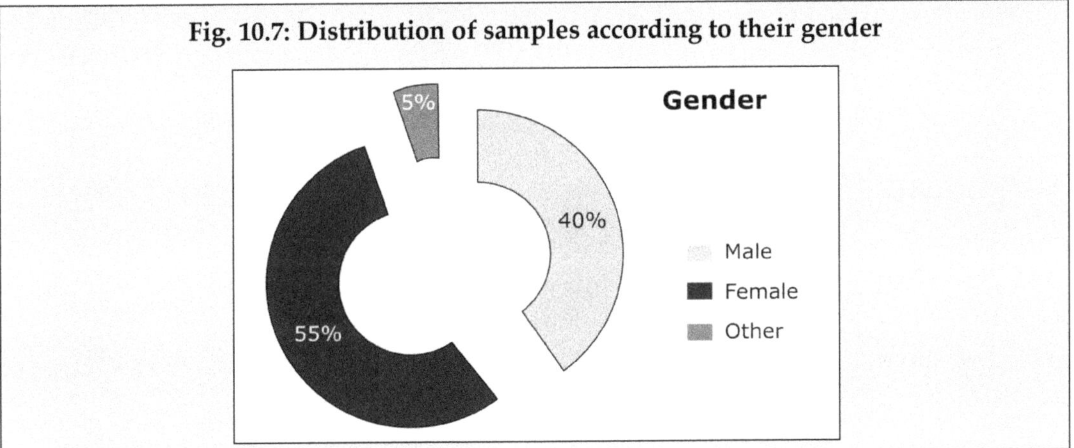

Advantage of Pie charts improve appearance of presentation but useful for single variable.

Disadvantage: cannot be used for comparing multiple variable and trends.

Fig. 10.8: Distribution of educational level

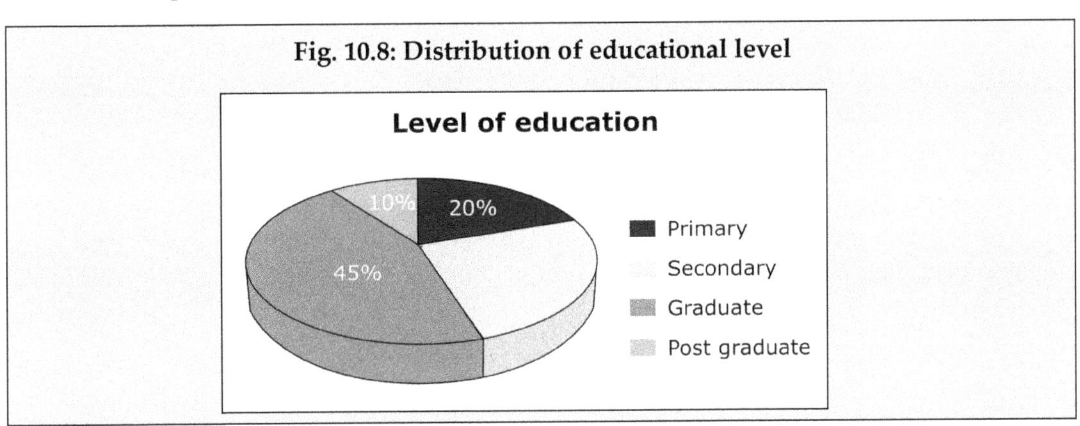

Fig. 10.9: Distribution of sample according to their age

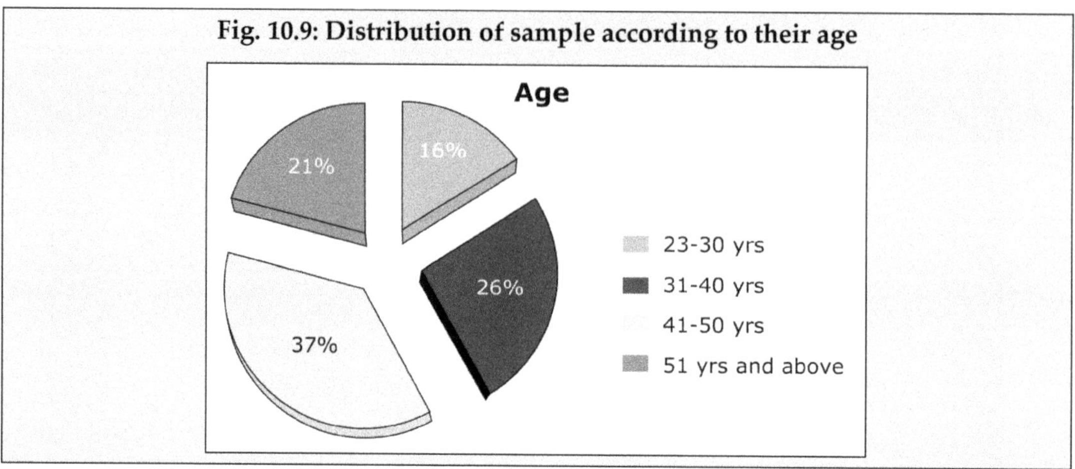

Line Graphs are series of values which are connected by a straight line, they show magnitude of the data. There are different types of line graphs used for presentation like **'simple line graph**' which depict trend and can compare categories, while simple line graph with markers is same except the value is highlighted. The other is presenting lines which are **stacked** on top of each other.

Fig. 10.10: Simple line Graph

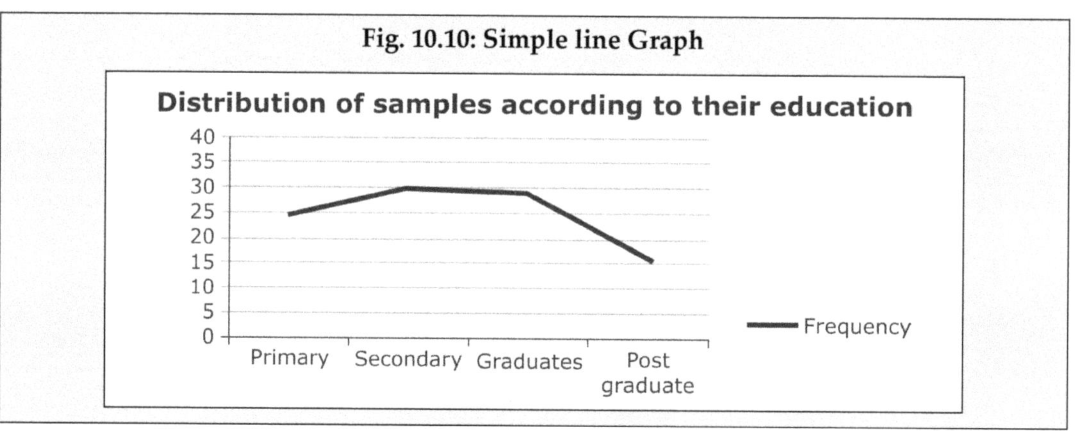

Fig. 10.11: Simple line graph with marker

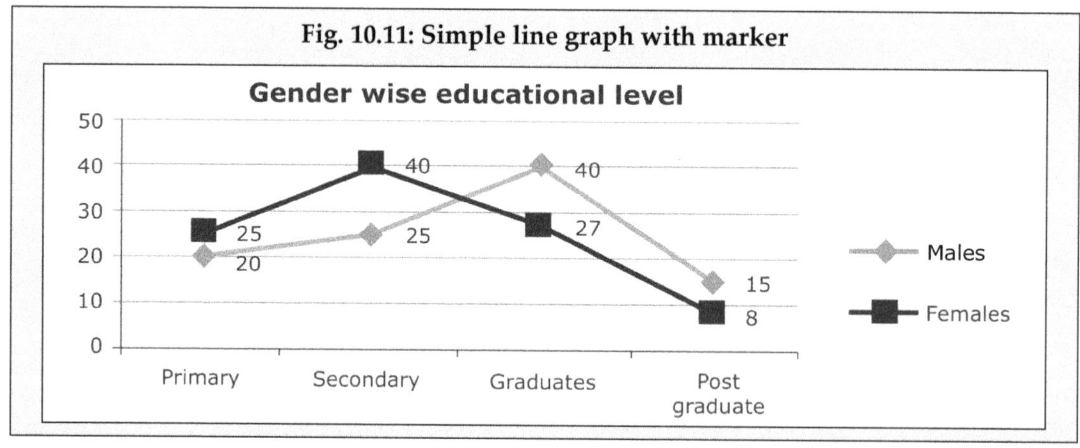

Fig. 10.12: Stacked line graph

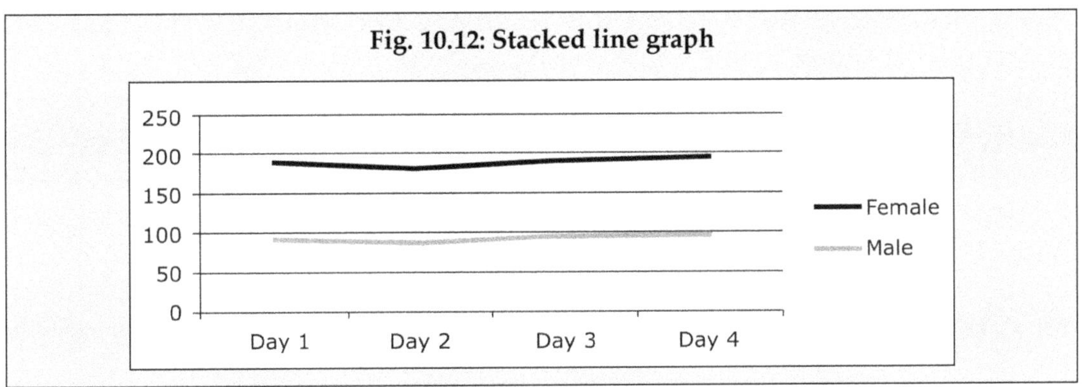

The inferential analysis is discussed in detail in chapter 14.

Qualitative data analysis: is a labor, intensive activity that requires insight, creativity, conceptual sensitivity and sheer hard work. Qualitative data analysing takes a loose form of data structure as when human beings communicate through their own native language, it's entwined with emotions, opinion, attitude, values and knowledge. Qualitative analysis is used to draw inference from qualitative data. This method uses text rather than number to draw patterns. Qualitative data is collected using a variety of person to person technique. The data collected is cumbersome as they are in text form. It has to be sorted, coded before analysing, if tried to be analysed in its raw form could cause lot of errors.

Purpose of data analysis is to organize, provide structure to, and elicit meaning from research data. Analysis usually occurs simultaneously, rather than after data has been collected. Search for themes and concepts begin from the moment data collection begins. Data collection stops once no new information, concepts or codes are available that means it reaches point of saturation.

Data in qualitative research may be **collected** through individual interview/ focus group discussion, conversations using open ended questions or analysing document (articles/essays/talks/books etc.) of any type.

Communication largely could be written as individuals can convince, motivate and manipulate through the use of various print medium. Large information is also communicated through television, radio, movies which influence individual's ideas, beliefs and values which could be analysed by the researcher based on his objective of what is to be explored or understood.

The qualitative analysis also presents demographic information of the participants of the study is presented in tabular form just like in quantitative study including all background information. After which the collected data constant read and re read to start sorting and coding the collected data.

Challenges in qualitative analysis: Qualitative analysis being subject and textual poses a challenge for 3 major reasons: (i) There is no universal rule for analysing qualitative data. (ii) There is enormous amount of work that is required. (iii) Concise data for reporting purposes.

Qualitative analysis process: Qualitative data is an active and interactive process, especially at the interpretive end of the analysis style of continuum. Researchers are required to carefully and deliberatively read data over and over for meaning and deeper understanding. For theories and insight to emerge the researcher has to become familiar with the data. Many research scholars state that qualitative research analysis is a way by which data is brought together to fit in like a jigsaw puzzle to draw links, make concepts or categories that were otherwise not visible to come into forefront tying the attributes so as to conjecture, verify modify and rectify to get a meaning from the collected material of information.

Fig. 10.13: Process of analysis

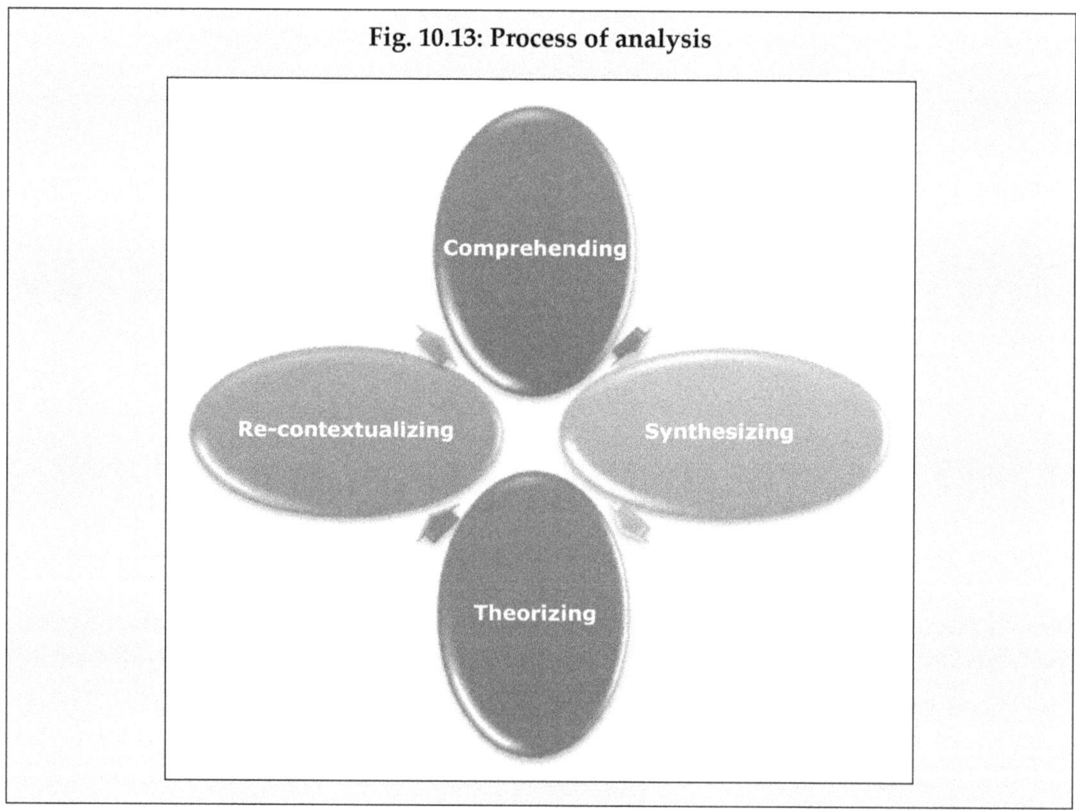

The 4 processes used in qualitative research for analysis are

1. **Comprehending:** is where the investigator goes through the data and makes sense out of it to bring out its meaning and richness of data.
2. **Synthesizing**: understands the data its features as to its typicalness and variation and to what extent generalization can be drawn regarding the phenomena understudy and the participants.
3. **Theorizing:** the research provides rationale regarding the phenomena under study in context of the data collected as they proceed to systematically categorization and derive answer.
4. **Re-contextualizing**: the researcher develops the theory in such a manner that it increases its applicability in different settings or individual groups.

Transcribing Qualitative data

In qualitative studies audio taped interviews and field notes are a major data source. Verbatim transcription is a critical step in preparing for data analysis and need to ensure that transcriptions are accurate and that they reflect the totality of the interviews experience. Transcribers have to indicate through symbols in the text who has said what, when there are gaps, sobs, or non-linguistic utterance and emphasis on words. Transcribing errors are almost inevitable hence one needs to check the accuracy of the transcribed data. Today there are soft wares which transcribe the data even high end mobiles used for recording and give a text version of the interview which reduces the effort of transcribing the recording. There is a variety of methods used for analysing data by researchers for conducting phenomological, ethnographic or grounded theory research.

Template Style: In which the ethnographic researcher prepares a template of words behavior, and then organize the collected data narratives according to

Fig. 10.14: Template style

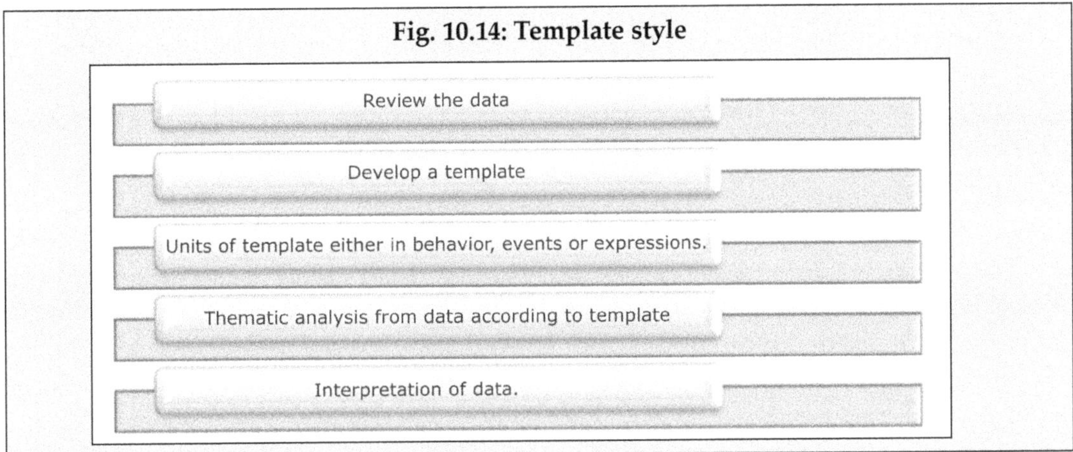

their behavior expression etc. then analysis after placing the content in themes and draws interpretation.

Editing style: While a researcher conducting a grounded theory would use editing style wherein researcher would pick meaningful segments and units to develop categories with codes to correspond it to organize and sort data to develop pattern and structure which connects to give a meaningful model.

Fig. 10.15: Editing

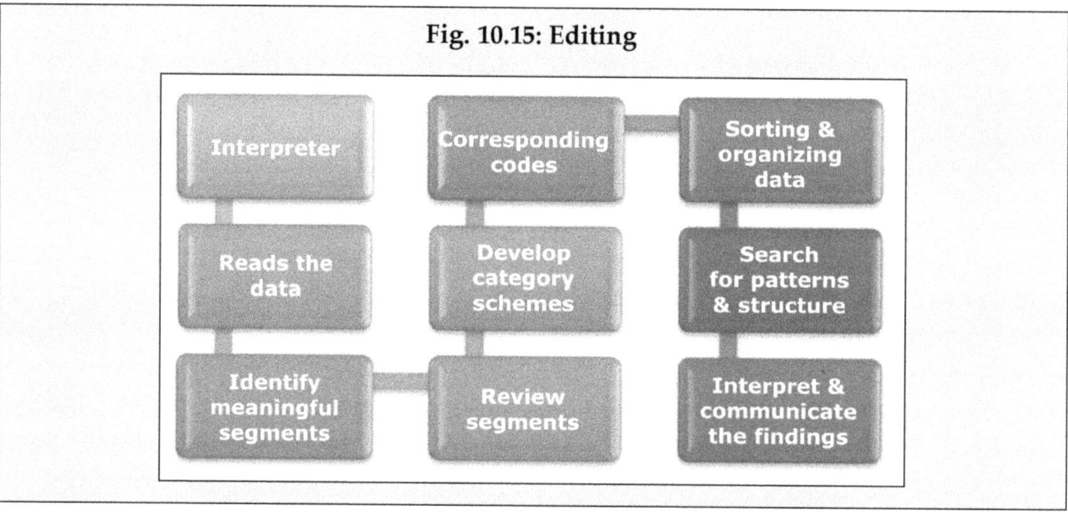

Researcher needs to immerse themselves in the data gathered so as to develop a crystal clear understanding of the data being analysed so as to interpret the findings and highlight ideas; concepts relationship affects the data is bringing forth meaningfully and it would contribute to new learning.

Researchers based on their understanding their own preconceived ideas sorts the data analysing its content for themes, words, key category (Fig. 10.16) so as to quantify where possible while interpreting data which uses a blend of statistics as the researcher describes the findings hence is referred to as "**Content analysis**" and use statistical approach which indicates a ***'Quasi Statistical style'***. Where the researcher may state as the data is being analysed related to primi gravid mother and their preterm babies.

"The mothers who were interviewed and participated in focus group interview were young mothers with less than 25 yrs of age with poor nutritional status. It was noted that 50% of the mothers who participated in the study gave birth to babies with low birth weight ranging from 900 gms to 1700 gms."

Fig. 10.16

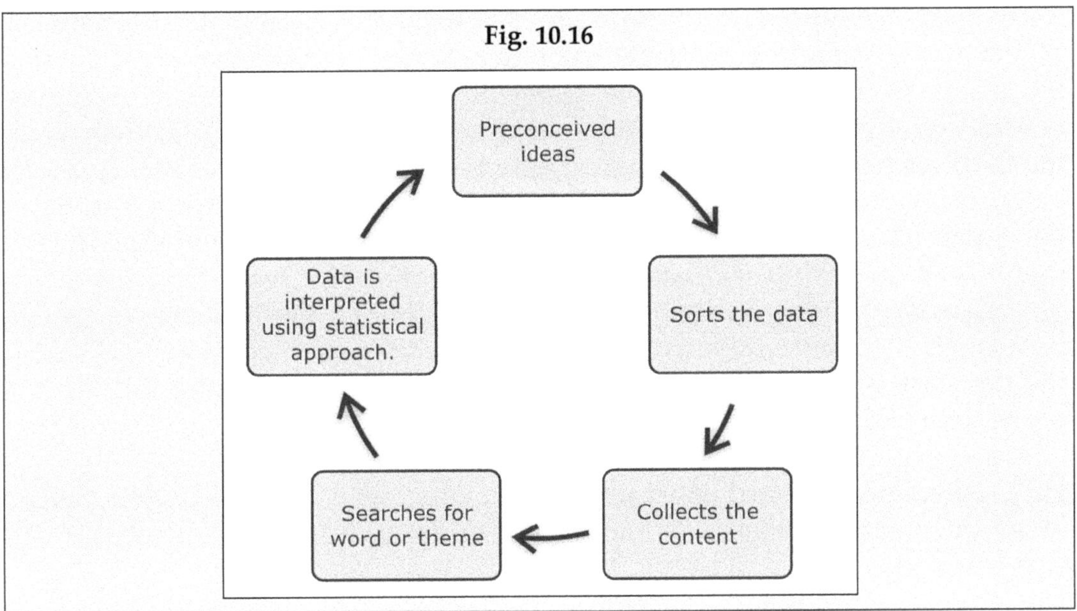

Content analysis as a method is mostly used by social researcher with aim to analyse the content, the document analysed may be a book, newspaper, magazine or any forms of written material.

In this method communication is referred to the material. Since content analysis is a technique using like any other methods of research to objectively, systematically and quantitatively describe what the content presents externally. It focuses on the subjective information like the value, belief, attitude, conduct, motive etc.. unlike the quantitative research which looks at the frequency or duration of an event occurring.

The researcher reads the content number of time to understand what is communicated which is not obvious; that is reads between the lines, for the tone, choice of words used and tries to infer what is the significance or hidden meaning. It also helps to identify concepts meaning and relationship of certain words or themes. The researcher can evaluate the language of the article to assess for partiality/bias or prejudice. It also draws meaning from the content in relation to the culture, background, the text is written and the audience to which it's being communicated to.

Content analysis is nothing but a technique to draw inference through systematic and objective method of dissecting a message for its characteristics.

Features of content analysis: according to Gardner (1975:598) there are four areas under which analysis would feature. (i) objectivity: where two or more individuals would obtain the same results from the same text/document. (ii) systematic: eliminating material supporting the research hypothesis which are being examined there by including and excluding material to applied criteria of selection of material for coding or categorizing. (iii) Generality: are the findings relevant since palin description of the attribute is of no significant value. (iv) Quantification: it refers to the number of times the anser is given or the numerical value given to the occurrence and stated in quantitative term that x% of individual stated from X individuals. But must remember that qualitativeness and quantitativeness are not dichotomous attributes but the lie on a continuum but inferences are drawn by the use of both methods due to the unnecessary weightage given to preciseness results in loss of the richness of the data and its significance.

How does one go about analysing: The textual data is coded broken further in to sub codes, categorised and code categories so that data can be well summarized.

How content analysis benefits: helps identify trends in organization, individual or group's focus area. During interview or focus group discussion helps elicit the attitudinal and behavioral pattern of conversation. Content analysis helps analyse focus group interview or may analyse open ended question included in structured questionnaire to complement data collected. They help in revealing pattern in communication from statements, words expressed by study sample or documents which revealing state of mind, emotions of the writer or respondent.

Content can be analysed using two methods analysing the **concept** and other is **relation**. In ***Conceptual analysis*** the researcher looks for concepts in the text. While in ***relational analysis*** goes deeper to identify the existence of relationship between identified concepts in the text. They contribute to draw meaning, interpret and draw conclusions.

Conducting concept analysis: The *first step* in conceptual analysis is read the text number of times for clarity, and then picking the concept/word or a term used and frequency of its appearance in the text or interview transcript. The word or term may be easy to understand or difficult one would require using their judgment as a lot of subjectivity may appear. The researcher may translate the terms from the language spoken by the respondent to English and back for clarity; may use dictionary grasp the essence and also see the term/word or sentence from contextual perspective. The research would have to analyses it from all angles and keep going back to research question. The researcher has to ensure that the right sample is chosen to gather information and would need to elicit as much data as possible this will ensure there is no gap or any thing missing. The second would be coding text and selectively reducing the content to coded categories so that it's simplified so that a pattern is developed which answers the research question.

The researcher would list the concept and count the number of times it appears. The frequency may be documented using descriptive statistics if researcher feels its importance.

Coding: Once the concepts are identified decide how each word will be differentiated, search for words that are similar yet communicate different meaning. After coding keep aside common words used in English relook at them if any essence or its implying anything. The researcher has to decide whether to code by hand or use computer software to code; though coding by hand helps recognize mistakes redoing rearranging codes, while in computer it may be autocorrected mistakes in terms of spellings but care has to be done by the researcher themselves. Researcher can assess and check for coding re-validates the categories and subcategories. Then start drawing conclusion and interpret the findings generalize where it's possible. Irrelevant or unwanted text material decide what to do or check if any codes are emerging if not then may be discarded. Carefully complete the process of interpreting, findings can be diagrammatically presented or in flow chart to depict pattern of concept.

Relational Analysis: after concept is analysed and identified the relationship between the identified concepts to *elicit meaning* as some concepts independently

Fig. 10.17: Steps of concept analysis

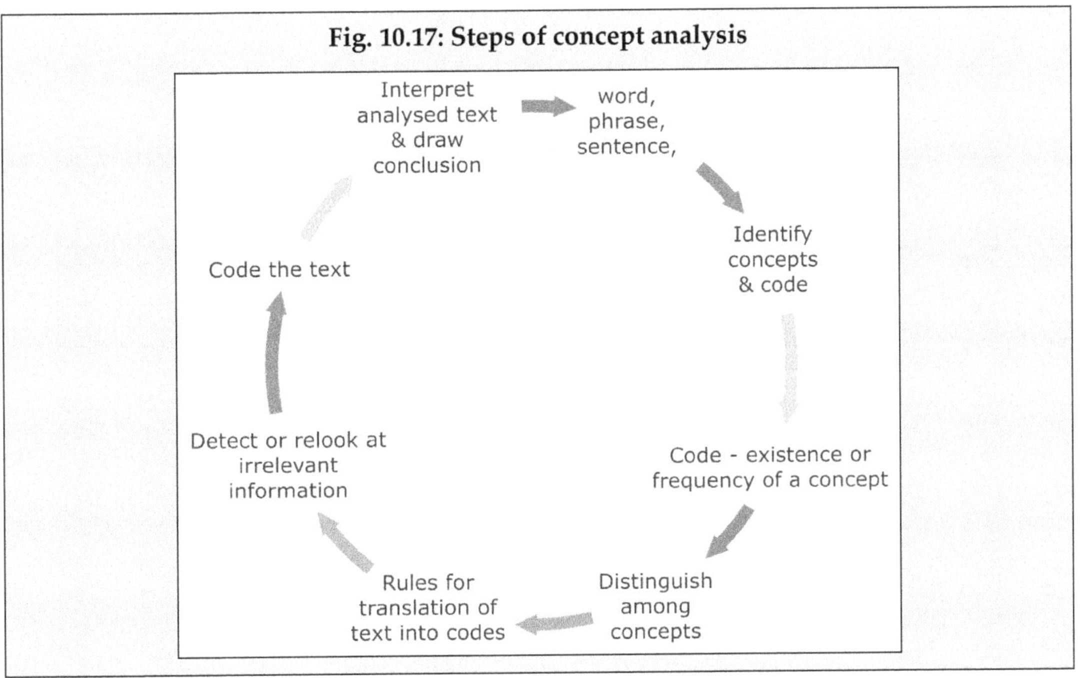

may not bring out any meaning or may not be significant, but its significance may be enhanced after relation between the identified concepts is drawn. When using relational analysis it's similar to content analysis the data in this method follows the similar steps, do **coding** after thorough reading of the text *identify and draw out* emotions, feelings, mental state of the participant, also consider the time frame and background of the participant. Analyse the word, sentence sense the word brings or theme appearing and code. Then prepare a *matrix* of the concepts and the interrelated/connected concepts which draws out the overall meaning or essence of the text or the conversation. Then diagrammatically *represent the concepts* and the *relationship* to provide a concept map or cognitive map to depict the relationship in a meaningful pattern.

Declare in the presentation the strength of the relationship between the concepts and the extent of the relationship, are the two or more concepts positively or negatively related. What is the type of relationship exhibited the two concept that is e.g. if 'A' affects 'B' or if 'B' is removed there are changes seen in 'A' or 'B' appears first and therefore 'A' is seen, what does it imply. The difference between conceptual and relational analysis is that the statement or relationship between concepts are coded. Keep looking out for relationship between identified concepts. To help understand the relationship between concepts create a concept map or flow chart depicting the relationship among the variables identified.

Reliability of content analysis: After content analysis is completed the data analysed showed be shown to another researcher or expert to identify errors or if anything has been overseen or missed out that is do *reliability*. Since its subjective data that is being analysed there is a possible of error or mistakes as the researcher is human. There should be focus on three aspects to ensure its *reliable* is if the coding has been done correctly and same or similar data has not been recoded differently which is possible when researcher is dealing with huge text or transcribed interviews and material is verbatim. Check if the other researcher or expert has coded the data in the same way or similarly; which means the codes can be reproduced by another researcher. Next see if the data categorized is matching the text to the given norm.

Having checked for reliability next *validity* needs to be assessed for it is the categories close which can be confirmed by getting many experts to arrive on agreement with the categories developed and it can be broadened to include implicit and synonyms in the variables. Secondly what conclusions have been drawn? Is there similarity in the findings with other studies; are the findings explainable using any other method. Identify difference in words if computer is used in coding as computer can give count of the words reappearing but may miss out the inherent meaning of the word used. This could divert the result and conclusion could lose its significance in relation to the issue being studied. End of analysis a theory if generated are the concepts clear enough to generalize to a larger context and clarity in the idea. This also further confirms the reliability.

There can be *risk of error* that can occur *deliberately, accidentally or unavoidable alteration* in the data being analysed.

Strength and weakness if content analysis: the *strength* is the unobtrusive method used in content analysis leaving no effect on the sample being studied as the researcher is in direct contact with respondent, leave no room for biases that could affect the research. Analysis provides insight in to human thoughts and language. It can be used to study documents when the individual is not available or event has occurred long ago. Also permits conducting cross cultural studies when not possible using other research methods or designs. It facilitates studying values both personal and social held by people from different cultural background. It's inexpensive though time consuming. It encourages participants in the study to be candid in sharing their views, opinion or thoughts by writing, rather than giving interview or responding to questionnaire. It adds richness to the study and permits replication.

Weakness is that it lacks spontaneity or required documents may not be available and it's susceptible to bias. Context producing the text may be ignored. As the content is being reduced to concepts, words or statement the bigger picture may get lost.

Qualitative data is analysed right from reading the material to identifying concept and clustering concepts. If one is studying families of suicide victim who have experienced their child committing suicide and its impact on their family? "Mother of victim said: I don't know why my child committed suicide. It's becoming difficult to accept for us to accept, everyone is asking our children why our daughter committed suicide, we all were disturbed. We attended counselling; it was difficult for us to go to work and children to go to school. Father of Victim: we told relative she was not well we don't know if she had any mental problem she used to be very quiet, no my child did not committed suicide she was not well…..".

Example: Codes developed could be from the interview with parents as shown below:

Activities code: activity and therapy of other children/adults in the family

Sibling code: behaviors of father, mother, siblings and extended family.

Event code: school, work place, physical environment at home.

Strategy Code: reality, mental health deficiency.

Feeling Code: feelings, ambivalence, silence, support.

After the codes are developed and categories made the codes, words can be linked and presented in diagrammatic flow chart.

CONCLUSION

Qualitative analysis is challenging, labor intensive activity, guided by few standardized rules. The data collected is organized and indexed by coding the content according to category or in to conceptual files. Which is today replaced by the use of computer. Data analysis begins by looking for themes and patterns. Metaphors are used to evoke a visual and symbolic analogy. At time the researcher to give meaning to data may use quasi-statistics which would involve Tables and frequency.

Though the qualitative analysis appears to look simple it's more difficult, yet the findings are easier to understand because of their story form and still difficult to analyse. The richness of the analysis depends on the ability of the researcher to capture the essence and draw the thematic pattern of the data. While quantitative analysis brings out the answers to the research questions which is analysed and presented in Tables and visually as figures.

BIBLIOGRAPHY

1. Gardner, Lindzey and Elliott, Aronson, The Handbook of social psychology, vol:2 (2nd ed),Amerind Publishing Co, New Delhi 1975.
2. Ram Ahuja, Research Methods, Rawat Publications, Jaipur. Reprint, 2011
3. Krippendorff, Klaus. Content Analysis: An Introduction to its Methodology. Beverly Hills: Sage Publications, 1980.
4. Rose Marie Nieswiadomy, Foundations of Nursing Research, 5th ed. Pearson education, published by Dorling Kindersley 2009 New Delhi
5. Hsieh HF & Shannon SE. (2005). Three Approaches to Qualitative Content Analysis. Qualitative Health Research. 15 (9): 1277-1288.
6. Anselm L. Strauss (1987) Qualitative analysis for social scientists. New York, Cambridge University press.
7. Charmaz, Kathy (1983). "The grounded method: An explication and interpretation," in Contemporary field Research: A collection of readings, Robert M. Emerson, ed., Boston, Little Brown and Company, 109-128.
8. Denise, Polit and Cheryl Beck (2008) "Nursing research", 8th edition, Lippincott Williams and Wilkians, Wolter Kluwer, New Delhi, 507-535.
9. Miles, M. B. Huberman, A.M. (1994) Qualitative data analysis: Logical analysis/matrix Analysis,2nd ed, Newbury park, Cal,: Sage Publications.

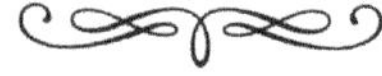

CHAPTER

11 Dissemination and Utilization of Research

Nancy Fernandes Pereira

Learning Objectives

This chapter helps the reader to –

- Document the research carried out.
- Follow a pattern to document and disseminate information generated.
- Critically evaluate the research report with view to improve.
- Use the appropriate way of writing references.
- Write abstract in an interesting manner without losing the essence.

Introduction

The Final Task that remains to be done after completion of the study is writing the research report and disseminating the research finding of the research process. It involves developing a research report for the purpose of disseminating the finding of the study to those interested. A research project cannot be considered complete until its results are effectively communicated to its users or consumers. Therefore disseminating the research finding is one of the essential and final steps of research process. When study has been carried out meticulously and careful records have been kept as the study progressed. All material needed for documentation should be at hand.

Even though the report writing is the capstone of the process it's often given least time and effort. Often the researcher is dazed by the thought of actually sitting down and putting the finding on a paper. Researcher usually spends more time getting started; with the result rushes to complete the project and takes the shortest route in writing the research report.

However if the nurse researcher feels lack of confidence in her skill of presenting the findings or may be overwhelmed by the idea of publishing her work, this could result in the information or findings lying in the draw or shelve even if the researcher intended to publish it or even disseminate the findings. Ultimately the findings which could be used to improve quality of nursing care gets lost. Not communicating the findings is considered a form of scientific misconduct on the part of the researcher. Since a study conducted could have a unique phenomenon described, a previously unrecognized relationship detected or effectiveness of an intervention determined. All of which could make a difference to nursing practice. Hence disseminating the finding is important, so that data/findings do not get shelved or lie in the drawer.

What is a research report?

Research reports are well crafted documented data giving first hand accounting for the research activity carried out by the researcher outlining the selected research design, process, analyzing the gathered information through a systematic scientific method.

Reports include documenting the "statement of the problem", Literature review, that provided the documentation or scientific rationale and background for the study, the statement of Questions to be examined or the hypotheses, the collected data, analysis of data, drawing conclusion and further Questions that have been raised which contribute to implantation of findings.

Purpose of a research report is to communicate what was done in the study to the particular group or individuals interested in the topic of the study. Communication of nursing research must be carried out for two Groups of people, other investigators, Consumers of research.

Other investigators need to be aware of the researches, as it relates to their own efforts of conducting researches. They may be interested in replicating the study or building on it and thus extending its value. A nurse researcher who has conducted a research having a unique phenomenon described, a previously unrecognized relationship detected or confirming the effectiveness of an intervention, this information might make a difference to the nursing practice.

Purpose of dissemination of research findings: To update individuals interested in the topic what was done in a particular study. To promote learning from newly acquired knowledge among professionals, helps increase the evidence for clinical practice. Need to refine the existing body of scientific knowledge to improve the health care outcome.

Benefit of Disseminating the Research Findings

Disseminating the findings has many benefit the researcher, nursing professional and consumers of nursing service. The researchers are able to advance the knowledge of the discipline, receive personal recognition, professional advancement, and psychological & financial compensation for their work. This also motivates researchers to continue conducting research in their respective discipline.

Disseminating the findings also promotes; opportunity for critique which facilitates improving quality of research. Gives other researchers a chance to replicate the studies and identify additional research problems. Using findings in practice, over a period of time the findings from number of studies get synthesized, and are evidences for clinical practice and support evidence based health care to patients. Stake holders for the research findings are Nurses, health care professionals, policymakers, health care consumers.

Challenges faced by researchers: Major challenges which continue to confront Nursing professionals are the ability to transfer research into practise in a timely and effective manner. As they require support from the management of the institution they are employed. This can be a hindrance for both conducting and reporting as the researcher may feel "any way who is interested". Protocols and rule of institutions could be hindrance for publishing their research work.

Criteria for Disseminating Research

The researcher should be selecting proper channel for disseminating and should be aware who are the takers/readers who would use the findings. Make a plan for writing the report which will hold attention of readers. Identify how the research findings would be disseminating to the professional world. Review the guidelines in which the research paper is to be published; carefully select a journal for publication of report. Research report of Ph.D. thesis or Masters Dissertation usually developed in depth to demonstrate the students understanding of the research problem and process to the faculty. Research report developed for publication in journal are concisely written to communicate findings efficiently and effectively to nurses and other health care professional.

Features of a research report

- A research report must have characteristics of conciseness, clarity, honesty, completeness and accuracy.
- It must cover all subjects' material of the topic under study and maintain interest among users.

- It must be written and presented logically.
- Presentation must be visually attractive.
- Report must reflect its originality

How Should the Research Report be Written?

Research report should be informative and not entertaining. It should be well organized and written in a readable style using clear, simple language. Technical phrases and words should be used only when they are clearly needed. If investigator finds it difficult to commence writing research report then it would be better to discuss their ideas with a colleague, a research interest group, support group or a mentor. Organization of the report is very important in presenting the research material well therefore should be probably started by making a tentative outline. Entries in the outline may become various subheadings of the report. Next step is to compose the first paragraph of the section by writing the problem statement studied. Report should be documented in past tense that is Literature review, study conducted, study findings all should be stated in the past tense.

Present tense may be used in reports and discussions of hypotheses, theories that are broadly accepted in the present time. Future tense is rarely used in 'Research report' except for making recommendation or for extrapolating implications for nursing Use of Passive voice may sometimes be necessary in the research report. The individual conducting the study may be termed as investigator or researcher. The researcher should be reading the research reports which will help the researcher to know what to do, and will point out what to avoid. Researcher should give credit to author of the material which is cited in the research report whether paraphrased, quoted, or referred to and discussed as it's usually copy righted when using quotations. Researches should check carefully for accuracy and indicate the source in a footnote or references at end of the chapter.

The original or first draft of the report is rarely the best, often unacceptable; more than one draft is required for the report to be in a polished form. It should be written in the third person, use terms with definiteness; if possible, in uncertain situation use terms such as probable, possible etc. It should be written in a manner to hold the interest of the reader. Writing the report requires skill and some amount for hold on the language to communicate the findings in an interesting way. It's believed that the researcher should have good journalism skill to document the findings of the research.

When writing report researcher should ensure:-

- **Conciseness**: The research report is concise and brief, yet thorough, it should save readers time as it avoid unwanted explanation or irrelevant content.
- **Clarity**: is lucidity of expression, the thought or meaning is easily understood.
- **Honesty**: is free from fraud. There is clear difference indicated between opinion and facts. Do not change the hypothesis but state it whether it is accepted or rejected.
- **Accuracy**: a quality of being precise and error free data should be exact, avoid broad generalization. Do not add pilot study findings in the main study to increase the sample size, it's neither fair nor accurate.
- **Completeness**: Researcher must report all the important details of the study, including all the information. To enlighten the reader only when the study is completely written it can be criticised.

The written report may use combination of phrases, visual presentation such as Tables, charts, graphs or flow charts so as to use visual aids to assist classify, meaning of information as well as improve the appearance and readability of the report. The basic objective in using this is to arrange statistical material in a manner to provide order, classification so that its meaning and significance is easily and quickly understood. Any visual, illustration other than Table is designated as figure. It includes graphs, maps, blue print of questions or the instrument, charts, photograph and diagrams. They are either numbered consequently in each section or throughout the report.

Outline for a Nursing Research Report

A. ***Preliminary Pages:***

Title Page: - It is the very first page of the thesis or research report indicating the topic of the research, the name of researcher, institution where research is conducted, if it's done as a part of academic requirement the course or degree being pursued and date of submission, name of the guide or supervisor and would also include institutional logo. Since it goes for evaluation the cover page may have only the topic, other details are included only after assessment is completed. Institutions would normally give the research scholar a guideline for the cover page.

i. **Abstract**: Is a short summary of the research work usually covering three pages which could be also concised approximately in 150 to 300 words.It is written once all the chapters are completed. It should include the main title of the study, objectives of the research, briefly highlight the methodology used, the key findings and end by drawing conclusions. Since the abstract short and briefly highlights the work done by the researcher. It is the first thing the individuals read hence it's important to get it right. Mentors or guides can help you in writing a strong and impressive abstract as one need to get the right impression to the readers..

ii. **Acknowledgment:** This section provides the researcher with the opportunity to thank all who have contributed and supported the research activity. It may include the guide, participants of the study, funding agency, if study was funded. The institution which provided the permission for conducting the study, researcher may also acknowledge the support of their family and all who have contributed directly or indirectly towards successful completion of the research project.

iii. **Table of content**: It includes list of all the chapters, subheadings with their page number, this allows the reader to navigate through the pages. It also provides with an overview of the structure of presentation and its flow, all key aspects should be included in the Table of content.

iv. **List of Table and Figs**: It includes numbered and titled diagram, pictures, and tabulated content as it appears the body of the research paper. A list of Table is separately included which is itemized and numbered.

B. Main body-

Chapter 1: *Introduction*: - It includes a brief introduction to the study area, purpose/need of the study, research question and objectives should be clearly stated, so that the readers get a gist of the study. The introduction provides a background and the context in which the study is carried out. It lays stress on the relevance of the research being conducted and scope of the study. The presentation in the introduction should be clear and hold the attention of the reader. The reader should get a clear picture as to what the study is about, why the researcher is interested in carrying out this study and how the study will proceed. It should focus on the importance of conducting this study and justify.

Chapter 2: *Review of literature:* It should reflect the literature review conducted before commencing the study done to develop insight in to the study area, also to become aware of the amount of work already done. Indicating the most relevant and recent researches reviewed from journals. Drawing connection to the present study and identifying gaps, and presenting a summarized version of the existing research studies. Researcher can develop an argument which would lead to provide a foundation to the present study. Would also focus on the theoretical methodology used to approach the topic? It also builds on the strength of the existing literature to find a path for solving unsolved problems or propose solution to the identified problem. It also helps to develop the theoretical frame work on which to base the study.

Chapter 3: *Research Methodology*: - This chapter describes how the researcher intends to proceed with the study. Provides the audience to understand the research approach utilized i.e. if it's qualitative, quantitative, Action research, experimental or ethnographic. The data gathering process and plan, what type of instrument was/would be used, interview schedule, questionnaire...e.tc. Also would specify the variable being examined/ manipulated to see its effect. It would allow the readers to draw their own validation. The chapter also indicates the plan for analysing the data gathered. The main focus of this chapter is to accurately report what was done by the researcher, at the same time letting the readers know this was the best method or approach to study the research topic or question.

Chapter 4: *Analysis and Interpretation*:-In this chapter the analysis is presented according to the objectives of the research and hypothesis to be tested. The content is organized in to sections and subsections. The content is woven with Tables and graphs too clearly and in a simple way to communicate the finding to the readers. In some research reports discussion is interwoven with interpretation while in some it's presented as independent chapter especially in doctoral studies. Qualitative research being largely analysed and describes the finding in words; is interwoven with discussions to add richness to the analysis. In qualitative data analysis it's better to present the interpretation and discussion separately to add more meaning and clarity to the findings. In the quantitative studies data is analysed using descriptive and inferential statistics and presented in Tables followed by its interpretation. The analysis should indicate whether the question in the objective is answered or not; whether the hypothesis is accepted or rejected/supports or not supported. The analysis should be clearly supported with Tables and figure/graphs to simplify the findings and help reads understand at a glance. Figures and illustrations should have numbering and caption below. Graphs provide a pictorial representation of a form of numerical data, a variety of representation can be used like line, bar, pie graphs and histograms. All the analysis which answer the research question should be presented even when finding are far from expectation. Additional calculations or Tables which are not essential to be included in the main body of the chapter may be included in the appendix. When documenting the findings it should be free of bias, speculation or manipulation of data to look impressive.

When writing the discussion emphasis should be laid as to why such finding was arrived at; what is the impact, is there any similarity in the findings with other previously conducted studies. What is the meaning of the findings, what is it trying to indicate, whether the intervention as in experimental study brought a change in the dependent variable and to what extent, was it a true difference or just by chance. How well does it fit in to the conceptual framework of the study included in the previous chapter. The researcher should indicate or state why the findings matter. If for some reasons the findings are deviant to the expectation, justification or rationalization should be given as to what might attribute to, should indicate to what extent the findings support the existing knowledge.

It should conclude with synopting the findings.

Chapter 5:-*Summary, Discussion, Implication & Recommendations*: This chapter mainly contains the key findings of the research study, it focuses on the central idea and emphasise on what the research contributes there by providing the reader a clear picture or understanding what has been done. Some researchers based on the frame work given for documentation of the research report would conclude and then discuss. This is the final chapter tying up or wrapping up the research report with highlight of the findings. The conclusion includes implication of the study which indicates how the findings can be beneficial or, how the findings matter to the researcher or readers who may be clinical nurses, student nurses, administrator or educators. The researcher also declares the limitation of the study as to what could not be done or was not foreseen barriers either in the data collection or methodology. This chapter also includes recommendation for future researches or use in clinical practice. This chapter leaves a clear impression for readers as to what is done and room for further investigation. The chapter also indicates what was known and what the new addition are being made.

C. Supplementary Pages:

- ***References and bibliography***: indicated the source cited in the study, and follows consistent pattern or style. Depending on which style is used it should be followed by the requirement. There is always confusion about the meaning of bibliography and references. A bibliography is a list of the sources used in the research report whereas a list of references sometimes includes other appropriate literature. References are usually citations of work that were referred but may or may not be quoted in the study.

  The common styles followed are APA and Vancouver, but each institution will state which style is to be followed. The reference or the bibliography should be developed side by side to ensure none are missed out, correctly format all citations. Bibliography which comes at the end is always arranged in alphabetical order while references are noted at the end of every chapter in the order of being quoted or cited in the body of the chapter. Librarian usually suggests use of citation generator.

- **Appendix** is placed at the end of the research report. It would include instrument in English, Translated Version, relevant Information and Statistical calculation which is not included in the body of the report, permission letters, Audio visual aids used like flash card or power point print outs, List of experts with their consent letter who validated the instrument for data collection and consent of participants of the study.

Types of Research Reports

i. **Dissertations:** Sometimes also referred to as thesis, dissertation is a research project submitted as a part of partial fulfilment to earn a postgraduate or doctoral degree, it is sometimes part of undergraduate assignment. The term dissertation is referred to research project submitted by masters student while thesis is referred to submission research report by doctoral student, the term may be used interchangeably by different universities. Whether it's thesis or dissertation they mark the end of research activity carried out as a part of requirement of the respective academic work. It provides opportunity for student to present their findings to the research question or problem they have chosen. It is carried out to test the research skills of the students; they would carry out the project independently under the guidance of their mentor or faculty.

   The document is presented in a formal way based on the pattern given by the respective institution. All dissertations are not written in the same pattern; it depends on the form your research takes and on the research design. The content or piece of work is original mean to add to or extend the body of professional knowledge. Dissertation is evaluated by experts if it meets the requirements the scholar is awarded the degree, if not is given opportunity to do the required correction and resubmit.

   The findings of the research carried out for the purpose of submitting for degree can also be published. The pilot study if carried out on a large sample may also be published independently. Dissertations carried out by students can be published following the rules/criteria given by the journal.

ii. **Monograph** is a specialized scholarly long article or a short book on a single topic written by a single author. e.g. Physiotherapy in patients recovering from Guillain-Barré syndrome. It is a book generated based on research project which can be used to educate on the current status or issue to update knowledge Monograms are mostly used in text based research like qualitative studies like ethnographic or grounded theory. Monogram is written in the same way as a research report which includes the topic methodology review of literature, findings and conclusion except there is more verbatim, quotes respondents, where required to make an impact. Monograms are important to disseminate scholarly work and stimulate debate.

iii. **Scientific paper:** It's a written original report of the research conducted, submitted for publication or available to the professional community after it has been reviewed by a peer team. It is often the first publication, provides opportunity to other researchers to replicate or draw their own inferences by retesting in a new setting and helps justify the findings. Large amount of the researchers available in peer reviewed journal are funded by government or non-governmental agency. These papers may be published in phases as it is completed so that findings can be implemented. It also includes publication of researchers conducted by scholars that is masters or doctoral projects. Scientific research paper may also be an action research carried out by the nurse practitioner who may be nurse educator, clinical nurse or nursing administer to find solutions to the problem at hand and to communicate their findings to other so that they implement or give their critical view.

iv. **New paper and magazine articles:** Research paper which originate in response to community/public/societal issues need to be disseminated as the primary beneficiaries is the members of society. e.g. "studies related to home management of osteoporosis". Or "causes of respiratory problem among individuals residing near factories emitting fumes" The dissemination of such researches would create awareness and help individuals to take required preventive measures. It should be disseminated in simple language which will be understood by the people without technical jargon. Publishing the findings in newspaper or as article in magazine ensures wide dissemination of the findings to stake holders. If also helps to have an impact on government agencies and policy makers. The most important is that it should be titled to hold attention of readers and published at the earliest after completing the project else it would become old news or similar content may be published by another researcher.

v. **Publication in Professional journals:** Research reports published in professional or subject specific journals which would be peer reviewed would require that the paper be original and brings forth a novel concept. The research paper has to provide details so that other researcher can replicate or stimulate further research. They have set of guidelines that require the author to follow. Mostly the papers published are by Ph.D. scholars or eminent professionals in their respective fields or by post graduate student who have worked under research guides. This would require appropriate acknowledgment of contributors. The paper is send to a panel of experts on the journal's board who would review for accuracy of the research methodology and documentation of report, before it's published if not up to the expected mark it's rejected or recommended to be reworked on for publication. Researcher should remember submission of the paper to the journal does not suggest their acceptance.

How to disseminate the findings of research: The research report needs to be developed and disseminated through presentation to audience of interest group it could be written report: published in journals, publication, Oral report can be presented in conferences.

Guideline for making oral presentation: be clear, simple and logical in presentation; focus on disseminating scientific facts, avoid unwanted floweriness. It is opportunity to show case the research work.

a) Talk to the audience, but before you start should be aware of the composition of the audience so you give what they want to hear and do not waste time of audience on irrelevant points.

b) Be concise and brief in your presentation. Provoke them to get a discussion rolling.

c) Treat the dais as a stage to make the presentation interesting, use anecdotes to catch and hold attention of audience but avoid overdoing as it could distract and take home message would be lost. d) Maintain a logical flow in the presentation with appropriate introduction the main content or body and conclude with a key message.

e) Practice and time your presentation so it will help a smooth flow. Support the presentation with visuals and avoid overcrowding of slides.

f) Do not forget to acknowledge the organizers for the opportunity to disseminate your findings before starting and those who have contributed to the presentation material.

Posters presentation are brief at a glance or snap shot yet they provide all the details of the research project and require very little time to explain. The poster should contain research title, objectives, abstract and methodology, findings presented as graphs or key Tables and conclusion in a line. Poster presentations do not carry much value but are used by institutions to give every novice researcher an opportunity to present their work.

Points for poster presentation: Remember it's an opportunity to sell your work to the viewers in ten seconds. It should be visually attractive and not crowded yet covering the content. Plan the lay out of the poster as many may view it from a distance. The poster should have a unique touch of your personality if it's not going to be evaluated can have a picture of the researcher so that those interested can find and interact to get more detail.

How to write references/bibliography/citations

There are basically two styles very commonly followed:

1. Vancouver,
2. APA style.

1. **Vancouver style**:

   A **reference** list includes the information of the material cited by the research scholar in their text, which may include material picked from books, journal, articles, pamphlets etc. The reference list appears at the end of the content of the report/article or chapter the reference entries should appear in the order that they have been cited in the text. Proper citing of source helps readers to go back to the source. References should be formatted and appear on a fresh page. Whereas **Bibliography** is different from reference as it's arranged in alphabetical order, it includes all material the researcher may have reviewed to build the study but may not have quoted in the text of the research document.

   Whether it's reference or bibliography have their own way of citing and spacing which may be 1.5 or double but best to follow instruction of the institution or publishing house. Examples of different sources are shown below.

   Book: For books a standard format is followed where one indicates; Author (s) of book. Title of book. Edition. Place of publication: Publisher; Year of publication. Chapter number: Chapter title; inclusive pagination. If author has written in edited book the format changes as shown in the example no. 3. Put comma between two authors and full stop after last author. If there is no author then title of the book will appear first as shown below:

   1. Murray PR, Rosenthal KS, Kobyashi GS, P Faller MA. Medical microbiology. 4th ed. St Louis: Mosby; 2002.
   2. Dillon PA. Nursing health assessment; a critical thinking, care studies approach. Philadelphia: Davis, 2003. Chapter 3: Approach to the physical assessment; p. 49-77.

3. MacDougall C, Chambers HF. Aminoglycosides. In: Brunton LL, Chabner BA, Knollman BJ, eds. Goodman & Gilman's the pharmacological basis of therapeutics. 12th ed. New York: McGraw-Hill; 2011. p. 1505-20. (edited book, authors name followed by editors)
4. Gilstrap LC, Cunningham FG, Van Dorsten JP, editors. Operative obstetrics. 2nd ed. New York: McGraw-Hill; 2002. (no authors but there are only editors)

On line E book:

1. Lee HC, Pagliaro EM. Serology: blood identification. In: Siegel J, Knupfer G, Saukko P, editors. Encyclopedia of forensic sciences [e-book]. San Diego: Academic Press; 2000 [cited 2005 Jun 30]:1331-8. Available from: https://www-sciencedirectcom. libproxy. murdoch. edu.au/science/article/pii/B0122272153004212.
2. Watson J. Nursing; the philosophy and science of caring [book on the Internet]. City: Publisher; Year. Chapter X: Caritas processes; extension of carative factors [cited 2013 July 28]; p.39-44. Available from: EBSCOhost eBook Collection.
3. *Benowitz NL. Antihypertensive agents. In.* Trevor AJ, Masters SB, Katzung BG. Basic & clinical pharmacology [book on the Internet]. 11th ed. New York: McGraw Hill Lange; 2009 [cited 2013 June 26]; p.167-89. Available from: EBSCOhost eBook Collection http://web.ebscohost.com/.

Journal: For journal articles a standard format is followed i.e. Author of article AA, Author of article BB, Author of article CC. Title of article. Abbreviated Title of Journal. Year; vol (issue): page number (s). For journal articles from e source it should be indicated i.e. e-journal, capitalization of the first letter and proper noun is done. Indicate the range of pg. nos. as 112-118 if a single pg. is referred only one pg. no. should be indicated like "Pg. no.456".

1. 21st century heart solution may have a sting in the tail. BMJ. 2002; 325 (7537):184. **(no author)**
2. Halpern SD, Ubel PA, Caplan AL. Solid-organ transplantation in HIV-infected patients. N Engl J Med. 2002; 347 (7):284-7. **(With more than one author)**
3. Gillespie NC, Lewis RJ, Pearn JH, Bourke ATC, Holmes MJ, Bourke JB, et al. Ciguatera in Australia: occurrence, clinical features, pathophysiology and management. Med J Aust. 1986; 145: 584-90. **(With more than six authors it should be followed with et al. {e.g. Smith AB, Jones CD, McDonald EF, et al}.)**

4. Diabetes Prevention Program Research Group. Hypertension, insulin, and proinsulin in participants with impaired glucose tolerance. Hypertension. 2002; 40 (5):679-86. **(Institution as author.)**
5. Banit DM, Kaufer H, Hartford JM. Intraoperative frozen section analysis in revision total joint arthroplasty. Clin Orthop. 2002; (401):230-8. **(with no volume)**
6. Abend SM, Kulish N. The psychoanalytic method from an epistemological viewpoint. Int J Psychoanal. 2002;83 (Pt 2):491-5. **(volume with part)**

Internet source:

1. Diabetes Australia. Gestational diabetes [Internet]. Canberra (ACT): Diabetes Australia; 2015 [updated 2015; cited 2017 Nov 23]. Available from: https://www.diabetesaustralia. com.au/gestational-diabetes

Conference proceedings: the standard format is "Editor (s), ed (s). Title of conference: subtitle of conference; Year, Month, Date of Conference; Location of Conference. Place of publication: Publisher; Year of Publication."

1. Luca J, Tarricone P. Does emotional intelligence affect successful teamwork? In: Kennedy G, Keppell M, McNaught C, et al, eds. Meeting at the Cossroads: Proceedings of the 18th Annual Conference of the Australasian Society for Computers in Learning in Tertiary Education, 2001 Dec 9-12; Melbourne: Biomedical Multimedia Unit, The University of Melbourne; 2001. P.367-76.
2. Muller S, ed. Proceedings of the 10th International Conference on Head Driven Phrase Structure Grammar; 2003 Jul 18-20; East Lansing (MI) [conference proceedings on the Internet]. Stanford (CA): CSLI Publications; 2003. [cited 2013 Jun 26]. Available from: URL: **http://csli-publications.stanford.edu/HPSG/4** . (if the conference proceedings was published on line.)

Newspaper articles: When citing articles cited from newspaper, it's similar to those cited from journals, they too follow a standard pattern, "Author. Title of article. Title of Newspaper (Edition). Year, Month, Day: Sect.: page (col.) ". and for online paper article its "Author. Title of article. Title of Newspaper (Edition) [newspaper on the Internet]. Year, Month, Day [date cited Year, Mon, Day]:Sect.:page. Available from:" as indicated in the example given below.

1. Harris G. FDA orders recall of intravenous pumps. New York Times (Washington Final). 2005 Jun 22; Sect. A:12 (col. 1).
2. Grady D. Jump in doctor visits and deaths in flu season. New York

Times [newspaper on the Internet]. 2008 Apr 18 [cited 2008 Dec 19]; Research:[about 4 screens]. Available from: **http://www.nytimes.com/2008/04/18/health/research/18flu.html?scp=7&sq=flu%20season&st=cse**

Points to remember: Remember to list all authors in the order they appear in the original document. In citation within the text the reference should be written in bracketed number (4) which can be superscript or subscripted though superscript is more often used, e.g. **Lalitha.**[(4)] Placement of citation numbers should be carefully done and number should be placed outside the full stop. If number of text are quoted from different references a commas should be placed between the numbers **e.g.2, 8.** If the text quoted is supported by number of references which appear continuously then **e.g.4, 5, 7, 9 or 4-9** if all reference support. If there is a difference between edited and edition, **edition** is denoted by ed. (i.e. 4th ed.); while **editors** is written after the names of individuals who have edited the book. Clearly indicate place of publication if multiple place of publication write the first, **e.g.: Texas (USA)/Palm Springs (CA) or publishers as e.g.: Williams & Wilkins.** Have the year of publication followed by page no. denoted as, '**p**'. e.g.: **2020, p122-127.** If cited from different pages then it should as follows 122, 124,126-127.In journals there is volume no. and issue no. to be included,which is written as follows volume is 3 and issue is 1, which is indicated as **2020;3 (1):122-127**. If the journal has a month and date then it will be

Mar 2020;3 (1):122-127.or **2020 Mar.5, 3 (1):122-127**. If the site visited has a URL it should be written as it is on the website, it may have a 'doi' number.

2. **APA style:**

The standard formatting of a book requires author's name, title of the book, publisher's name, and date of publication. If it does not have author but it is edited then name of editors will replace the author in its place. See example of Book for referencing.

Book referencing

- Author, A. A., & Author, B. B. (year). Book title. Location: Publisher.
- Author, A. A., & Author, B. B. (year). Book title. Retrieved from http://www.xxxxxx.
- Author, A. A., & Author, B. B. (year). Book title....
- Editor, A. A., & Editor B. B. (Eds.). (year).
- Editor, A. A. (Ed.). (year)....

1. LaRue, F. (2007). *My fabulous life: Parisian flings and other things*. LaPlume.

2. Dactyl, T. A. & Saurus, B.T. (2011). *The jury's still out on Jurassic Park.* Altamira Press. (Two author's)
3. Anklet, T. M. (Ed.). (2001). *Big bruisers.* Strange Brew Press. (no author only editor)
4. Snodgrass, F. (2007). [Review of the book *My fabulous life: Parisian flings and other things*, by F. LaRue]. *Parisian Personnae, 37* (2), 132. (**Book which is a review..)**

Book: Print

Author/Editor (if it is an editor always put (ed.)..., Title (this should be in italics)

Series title and number (if part of a series), Edition (if not the first edition)

Place of publication (if there is more than one place listed, use the first named), Publisher.

Year of publication

Example: Anklet, T. M. (Ed.). (2001). *Big bruisers.* Strange Brew Press. (**no author only editor**)

Online book:

1. Freud, S. (1953). The method of interpreting dreams: An analysis of a specimen dream. In J. Strachey (Ed. & Trans.), *The standard edition of the complete psychological works of Sigmund Freud* (Vol. 4, pp. 96-121). Retrieved from http://books.google.com/books (Original work published 1900)
2. Thomas, N. (Ed.) (2002). *Perspective on the community college: A journey of discovery* [Monograph]. Retrieved from http://eric.ed.gov/
3. American Psychological Association. (2010). *Publication manual of the American Psychological Association* (6th ed.). Washington, DC: Author. **(Book with corporate author)**
4. U.S. Department of Health and Human Services, National Institutes of Health, National Heart, Lung, and Blood Institute. (2003). *Managing asthma: A guide for schools* (NIH Publication No. 02-2650). Retrieved from http://www.nhlbi.nih.gov/health/prof/lung/asthma/asth_sch.pdf (Govt. report on line)

Journal: Basic order for referencing a journal article

Author or authors.....Year of publication of the article (in round brackets). Article title.

Journal title (in italics). Volume of journal (in italics). Issue of journal (no italics). Page range of article.

1. Beal, M. F. (2003). Mitochondria, oxidative damage, and inflammation in Parkinson's disease. Academic Science 991. 120-13 . *Health Informatics Journal, 13* (2), 155-6.
2. Chase, M. H. (1999, September 24). Too often the elderly don't get the drugs or care they need. *Wall Street Journal*. 31. (**includes month and date of publication**)
3. Jakupcak, M., Luterek, J., Hunt, S., Conybeare, D., & McFall, M. (2008). Post-traumatic stress and its relationship to physical health functioning in a sample of Iraq and Afghanistan war veterans seeking post-deployment VA health care. *Journal of Nervous and Mental Disease, 196,* 425-428. **(includes more than one author)**

Internet source:

a. Cybernaught, C.B. (1995, April). Hyper over hypertext. *World Wide Wanderer, 39* (4). http://www.ccu.edu/wwwander/
b. Cremedelacreme, C. (2008). An examination of gastronomic imagery in the later poetry of Fifi LaRue. *Poetry Parisienne, 13* (2), 23-43. https://doi.org/29.1027/00013-2893.13.2.23 **(with doi listing)**
c. Buttons, R. (2006). Send in the clowns: Political misadventures of 21st century America. *Political Profundity, 3* (2), 47-62. http://www.polprof.com/**(on line full text data base with URL)**

Conference proceedings

1. Family name, INITIAL (S) (of the presenter). Year. Title of the presentation. Title of **conference**, date of **conference**, location of **conference**.
2. Title of **Conference** [**Internet**]; Date of **conference**; Location of **conference**. Place of publication: Publisher's name; Date of publication [**cited** YYYY, Mon, DD]; p. page numbers. Available from: URL or Database Name. **(on line conference citing in the reference or bibliography)**

Newspaper articles: Author or authors. The surname is followed by first initials. Year and publication date. **Article** title. **Newspaper** title (in italics). Page number (if available). URL.

The first line of each **citation** is left adjusted. Every subsequent line is indented 5-7 spaces.

Conclusion

Disseminating the findings of the research is the ultimate outcome of research process. The research task is not completed until the report has been written. Dissemination of research finding serves to create awareness among the scientific, professional and public body.A timely documented and disseminated finding of research study through presentation-orally, in journal, as an article. This has importance in nursing practice and adds to the body of nursing knowledge, updates nurses thereby contributes to provide evidence based nursing practice.

WRITING AN ABSTRACT FOR RESEARCH PAPER

An abstract is a short summary of the research paper, usually about a paragraph. (6-7 sentences, 150-250 words long.) For research thesis as a part of research project should not exceed 2 to 3 pgs maximum approximately 1000 words. (Published or unpublished)

Purpose of Abstracts

A well-written abstract serves multiple purposes:

- an abstract lets readers get the gist or essence of the research paper or article quickly, which allows to decide whether to read the full paper,
- an abstract prepares readers to follow the detailed information, analyses, and arguments in the full paper;
- and, later, an abstract helps readers remember key points from the research paper if they wish to implement.

It's also worth remembering that search engines and bibliographic databases use abstracts, as well as the title, to identify key terms for indexing the published paper. What is included in the abstract and in title of research paper is important for other researchers to locate the paper or article.

When writing an abstract for a course paper, the professor/institution would provide specific guidelines as to what needs to be included and how to organize the abstract. Various academic journals have specific pattern for submitting abstracts.

The Contents of an Abstract

Abstracts should contain the following information in brief. The body of the paper will develop and explain the idea more fully. The abstract should give adequate weightage to every information and should flow in a sequence but it all depends on the nature of the genre of the research paper that is being summarized; the information may be implied or stated explicitly presented.

Some of the reputed journals provide specific guidelines indicating what to include in the abstract for different kinds of papers like for empirical studies, literature reviews or meta-analyses, theoretical papers, methodological papers, and case studies.

Key aspects expected by most journals in their abstracts are:

1. The context or background information for the research; the general topic under study; the specific topic of research,
2. The central questions or statement of the problem the research addresses,
3. What is already known about the research question, what has previous research done or shown (brief highlight of literature review or gap in existing literature)
4. The main reason (s), the exigency, the rationale, the goals of the research—Why is it important to address these questions? Is a new topic being examined? Why is this topic worth examining? Is the present study filling a gap in previous research? Is a new method applied? Or fresh approach taken to look at existing ideas or data? Is it a solution to a dispute within the literature in the field?
5. Research methodology used.
6. Key findings, results, or discussion or arguments
7. Significance or implications of the findings for academic/administrative or clinical practice.

Abstract should be intelligent and provide insight on its own, without a reader has to read the entire paper. Abstract will describe what the researcher has studied in their research and what they have found and what is argued in the research paper. In the abstract there is no citing of references may be any literature that supports the study may be cited. The main focus is the present study findings and justification of conducting the study.

When to Write the Abstract

It is the last step of the research process once the full research document has been drafted; it provides the author with an idea of how to go about summarizing. Writing abstract for publishing in journal once the research has been accepted by the evaluating body.

Choosing verb Tenses within Abstract

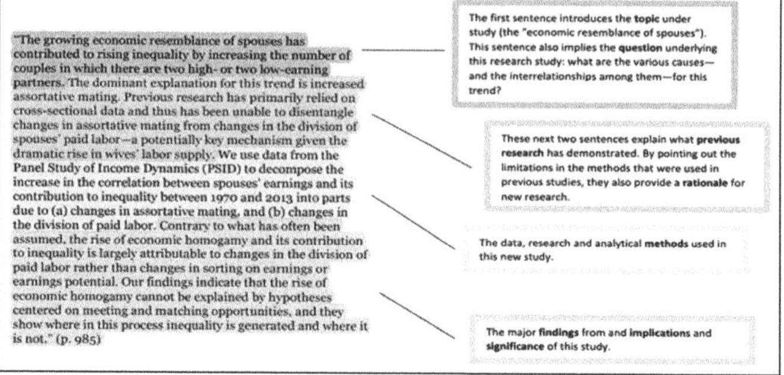

Example: in the **social science** paper quoted it can be noted present tense was used to describe general facts and interpretations that have been and are currently true, including the prevailing explanation for the social phenomenon under study indicating reason for increasing economic homogamy among spouse. That abstract also uses the present tense to describe the methods, the findings, the arguments, and the implications of the findings from the new research study. The authors use the past tense to describe previous research. (Gonalons-Pons, Pilar, and Christine R.Schwartz "Trends in economic Homogamy: changes in Assortative Mating or the Division of labour in Marriage? Demography,vol.no.3,2017,pp.985-1005)

"The growing economic resemblance of spouses has contributed to rising inequality by increasing the number of couples in which there are two high- or two low-earning partners. The dominant explanation for this trend is increased assortative mating. Previous research has primarily relied on cross-sectional data and thus has been unable to disentangle changes in assortative mating from changes in the division of spouses' paid labor—a potentially key mechanism given the dramatic rise in wives' labor supply. We use data from the Panel Study of Income Dynamics (PSID) to decompose the increase in the correlation between spouses' earnings and its contribution to inequality between 1970 and 2013 into parts due to (a) changes in assortative mating, and (b) changes in the division of paid labor. Contrary to what has often been assumed, the rise of economic homogamy and its contribution to inequality is largely attributable to changes in the division of paid labor rather than changes in sorting on earnings or earnings potential. Our findings indicate that the rise of economic homogamy cannot be explained by hypotheses centered on meeting and matching opportunities, and they show where in this process inequality is generated and where it is not." (p. 985)

The first sentence introduces the **topic** under study (the "economic resemblance of spouses"). This sentence also implies the **question** underlying this research study: what are the various causes—and the interrelationships among them—for this trend?

These next two sentences explain what **previous research** has demonstrated. By pointing out the limitations in the methods that were used in previous studies, they also provide a **rationale** for new research.

The data, research and analytical **methods** used in this new study.

The major **findings** from and **implications** and **significance** of this study.

In study related to **Humanities** past tense has been used in the example to describe completely the events in the past, uses the present tense to describe what is happening in the texts, to explain the significance or meaning of those texts, and to describe the arguments presented in the article. (Emily Callaci."Street Textuality: Socialism, Masculinity, and Urban Belonging in Tanzania's Pulp Fiction Publishing Industry,1975-1985." *Comparative studies in Society and History,* vol. 59,no.1,2017,pp.183-210)

"From the mid-1970s through the mid-1980s, a network of young urban migrant men created an underground pulp fiction publishing industry in the city of Dar es Salaam. As texts that were produced in the underground economy of a city whose trajectory was increasingly charted outside of formalized planning and investment, these novellas reveal more than their narrative content alone. These texts were active components in the urban social worlds of the young men who produced them. They reveal a mode of urbanism otherwise obscured by narratives of decolonization, in which urban belonging was constituted less by national citizenship than by the construction of social networks, economic connections, and the crafting of reputations. This article argues that pulp fiction novellas of socialist era Dar es Salaam are artifacts of emergent forms of male sociability and mobility. In printing fictional stories about urban life on pilfered paper and ink, and distributing their texts through informal channels, these writers not only described urban communities, reputations, and networks, but also actually created them." (p. 210)

The first sentence introduces the **context** for this research and announces the **topic** under study.

The remaining sentences in this abstract interweave other essential information for an abstract for this article. The implied **research questions**: What do these texts mean? What is their historical and cultural significance, produced at this time, in this location, by these authors? The **argument** and the **significance** of this analysis in microcosm: these texts "reveal a mode or urbanism otherwise obscured . . ."; and "This article argues that pulp fiction novellas. . . ." This section also implies what **previous historical research** has obscured. And through the details in its argumentative claims, this section of the abstract implies the kinds of **methods** the author has used to interpret the novellas and the concepts under study (e.g., male sociability and mobility, urban communities, reputations, network. . .).

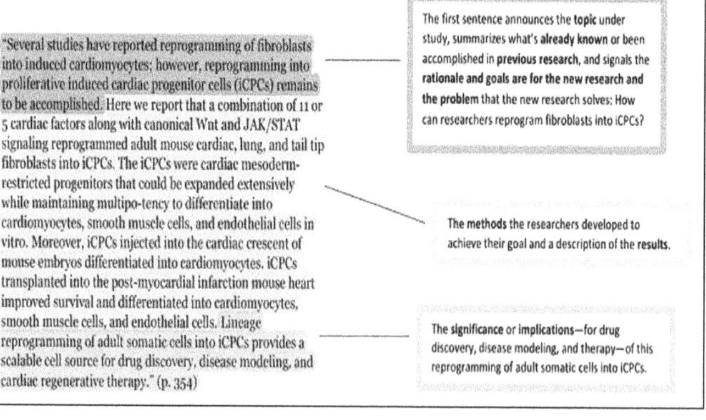

Science based studies use past tense to describe findings of previous research studies including the methodology,

"Several studies have reported reprogramming of fibroblasts into induced cardiomyocytes; however, reprogramming into proliferative induced cardiac progenitor cells (iCPCs) remains to be accomplished. Here we report that a combination of 11 or 5 cardiac factors along with canonical Wnt and JAK/STAT signaling reprogrammed adult mouse cardiac, lung, and tail tip fibroblasts into iCPCs. The iCPCs were cardiac mesoderm-restricted progenitors that could be expanded extensively while maintaining multipo-tency to differentiate into cardiomyocytes, smooth muscle cells, and endothelial cells in vitro. Moreover, iCPCs injected into the cardiac crescent of mouse embryos differentiated into cardiomyocytes. iCPCs transplanted into the post-myocardial infarction mouse heart improved survival and differentiated into cardiomyocytes, smooth muscle cells, and endothelial cells. Lineage reprogramming of adult somatic cells into iCPCs provides a scalable cell source for drug discovery, disease modeling, and cardiac regenerative therapy." (p. 354)

The first sentence announces the **topic** under study, summarizes what's **already known** or been accomplished in **previous research**, and signals the **rationale and goals are for the new research and the problem** that the new research solves: How can researchers reprogram fibroblasts into iCPCs?

The **methods** the researchers developed to achieve their goal and a description of the **results.**

The **significance** or **implications**—for drug discovery, disease modeling, and therapy—of this reprogramming of adult somatic cells into iCPCs.

rationale for the study or justification for the study. They also indicate the gap i.e. what remains to be studied.... This is written in present tense. The study which is being published is introduced using present tense i.e. here its reported..., though most journals prefer past tense as study is completed and then information is being disseminated. The author is also expected to indicate the significance of the study.

(Lait, Pratil. A, Max R. Salick, Daryl O. Nelson,Jayne M. Squirrell, Christina M Shafer, Neel G.Patel, Imaan Seed, et al. " Lineage Reprogramming of Fibroblasts into Proliferative Induced Cardiac Progenitor cells by Defined Factors." Cell Stem Cell, Vol.18, 2016, pp. 354-367.)

The next example is from pediatric journal.... "effectiveness of antibiotic therapy in managing acute bacterial sinusitis, from a rigorously controlled study." Authors are required to present the abstract fewer than four sections yet maintaining the word limit so that it's self-explanatory.

Objective: the role of antibiotic therapy in managing acute bacterial sinusitis (ABS) in children is controversial. The purpose of this study was to determine the effectiveness of high dose amoxicillin/potassium clavulanate in the treatment of children diagnosed with ABS.

Methods: This was a randomized, double–blind, placebo-controlled study. Children 1 to 10 years of age with a clinical presentation compatible with ABS were eligible for participation. Patients were stratified according to age (<6 or ≥6 years) and clinical severity and randomly assigned to receive either amoxicillin (90 mg/kg) with potassium clavulanate (6.4 mg/kg) or placebo. A symptom survey was performed on days 0, 1, 2, 3, 5, 7, 10, 20, and 30. Patients were examined on day 14. Children's conditions were rated as cured, improved, or failed according to scoring rules.

Results: Two thousand one hundred thirty-five children with respiratory complaints were screened for enrolment; 139 (6.5%) had ABS. Fifty-eight patients were enrolled, and 56 were randomly assigned. The mean age was 6630 months. Fifty (89%) patients presented with persistent symptoms, and 6 (11%) presented with non-persistent symptoms. In 24 (43%) children, the illness was classified as mild, whereas in the remaining 32 (57%) children it was severe. Of the 28 children who received the antibiotic, 14 (50%) were cured, 4 (14%) were improved, 4 (14%) experienced treatment failure, and 6 (21%) withdrew. Of the 28 children who received placebo, 4 (14%) were cured, 5 (18%) improved, and

19 (68%) experienced treatment failure. Children receiving the antibiotic were more likely to be cured (50% vs 14%) and less likely to have treatment failure (14% vs 68%) than children receiving the placebo

RESEARCH UTILIZATION

Research utilization process was developed to address the problem of using the research findings in nursing practice. It is a process by which the generated data is assimilated and disseminated to assess for its impact or improve the quality of nursing practice making it evidence based.

Utilization of Nursing Research: It requires nurses to incorporate the research findings in to daily clinical practice. In recent days in nursing the need for research based practice is widely accepted but unfortunately many existing nursing interventions are based on traditional practice rather than science. Today's the consumers are conscious of time and cost and quality of health care, nurses cannot afford to spend time on unnecessary or ineffective procedure/ interventions. Nurses are hard pressed with time managing complicated and demanding patients, they strived to reduce the hospital stay, as many can get benefit of health care. There is a need for nurses not merely to work hard but to work smartly which is possible if they utilize the research finding and stay a step ahead by regular reading of scientific material.

Hindrances in Utilization research findings: Nurses lack time to actively participate in conducting and implementing research. Do not understand the importance of research. It is a minute and difficult component of UG program. Our health care scenario pays little attention to research. Staff nurses may not read nursing research journals. Research reports are presented to researcher at conference but for many bedside nurses the reports do not reach them who can practically use these new ideas.

Strategies in Facilitate Utilization of Nursing Research: When clinical problems or issues are identified; nurses should be encouraged to be utilized research findings. Clinical nurse or nurses working at the bed side may not have adequate time to visit the library to reach for appropriate research findings to implement, to overcome this barrier nurse educators form the clinical side, can work in collaboration with nursing faculty administrators to make clinical practice evidence based, also regularly they can update nurse through in-service of the latest research findings.

Nurse educators or faculty from the academic area may integrate the research findings in their lectures. They may also motivate students to incorporate research findings in their assignment or presentations. Nurse educators may motivate student nurses to carry out small researches projects in groups.

Clinical nurse practitioner: requires stay updated with research findings and conduct literature review. Has commitment to continuously increase knowledge and involve in continuing education programs, pursue higher education. Participate in clinical research or action research carried out in the nursing department to improve practices or solve issues related to patient care. If the hospital has a research department she can work collaboratively with them to focus on issues and in disseminating the findings to nurses at the bedside and in revising the care protocols.

Nurse researcher: delineate the implications for nursing practice. They focus on the research activity which exists in the clinical area and try to disseminate the findings at the earliest. Dissemination may be done at the local, national or internationally through publication in journal. They would also try to disseminate through oral presentation so that nurse can implement the findings.

Nursing Administrators: focus on creating a research based practice, and support continued nursing education. Some of the nurse administrators would include research as a part of the nurse's job so that there would be ongoing research climate. The administrators can all stimulate debates to critically evaluate clinical practice so that routine and meaningless traditional practices can be replaced with innovative research based practice. The administrators can support researches and reward those attempting to conduct research to improve clinical practice.

CRITIQUING RESEARCH

Critique is an essential process in the development of body of knowledge though it's poorly understood process related to research. The word "Critique" often linked with the word "Criticize" which has a negative connotation and is considered un-therapeutic in nursing and leads to feeling of inadequacy and rejected. To criticize another is thought to be unkind, mean and self-centered and is often interpreted as a personal attack. In 'Art' and 'Science', however, criticism takes on another meaning.

Critique is associated with critical thinking and appraisal requiring intellectual skill. Hence referred to as intellectual Critique, it is directed not at the person who created but the product of creation.

'Intellectual Critique' of research involves a systematic, unbiased, careful examination of all aspects of a study to judging the merits, limitations, meaning & significance in light of previous research experience and knowledge of the topic. It is essential for the development and refinement of nursing knowledge base and the use of research evidence in practice.

This judgment is made in light of experience with previous objects conducting a critique requires both a thorough background in critical analysis and skill in logical reasoning process.

Research critique is a planned activity to evaluate the research paper for its strength and weakness against set criteria, and provides constructive comments about the research.

In nursing Critique is often seen as the first step in learning the research process. It focuses on improvement of practice, broaden understanding and provide a base for conducting future studies. The notion that the research study was 'poor' if the hypothesis was not accepted is wrong. All research has value and any subjective statement of worth must be regarded even if a hypothesis is rejected, something is learned from that data. That is why it's important to learn what is 'not true' as much as to learn what is 'true'.

Who Does Critiquing and How Does it Benefit

In nursing critiquing may be done by nursing students, practicing nurses, nurse educators, and nurse researchers. If a research paper is submitted for competition it's then done by a panel of research experts. For '**students**' it's a learning step in research process and helps strengthen their knowledge base and increase their use of research findings in practise. Skill involved in critiquing is increased as their knowledge of 'Research' expands. For' **practicing or clinical nurses**' it is essentially for implementation of evidence based nursing care. They need to question the quality of the studies, credibility of the findings and share their concerns with others nurse's like in journal club or during nursing discussions. They can synthesize the most significant finds and implement in nursing practice.

'**Nurse Educators**' would do critiquing to expand their knowledge and incorporate in their teaching the evidences. Educators can revise or make changes in the curriculum both in theory and practice/clinical area. They can encourage students to integrate research findings in their case study presentation. They can be role model to students by participating in research critiquing. While critiquing helps '**Nurse Researchers**' to update their knowledge, plan and implement studies. They themselves can influence the selection of a new research problem and develop methodology and draw interpretation of the findings as in met analysis. Critiquing can be done while conducting review of literature.

When is Research Critiquing Done?

Critiques are often conducted after verbal/oral presentations of the studies, after published research report, for abstract or article selection and for evaluating research proposal.

Purpose: Identify strength and weakness of the study. To provide suggestions related to the research methodology if any mistakes are noted in the work of novice researcher, to judge the merit of student research and their understanding of research. To decide based on the evaluation if the work is worth publishing in journal.

Nurses need skills to examine the meaning of study findings. To ask following questions: are the findings accurate reflection of reality, are they providing clarity of the phenomena being studied, are the findings consistent with previous studies. Can the findings be implemented by the clinical nurses and is it worth replicating this study in another setting.

What Should be Focused on When Critiquing a Research Report?

Critique of research report includes comments on the information provided as well about omissions that should not have been made. It could include most of the topic covered in the document. The drawback, if it was too lengthy. The length of critique is limited by its purpose and the amount of time available for the task.

Critiquing follows different guidelines for quantitative and qualitative researches, the critique requires special skills to question and examine all aspects of research document beginning from the research problem, purpose of the study, concept, review of literature, hypothesis, and assumption, design of the study, methodology, analysis of the data, conclusions, implications, recommendations for further study, bibliography and other references used. Need to also evaluate the language/writing style, grammar and the abstract as it reflects good journalism skill. Need to critically look at the reasoning both logical and rational, how the study was planned and implementation. Need to identify the flaws in the study if present they may skew the findings and affect the interpretation. The studies may have a flaw that does not mean study should be discarded. If studies are discarded there would be lacunae/dirt of scientific knowledge on which to base nursing practice. One needs to remember science itself is flawed as no single study studies all aspects of a situation or topic, there would be some dimension or the other that would be missed and complete control of variables is not possible in experimental studies also to do a perfect prediction.

Points to be kept in mind before critiquing: The document should be read carefully and understand before carrying on the appraisal. When writing the critical assessment report should avoid vague comments, maintain balance of both strength and weakness. Be focused on objective and be sensitive when framing comments especially negative ones should be supported with an example for clarity to the researcher.

Chapter wise review: The reviewer or critique should look at the 'Problem' was it clearly stated, is differentiated between specific i.e. local or personal problem General i.e. national or universal problem.

Guidelines for conducting Quantitative & Qualitative Research Critiques.

Quantitative research:

1. Read & Critique the entire Study:- If research critique requires identification & examination of all steps of the research process. (Comprehension)
2. Examine the research, clinical & Educational background of the authors: - authors need a clinical & scientific background that is appropriate for the study conducted. (Comprehension)
3. Examine the organisation & presentation of the research report:- title of research need to clearly indicate the focus of the study. The report usually include abstract, introduction method, results, discussion & reference. Abstract of the study needs to present the purpose of the study clearly & highlight the methodology & major results.

   Body of the report needs to be concise, complete, clearly presented & logically organized reference needs to be complete & presented in a consistent format. (Comparison)
4. Identify the Strength & weaknesses of a study:- all studies have strength & weaknesses Q's can be put to facilitate identification of them.

   Address the quality of the steps of research process & the logical links among the steps of the process. (Comparison & analysis).
5. Provide specific examples of the strengths & weakness of a study: eqs provides a rationale & documentation for your critique of the study. (Comparison & Analysis)

6. Be objective & realistic in identifying a studies strength & weaknesses:- try not to be overly critical when identifying a study's weakness or overly flattering when identifying the strengths
7. Suggest modifications for future studies:-modifications should increase strengths & decrease the weaknesses in the Study.
8. Evaluate the study:-Indicate the overall quality of the study and its contribution to nursing knowledge.

   Discuss the consistency of the findings of the study with those of previous research. Discuss the need for further research & the potential to use the findings in practise. (Evaluation)

Qualitative Research process includes:- (for Critique)

- Comprehension
- Comparison
- Analysis
- Evaluation & Conceptual clustering.

Comprehension- involves understanding terms & concepts in the report as well as identifying study elements & grasping its nature, significance & meaning of those elements.

Comparison: involves knowledge of each step of research process as to what it should be like. The ideal is compared with real, examine the extent to which the research followed the rules of ideal study & how well the study situation is grasped & expressed.

Analysis:- involves critique of the logical links connecting one study element with another. Overall flow of logic in the study.

Variables identified need to be consistent in the study purpose, research objectives, questions or hypotheses need to be conceptually defined, operationally defined study design & analysis need to be appropriate for the investigation

Limitation in the study arise from breaks in logical reasoning during analysis the process moves into examining abstract dimension of the study & skill required in abstract reasoning.

Evaluation:- involves determining the meaning & significance of the study by examining the links between the study process, study findings & previous studies.

Evaluation in light of previous studies & present study in terms of Hypothesis, design, methods of measurements, findings evaluation in build on conclusions, reached during the 1st 3 stages of critique & provide basis for conceptual clustering.

Conceptual clustering:- is the final step: it involves synthesis of study findings to determine the current body of knowledge in an area.

Integrated view of research on a variety of topics relevant to nursing is provided. Qualitative Research critiques process includes.

- Content flexibility
- Inductive reasoning
- Conceptualization, theoretical modelling & theory analysis
- Transforming ideas across levels of abstraction.

1. Content Flexibility:- is capacity to switch from one content or world wide view/to another, to shift perception, to see things from a different perspective.

   Switching of context requires investing time & energy to learn more about the pt and setting aside personal, sometimes strongly held views.

   Scholarly work requires a willingness & ability to examine & evaluate works from different perspectives.

2. Inductive reasoning:- The transformation process used in data analysis in qualitative research is based on inductive reasoning. The logic is revealed in the systematic move from the concrete description in a particular study to the abstract level of science.

3. Conceptualization, Theoretical Modelling & Theory Analysis:-

   — The study is oriented to works theory construction

   — Need skill in conceptualization, theoretical modelling & theory analysis.

   Theoretical structure is developed inductively & expected to emerge from the data, follow logical flow of thought, analyse & evaluate the adequacy of resulting theoretical scheme & its connection to theory development within the discipline.

4. Transforming idea across levels of abstraction:- review of literature → organizes ideas from review & then again modifies those ideas in the process

of developing a summary of the existing body of knowledge-involved in the transformation of ideas

Standards recommend to evaluate qualitative studies include:-

1. **Descriptive vividness**: or validity refers to the clarity and factual accuracy of the researcher's account of the study.
2. **Methodological congruence**: reviewer as well researcher need to have knowledge of the philosophy and the methodological approach and cite sources where the reviewer can obtain further information through four dimensions i.e. Rigor in documentation, procedural rigor, ethical rigor and auditability.
3. **Analytical preciseness**: involves a series of transformations during which concrete data are transformed across several level of abstraction.
4. **Theoretical connectedness**: requires that the theoretical scheme developed from the study be clearly expressed, logically consistent reflective of the data and compatible with the knowledge base of nursing.
5. **Heuristic relevance**: value is reflected in the reader's capacity to recognize the phenomena described in the study, its theoretical significance it's applicable to nursing practice situations and its influence on future research activities. Heuristic relevance includes intuitive recognition, relationship to the existing body of knowledge and applicability.

CONCLUSION

Critiquing is a Complex valuable mental process for beginning researchers that is stimulated by raising Questions. It helps them to gain understanding of the investigative process. Research is critiqued to broaden, understanding summarize knowledge for use in practise. Critiquing of previous studies help determine their limitation & study findings need to be interpreted in light of the limitation. Limitation can lead to inaccurate data, in accurate outcome of analysis & decrease ability to generalize the findings. Recognition of strength is also critical to the generation of scientific knowledge & use of study findings in practise. If only weakness are identified nurse might discount the value of the study & refuse to invest time in Examining Research. Critiquing process is followed for both "Quantitative" and "Qualitative" research. While conducting critiquing would use Comprehension, Comparison, analysis, evaluation, and Conceptual clustering. Critiquing should never become faultfinding but evaluation should teach researcher new technique and methods. So that the process of critiquing does not become a traumatic and unpleasant experience which would demotivated the novice researcher who would give up before getting started.

BIBLIOGRAPHY

1. Brockopp Dorothy Y, Hastings Tolsma Marie,Fundamental of nursing research, 3rd ed. Boston: Jones & Bartlet:2003.
2. Polit Denis F,Cheryl Tatano Beck, Nursing research 8th ed, Philadelphia: Lippincott William & Wilkims, A Wolters Kluwer company: 2007;327,367-414,517.
3. Bourne PE. Ten simple rules for making good oral presentations. *PLoS Comput Biol.* 2007; 3:e77. doi: 10.1371/journal.pcbi.0030077. [PMC free article] [PubMed] [Google Scholar] cited on 22.4.2021
4. Vancouver - Referencing Guide https://libguides.murdoch.edu.au/Vancouver/sample cited on 18.4.2021
5. https://guides.library.uq.edu.au/referencing/vancouver/reference-list cited on 22.4.2021
6. Vancouver Referencing Guide: Book chapters. https://wilkes.libguides.com/c.php?g=191948&p=1266862 cited on 22.4.2021
7. Farley library research guides https://wilkes.libguides.com/c.php?g=191948&p=1266585 cited on 15.4.2021.
8. The University of Queenlands Australia https://guides.library.uq.edu.au/referencing/vancouver/reference-list cited 23.4.2021
9. Murdoch University library, Vancouver Referencing Guide https://libguides.murdoch.edu.au/Vancouver/all cited on 23.4.2021.
10. Citation styles: A Brief Guide to APA,MLA and Turabian.https://libguides.unf. edu/citation guide/apasample.

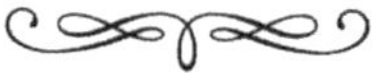

CHAPTER

12 Research Proposal Preparation and Use of Computer in Research

Swati Kambli

Learning Objectives

This chapter helps the reader to –

- Understand the meaning of the term research proposal
- Explain purposes of research proposal
- Develop skill in writing research proposal & present it
- Discuss the difference between references & bibliography & write it in research report/articles.
- Understand the importance of using computer in research.

A written research proposal plays an important role to conduct research study successfully & accurately. A research proposal is a written plan & an outline of research to be conducted. It specifies what is to be done, who will do it & why it is to be done. It begins with identification of good feasible research problem. It also gives a good direction to conduct research study successfully. A research proposal need to be approved by research & ethical committee & funding agency financing the research project. Research proposal is also known as synopsis.

Meaning of Research Proposal

A research proposal is well planned document in writing, focusing on what researcher proposes to study.

A written research proposal communicates the research problem, its significance & a clear problem solving strategy to the interested party. The party may be funding agency, an institutional research committee/ethical committee, depending on circumstances.

Purposes of Research Proposal

- It gives a clear direction to the researcher about conducting a research study.
- After presenting it to the experts i.e. research & ethical committee or funding agency, the investigator will get suggestions to improve/refine it.
- Good research proposal economizes the resources required for research study.
- It helps in minimizing errors when actual research study is conducted.
- It serves as a contract between researcher, guide, university & funding agency.
- It is also submitted to scholarship committee or other funding agency to seek the financial grants for conducting research.

Steps of Developing a Research Proposal

Development of research proposal involves following steps-

- Selecting & specifying a topic
- Developing objectives/questions for analysis
- Identifying current, relevant literature related to topic
- Planning for research methodology which includes research approach, design & other significant things
- Preparing a plan for data analysis
- Planning for deadline to complete research study
- Developing budget & planning for required resources for the project
- Locating & organizing references & bibliography

Writing research proposal is a time consuming process. It requires various skills i.e. writing skills, locating & identifying literature review, specifying a knowledge gap which can justify the need to conduct research study. It also helps in measuring progress being made by referring back to research proposal.

Format of Research Proposal

There are different formats or guidelines used by different institutions/ funding agencies. A researcher has to follow the format in developing research proposal. It should be compiled. For a neophyte researcher it is a difficult task so researcher should take help from various resources to develop it. It should give an insight to the researcher that problem to be studied is really significant with good justification for it. A written research proposal should be done in a logical format specifying how to conduct a research study. The format includes the following areas-

- **Study title** - Developing title is a challenging task. It must be interesting, specific & precise e.g. The effect of using mask, social distancing & hand hygiene on prevention of covid 19 infection in the community.

  The title should include the following-

  - What will be researched
  - Who will carry out the investigation
  - Where will it be done
  - When will it be done
  - How will it be done
  - What will be an outcome

- **Investigators** - up-to-date curriculum vitae of each of the investigators & co-investigators to be provided.
- **Information** about institutions under whose umbrella the research study will be conducted should be given clearly.
- **Introduction** - should include data emphasizing extent of problem area. It should be interesting.
- **Need for study** - should include review of recent literature, being published in the past 5 to 10 years at most. Number of research studies included should justify need for conducting research.

  Depending upon level of learning number of studies included in the literature should be more. Considering cultural & other differences, studies from the countries where research to be conducted, need to be included. Also unpublished material & clinical observations also can be included.

- **Rationale or justice for research project** - A good justification including a knowledge gap identified from literature review should be given to explain how this research study will be benefitting the subjects.
- **Objectives of the study** - there can be main/primary objective & specific/ secondary objectives.

- **Operational definition** - in quantitative research study, concepts should be defined in such a way that it can be measured during study.
- **Number of hypothesis** depends upon the problem area selected for the study.
- **Methodology** - it should be specific & in detail on the following aspects –
  - **Research approach & research design**
  - **Study setting** - where the study will be conducted should be mentioned with good justification of adequacy of sample & availability of other resources.
  - **Study population** - overall characteristics of the groups of people from which sample is derived should be mentioned e.g. all patients admitted with diagnosis of type2 diabetes in all hospitals of Mumbai city.
  - **Sample size** - Calculation with justification is stated. Type of sampling selected to be mentioned. Inclusion, exclusion criteria of sample selection is clearly mentioned.
- **Data collection** - details to be provided like what information is to be collected, how to collect the information will be clearly stated. Who will collect data should be specified & orientation needed for collection of data to be mentioned.
- **Data management & Analysis** - Details on data analysis, such as computer package to be used in data entry & analysis is to be given e.g. SPSS 25, API-INFO etc.
  - Results presentation - like types of graphs used, Tables etc to be mentioned.
- **Dissemination of the results** - Plan for dissemination to be included whether in conference, publishing paper, writing report etc. to be included in proposal.
- **Ethical justification** - Ethical issues need to be addressed clearly. The risk & benefit ratio, informed consent form signature, permission from concerned authorities to be mentioned clearly.
- Details about all required resources to be provided.
- Budget is to be clearly prepared so that funding agency is convinced to provide finance required for study.

- Supporting material included like references, tools, initial drafts, protocols if any, patient information sheet & consent form.

Computers in Nursing Research

Advancement in technology is a blessing to carry out research activities very accurately. It economizes time as manual work in research is very much time consuming. Computer in research is used at all stages of research study, right from preparation of research proposal to the presentation of findings.

Major uses of computer in nursing research are as follows:

- A good presentation of research proposal is possible.
- A large amount of research data helps in identifying recent, relevant literature to justify or support why a research is needed in a particular area/aspect.
- Artificial intelligence based search engines help in identification of literature very quickly.
- Conceptual/theoretical framework can be easily prepared with the help of visual display software.
- Research design - Access with database helps in the selection of research design very accurately.
- Sampling - Computerized Table of random number generators such as Fortuna or Yarrow can be used to generate true random numbers selection to facilitate random sampling for experimental research designs.
- Research instrument & data collection - Standard validated tools which are available online can be used for data collection. Online data collection can be done using webforms or other soft wares. Virtual meeting can be used to collect data about sensitive issues like sexual abuse etc.
- Informed consent - A downloadable file can be used through email. Consent form can be created by using word processing program.
- **Data Analysis methods** - Traditionally research data was handled manually involving laborious work. It was very much time consuming. Presently several computer packages are available, which can be used for statistical analysis in quantitative & qualitative research studies. There are a large numbers of tools used in health science research. These tools get the job done in similar ways, but differences lie in ease of use & presentation as differences in licensing, interface & cost. These tools handle the processes like collecting, organizing, analysing & interpreting

statistical data. There are top ten tools used by various researchers. These are **- STATA, R, GRAPHPAD PRISM, SAS, IBM SPSS, MATLAB, JMP, MINITAB, STATISTICA, EXCEL.** (kolabtree.com/blog/top-10-statistical-tools-used in medical research cited on 2021-July-9)

- **SPSS** - Originally known as Statistical Package for Social Sciences, developed in 1960 at Stanford University. It is made & sold by IBM. It is comprehensive, flexible & can be used with almost any type of data file. It can be used to generate tabulated reports, charts, as well as generate descriptive statistics such as means, medians, modes & frequencies. In addition to more complex statistical analyses like regression models. It is also simple & easy to enter & edit data directly into program. Its drawback is the limit on numbers of cases one can analyse (thought.com/quantitative.analysis-softwarereview-3026539 cited on2021-7-9). More information is available about it at the website www.spss.com.
- **SAS -** The Statistical Analysis System is developed by North Carolina State University. This system contains a very large variety of statistical methods. The more useful components of SAS are BASE SAS, SAS/STAT, SAS/GRAPH etc. More information about it is available at the website www.sas.com.
- **Minitab** - This package is designed to use it for teaching of statistical methods by using computer. It is very user friendly product. To get more information about it one needs to visit the website www.minitab.com.
- **Ms Excel-** is very popular & useful spreadsheet program that can be used for data entry & analysis. It has a capacity to generate random numbers, & it can be used for the computation of many standard statistical applications like computation of mean, range, standard deviation etc. There are certain problems in the algorithms of some version of this program so it is better to use other packages like spss or sas for analysis purpose.
- There are **qualitative data analysis softwares** also available which help in the form of explanation, understanding or interpretation of the people & situations to help in the meaningful & symbolic content of qualitative data. The data in qualitative research can be analysed using some of the special soft wares as **QSR'Sn6 & NVitro, WEFTQDA, Atlasti, Hyperresearch 2.6.**
- Discussion of findings, recommendations & summary - can be typed by using word processing Microsoft Office.
- References & Bibliography - References & bibliography can be formatted

correctly by using common citation styles, such as Vancouver, APA, Harvard etc.

Writing References & Bibliography

To support & justify research work, at the end of report, references & bibliography is recorded. In health sciences, Vancouver style of references is commonly used. This chapter explains about Vancouver & APA style of referencing. There are soft wares available to do this job.

- **Differences between References & Bibliography**

  Bibliography & references are different & used in different contexts in article/book. Bibliography enlists all materials that has been referred to while writing an article or research report. It is listed at the end of the text. It may or may not be cited in the text. It contains books, articles, websites & so on. These resources are used but not cited in the text/write up.

  - References are those that have been referred to or referenced in article/book. It contain a source of material like quotes or texts, which has been actually used when writing a report/book.

  - Both bibliography & references appear at the end of the text but bibliography is listed after the references. Bibliography is arranged alphabetically, but references are arranged in numerical style, means arranging references according to the numbers in the text. Commonly used referencing systems/styles of writing references are- Vancouver, & APA. Among these styles Vancouver style is commonly used in health science research.

  - **Vancouver style** is based on an American National Standards Institute (ANSI) adapted by National Library of Medicine (NLM) for databases, such as Medline. It was developed in Vancouver in 1978 by editors of medical journals, who now meet annually as the International Committee of Medical Journal Editors (ICMJE). Most journals in health sciences use this style to write references. A reference number is given to the reference in the list. References are numbered consecutively in the order they are first mentioned in the text. If the same reference is used again, the original number is reused. If a direct quote is necessary, quotation mark is placed around the quote & reference is numbered as usual.

  - **APA** - This style is devised by American Psychological Association. The style guide called as "publication manual of the American Psychological Association" was first published in 1929. Thereafter it was published in 2009. This style was previously used in nursing & education. In this style the reference list is written at the end of the report/article. The order of the reference list is prepared by arranging all entries in alphabetical order by the surname of first author followed by initials of the author's given name.

- **Harvard Style** - This system follows author & date system. This system places the authors & date of work being referred to at the appropriate point in the text rather than using a number. This is called a "citation". All the works cited are then listed at the end of the report/article in an alphabetical order according to the authors surname. The reference list must contain all the works cited in the text.
- Examples of the abovementioned first two styles which are commonly used in health science research shown in Table 12.1.

Table 12.1: Format of writing the references using Vancouver & APA style

Style	Vancouver	APA
Type of source	format	format
Book	Author's surname, author's initials. Book title, Edition, Place of publication, Publisher; year, Page numbers	Author's surname, author's initials, Year of Publication, Title of book, Publisher city, State. Page numbers
E - Books	# Author's names. Title of E Book, Place of Publisher, Date of original publication (cited year, abbreviated month, date) available from source. URL	Author's surname, initials, (year of publication). Title of book (E reader version). Retrieved from URL.
Journal article	Author's surname & initials. Title of article. Title of Journal or title abbreviation. Year, volume (issue):Page (s).	Author's surname & initials. (year) Title of the article. Title of Journal. Volume (issue) page numbers
E Journals	Author's surname & initials. Title of article. Abbreviated title of journal, year (cited year abbreviated month, date); vol. (No) Page nos. Available from: database name URL.	Author's surname & initials. (year). Title of article. Abbreviated title of journal (cited year abbreviated month & date);vol. (no): Page nos. Available from: database/URL.
Dissertation/ Master's thesis	Surname & initials, Title. Type of Publication. Place: Publisher; year	Surname & initials. Title (year) Type of publication. Place: Publisher; URL

(Continued...)

Style	Vancouver	APA
News papers & popular magazines	Author's surname & initials. Article title. Newspaper title. Date, year: page	Author's surname & initials. (Year, month, date of publication) Article title. Newspaper/ magazine title. Page nos.
Online newspaper/ internet documents	Author's surname & initials. Webpage name, source/production information. Date of internet publication (cited year, month, date). Available from URL	Author's surname & initials. (year, month, date of publication). Article title. Newspaper title. Webpage name (cited year, month, date). Available from: URL.
Conference paper	Author's name & initials. Paper title, name of conference where paper is presented. Date, place.	Author's name, initials (year) paper title, name of conference where paper is presented. Date, place of publication, publisher
Government agency	Author's name, initials. Name of organization/agency. Title. Place of publication: publisher; year of publication.	Author's surname & initials/ Government name. Name of Government agency. (year) Title: subtitle (report no. if available). Place of publication: Publisher.

SUMMURY

- A research proposal is a well thought out plan in writing to conduct a research study.
- It gives a clear direction to the researcher to conduct a research study.
- Research proposal must be framed as per the guidelines provided by institute.
- It is to be refined after presenting it to various experts from research & ethical committee with their suggestions.
- Advanced technology is a major blessing to carry out research accurately. It helps in the preparation of research proposal till successful completion of research study.
- Research study conducted is to be supported & justified at each stage with good review of literature. Reviewed literature should be recorded appropriately. Commonly used referencing style in health science related research is Vancouver style.

BIBLIOGRAPHY

- Clement Nisha. Textbook of Nursing Research & Statistics. Published by Emmess publishers, Benglore. P. 353-356.

- Dr. Sharma Suresh. Nursing Research & Statistics. Publication Elsevier RELX India Pvt Ltd. 2019. P.397, 398, 428.
- Kolabtree.com/blog/top-10-statistical-tools-used in medical-research cited on 2021-9-7.
- Publication manual of the American Psychological Association 6th edition, Washington, D.C.: American Psychological Association, 2010.
- Roberts K, Taylor, B. Nursing Research Process: An Australian Perspectives; 2nd edition, pub. Thompson, Nelson Australia Pty Ltd.; 2002.
- Thought.com/quantitative-analysis-software review-3026539 cited 2021-7-9.
- Olk, H. How to write a research proposal. In Dentcher Academicscher Austausch Dienst (DAAD; 2009.

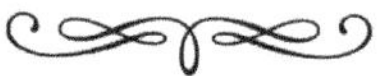

Section II

Statistics

CHAPTER

13 Descriptive Statistics

Pradnya Wakpainjan

Learning Objectives

This chapter helps the reader to –

- Identify different types of data
- Organize & tabulate data
- Present data in a graphical form
- Prepare Frequency distribution Table
- Explain measures of central tendencies, variability and dispersion.

INTRODUCTION

The statistics is the science in which we study the methods and techniques used in collection, organisation, presentation, analysis and interpretation of numerical data. The data analysis is an extremely important step in research. The data collected need to be organized systematically before one starts its analysis. The data is obtained from the surveys, experimental studies and records. The experimental researches are carried out with the intention to bring about change while surveys are conducted to study the trends and existing situation. For example in experimental research the programme can be developed to enhance the knowledge about organ donation and study if the program is found to be effective. While in descriptive type of research the researcher will study the extent of the knowledge about organ donation among people.

DATA, INFORMATION & KNOWLEDGE

There are terms like information, data and knowledge widely used in the research. Let's understand the relationship between these terms in the context of research.

Fig. 13.1: DIK model

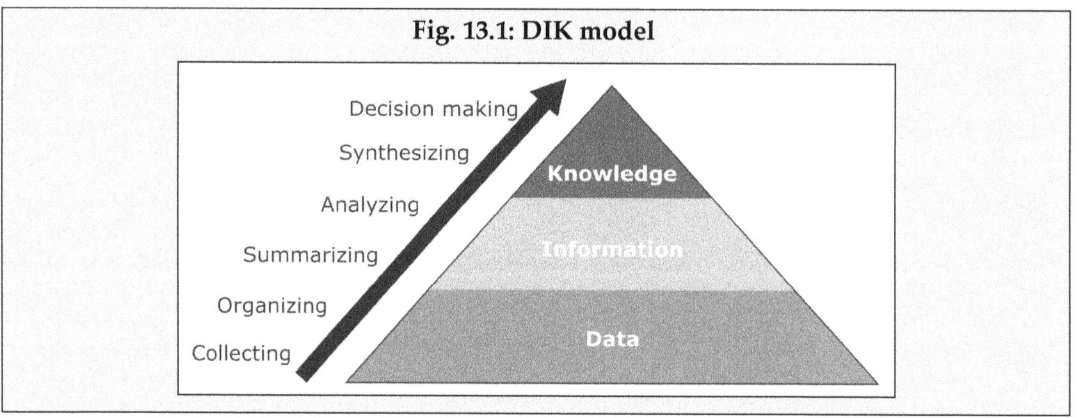

Fig. 13.2: Understanding the relationship between data, information & Knowledge

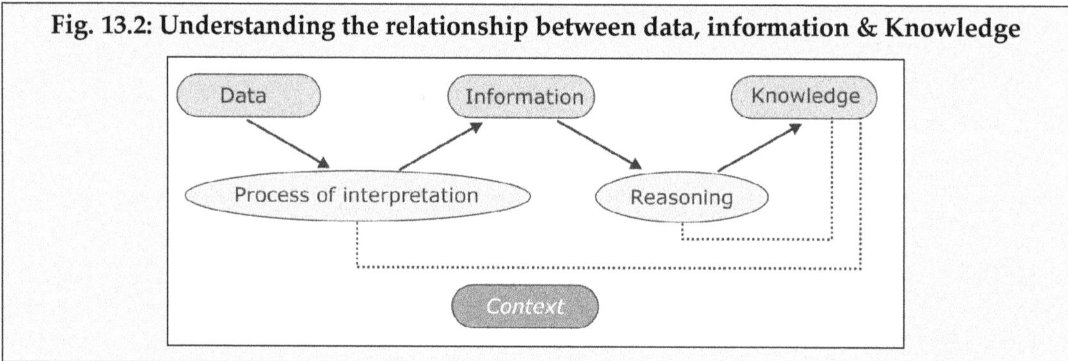

The above figure indicated the relationship between data, information, and knowledge. It means the data when processed for interpretation then it becomes the information and when this information is understood with reasoning in the context then it creates knowledge. The terms that are used for data are collecting and organising that is then process for interpretation and thus it is information and in the knowledge it's synthesizing and decision making wherein researcher generalize the results.

In other words we can say that Information is processed data so that it becomes useful and provides answers to questions such as "who", "what", "where", and "when". On the other hand knowledge is an application of information and data, and gives an insight by answering the "how" questions. Knowledge is also the understanding gained through experience or study.

For example there is a data of salary of people working in the organisation. When you try to interpret you will ask the question who gets more salary? What is the difference in the salary on the basis of positions/designation? When was the last increment given? Etc. Further the questions related to how the salary is related to investment? What is the pattern of investment in relation to the salary? and so on.

Types of Data

The researcher uses different type of data as per the objectives of the study. The data has been classified in various ways as follows:

1. **Quantitative data**

   Quantitative data is the one that answers key questions such as "how many, "how much" and "how often". It is the data that can be quantified or expressed as a number. In other words it can be said that it can be measured by numerical variables. It can be easily managed represented by a variety of f graphs and charts such as line, bar graph, scatter plot, etc.

   Examples of quantitative data

   Students' Scores on tests in exams e.g. 85, 67, 90, etc.

   The weight of a person in Kg 65, 75, 45, 56 etc.

   There are 2 general types of quantitative data: discrete data and continuous data that is discussed later.

2. **Qualitative data**

   When the data is in various forms like words, pictures, and symbols etc. When the researcher try to find out the answer for the questions like "how this has happened" or and "why this has happened" then the Qualitative data can answer questions using textual form. Qualitative data is also called categorical data because the information can be sorted by category, not by number.

   Examples of qualitative data

   Ethnicity, Religious affiliation or if someone explaining what happened.

3. **Nominal data**

   When the researcher wants a data that is used just to label variables, without any type of quantitative value then it is nominal data. The word 'nominal' derived from the Latin word 'nomen' which means 'name'. The nominal data is just name a thing without applying it to order. Thus, the nominal data could be called 'labels'.

   Examples of Nominal Data: Gender (Women, Men), Marital status (Married, Single, Widowed)

4. **Ordinal data**

Ordinal data is data which is placed into some kind of order by its position on a scale. This order is not used for calculation purpose. In other words, the ordinal data is qualitative data for which the values are ordered and one can see the sequence. Ordinal variables are considered as "in between" qualitative and quantitative variables. One can assign numbers to ordinal data to show their relative position like first, second, third...etc.

Examples of Ordinal Data

The first, second and third person in a competition.

Grades obtained by students: A, B, C, D, F etc.

Economic status: low, medium and high.

5. **Discrete data**

Discrete data is a count that involves only integers. The discrete values cannot be subdivided into parts. In other words, discrete data can take only certain values and cannot be divided into smaller parts.

For example, the number of children in a class is discrete data. You can count whole individuals. You can't count 1.5 kids. The number of workers in an organization, the number of test questions you answered correctly are few examples

6. **Continuous data**

When the data is meaningfully divided into finer levels, it can be measured on a scale or continuum and can have almost any numeric value. Such data is in a continuous form

For example, you can measure your height at very precise scales – meters, centimeters, millimeters, etc. For various measurement like width, temperature, time, etc. the same logic can be applied.

7. **Ungrouped data**

Ungrouped data is the data you first gather from an experiment or study. The data is raw data that is, it's not sorted into categories, classified, or otherwise grouped. An ungrouped set of data is basically a list of numbers. For example Students marks in science: 45, 40, 32, 23, 34, 25, 44, 21, 37, 33 etc.

7. **Grouped data**

When the raw data is grouped in a systematic way it is known as grouped data. The frequency Table is prepared to group raw data that can be further used for descriptive analysis

Data Organization

As it is discussed in figure 1.2, the raw data needs to be converted into information and this is possible only when the appropriate Statistical Techniques are used and the results are interpreted. In order to do so the first step is the organisation of data. Data organisation is the practice of categorizing and classifying the data to make it more usable. In research, when researcher wants to organize data, it is important to keep in mind the objectives of the research study. Now a days, data is organized using Microsoft Excel.

For example, Researcher wants to study the cultural competence of nurses. And further to compare cultural competence on the basis of gender age experience and type of hospital. The research will collect the data using personal data sheet and the cultural competence scale. The data can be organised as given below (Table 13.1).

,

Table 13.1

S.N.	Cultural Competence score	Gender	Age	Experience in years	Type of hospital
1	34	M	40	15	Government
2	40	F	34	12	Private
3	29	F	32	10	Private
4	37	M	26	4	Government
5	30	F	29	7	Private

After the preparation of Master sheet the data needs to be grouped in order to group the data frequency distribution Tables are prepared.

Frequency Distribution

Data collected from the respondent using different tools may have little meaning until it is arranged or classified in some systematic way. Therefore the first task is to classify scores into classes and that is known as preparation of frequency distribution Tables.

Frequency distribution of ungrouped data

Given below are marks obtained by 50 students in Math out of 50.

Consider the marks of 50 students of class VII obtained in an examination. The maximum marks of the exam are 50.

23, 8, 13, 18, 32, 44, 19, 8, 25, 27, 10, 30, 22, 40, 39, 17, 25, 9, 15, 20, 30, 24, 29, 19, 16, 33, 38, 46, 43, 22, 37, 27, 17, 11, 34, 41, 35, 45, 31, 26, 42, 18, 28, 30, 22, 20, 33, 39, 40, 32.

If we create a frequency distribution Table for each and every observation, then it will form a large Table. So for easy understanding, we can make a Table with a group of observations say 1 to 10, 10 to 20 etc. To prepare frequency Table the following steps can be followed.

Step 1: Determine the range: Take out the difference in the highest score and lowest score in the distribution.

Range = 46-8 = 38

Step 2: Divide the range by the number of groups you want and then round up. Suppose you want 6 classes then divide the range by 6 and you will get the class length

38/6 = 6.33. The length of your class will be 7 (round off)

Step 3: Use the class width to create your groups

I'm going to start at the smallest number we have, which is 8, and count by 7 until I have my 6 or 7 groups. For example, my first group will be 7 to 14. Next group will be 14 to 21 and so on.

Table 13.2

Class interval	Tally	Frequency
42-49	|||||	5
35-42	|||||||||	9
28-35	||||||||||||	12
21-28	||||||||	8
14-21	|||||||||||	11
7- 14	|||||	5

Step 4: Find the frequency for each group

Calculate the tally you have for each score and prepare Table as given above. Once the frequency Table is prepared one can proceed with the calculation of measures of central tendency, measures of variability & measures of dispersion

Descriptive Analysis of Data

In most of the researches conducted on groups of people, you will use both descriptive and inferential statistics to analyse your results and draw conclusions.

Descriptive statistics or descriptive analysis of data helps to describe, show or summarize data in a meaningful way. Descriptive statistics does not allow us to make conclusions beyond the data we have analysed or draw conclusions regarding any hypotheses. It is simply a way to describe our data. The descriptive analysis is very helpful for the researcher to make decision about the inferential statistics technique to be used.

Descriptive statistics are very important because if one presented raw data it would be hard to visualize what the data was showing, especially when data is huge. Descriptive statistics therefore enables us to present the data in a more meaningful way, which allows simpler interpretation of the data. If researcher is interested in the distribution or spread of the scores then the descriptive statistics allow us to do this. Typically, there are two general types of statistic that are used to describe data:

Measures of central tendency: these are ways of describing the central position of a frequency distribution for a group of data. Measures of central tendency/ average includes Mean, Median, Mode.

Measures of variability: these are ways of summarizing a group of data by describing how spreaded out the scores are. For example, the mean score of our 100 students may be 65 out of 100. However, not all students will have scored 65 marks. Rather, their scores will be spreaded out. Some will be lower and others higher. Measures of spread help us to summarize how spread out these scores are. To describe this spread, a number of statistics are available to us, including the range, quartiles, absolute deviation, variance and standard deviation.

MEASURES OF CENTRAL TENDENCY

There are several measures of central tendency, out of which the most commonly used are Mean, Median and Mode. Let us now focus on the most commonly used measures of central tendency as mentioned below:

Mean

Mean is defined as the sum of values in the dataset divided by the number of observations or values. This is the most commonly used measure of central tendency and also called the arithmetic mean. It is calculated by using formula:

$$M = \frac{\Sigma X}{N}$$

X1 + X2+ X3 +.................. + XN/N

There are two types of arithmetic mean like arithmetic mean of ungrouped data and arithmetic mean for grouped data.

For example, A montly income of 4 family is 1600, 1400, 1300, 1200. Find the average income of the family.

Solution: Given, 1600 + 1400 + 1300 +1200
= 1600 + 1400 + 1300 +1200/4
= 1375
Therefore, an average monthly income of family is Rs. 1375.

Table 13.3: Calculation of mean by short method

Class intervals	Mid-point	f	x′	fx′
195-199	197	1	5	5
190-194	192	2	4	8
185-189	187	4	3	12
180-184	182	5	2	10
175-179	177	8	1	8
170-174	172	10	0	0
165-169	167	6	-1	-6
160-164	162	4	-2	-8
155-159	157	4	-3	-12
150-154	152	2	-4	-8
145-149	147	3	-5	-15
140-144	142	1	-6	-6
		N = 50		Σfx′= **-12**

Formula: Mean = A.M. + Σfx′/N * (i)
Where A.M = Assume mean
f = frequency
fx′ = frequency multiplied by the deviation
N = sample size
i = Class length

Steps

1. Calculate the mid-point of each class interval by adding the upper and lower limit and divide by 2. e.g. 140 + 144 = 184/2 = 142
2. Locate the assume mean in a Class interval in which your frequency is maximum. Here it is in C.I. 170-174. In x′ in front of this CI write 0 and then towards upward +1, +2 etc and -1, -2 etc.
3. Calculate f multiplied by x′ and then sum that will be Σfx′ Here it is -12

   Divide Σfx′ by N. here it is 50. Here it is -12/50 = -0.240
4. Calculate class length. Here it is 5 (from 140 to 144 is 5)
5. Put all values in formula

   Mean = 172 + (-0.24*5)
   = 172-1.2 = 170.8

   Mean = 170.8

When to use Mean

Mean is the most accurate & reliable measure of central tendency

It is very stable and less fluctuating therefore when we want most reliable and accurate measure of central tendency

When researcher wants to go for further calculations like standard deviation, t-test etc

Median

It is defined as the value that divides the distribution into two halves. One part of the values is greater or equal to median value and the other is less than or equal to it. You can calculate median by arranging the data in ascending order.

For example, Arrange the data 5, 7, 6, 1, 8, 10, 12, 4, and 3 in ascending order and find out its median.

1, 3, 4, 5, 6, 7, 8, 10, 12

The middle value of the data is 6. Here, half of the numbers are greater than 6 and the other halves are smaller.

In case, the middle value have two numbers in the data, you calculate by using the formula mentioned below:

1, 3, 4, 5, 6, 7, 8, 10, 12, 13

This can be calculated by adding two median value divided by the number of observations. For example, 6 + 7/2 = 9.5

Therefore, the median value is 9.5.

Table 13.4: Median Calculations

C.I.	f	CuF
195-199	1	50
190-194	2	49
185-189	4	47
180-184	5	43
175-179	8	38
170-174	10	30
165-169	6	20
160-164	4	14
155-159	4	10
150-154	2	6
145-149	3	4
140-144	1	1
	N = 50	

Steps

1. Calculate Cumulative frequency (F)
2. Calculate N/2
3. Locate C.I. in which your N/2 value lies

   N/2 = 50/2 = 25
4. Locate the frequencies of the cumulative and within the same class

Formula of Median:

Mdn = l + (N/2 – CuF)/f *i

l = Exact lower limit of C.I. upon which the median lies

N/2 = Value obtained for half of total sample or frequency

CuF = Sum of the scores (f) on all intervals below l

f = Frequency within the C.I. upon which median lies

Here, l = 169.5

N/2 = 25

i = 5

f = 10

CuF = 20

Mdn = 169.5+ (25 – 20)/10*5

= 169.5+ (0.5) *5

= 169.5+2.5

Mdn = 172

When to use Median

When we want to calculate the exact mid-point of the distribution

When the series contain extreme scores then the median is the most representative central tendency

When it is impossible to calculate mean

Mode

Mode is the frequently observed score in the data.

Mode = 3 Mdn – 2 Mean

= (3*172) – (2*170.8)

= 516 – 341.6

Mode = 174.4.

When to use Mode

When we want quickest & approximate measure of central tendency

When we want most often recurring score

When we have information in graphical form

MEASURES OF VARIABILITY

The measure of Central tendency help us understand the mean, median, mode of the distribution. However you can see that the groups have the same mean but they differ in their composition.

Suppose a test on science has been administered to a two groups one of which is 60 boys and to a group of 60 girls. The mean scores are, boys, 34.6, and girls,

34.5. If you see the mean values then we may say there is no difference in the performance of the two groups. Further, if see the distribution, the boys' scores are found to range from 15 to 51 and the girls scores from 19 to 45. The range for boys is 36 while for girls is 26.

This difference in range shows that in a general the boys "cover more territory," are more variable, than the girls. This cannot be inferred through mean. If a group is homogeneous, that is, made up of individuals of nearly the same ability, most of its scores will fall around same point on the scale, the range will be relatively short and the variability is small. While the heterogeneous group will have larger variability.

The standard deviation is a technique that helps us to understand the deviation of the scores from the mean. Following is the example that depict the mean value is same but one group is homogeneous and other group is heterogeneous.

Fig. 13.3: Relation between mean and standard deviation

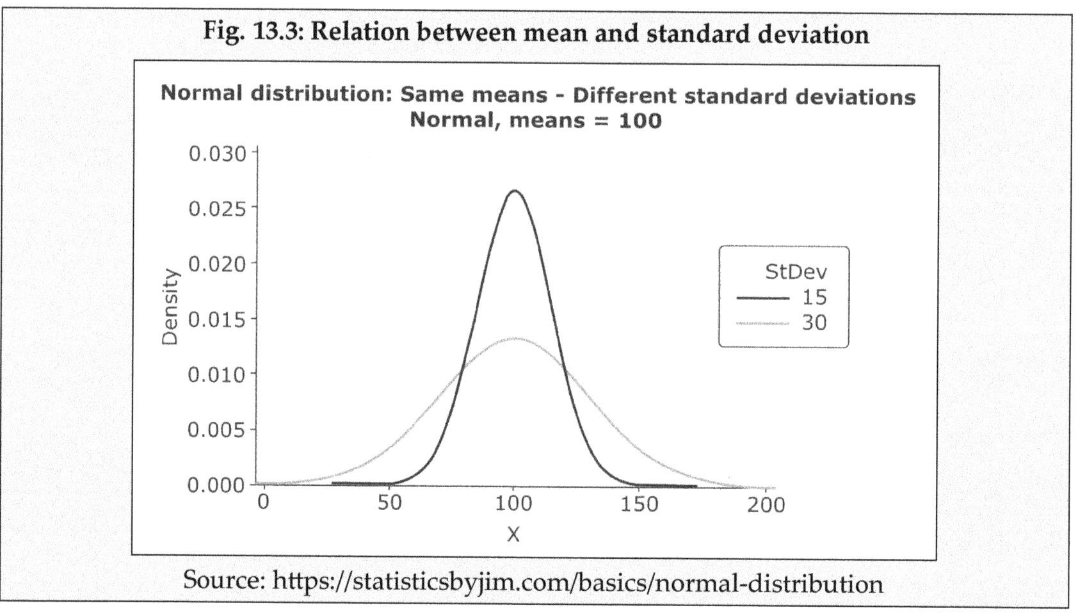

Source: https://statisticsbyjim.com/basics/normal-distribution

The above graph indicates that the mean of both values the groups are same that is 100 but group one (indicated with blue line) is more homogeneous while the other group (dotted red line) is heterogeneous. In other words, it can be said that the scores in group one are not far away from mean value while the scores are away from mean in second group. Therefore it is necessary that researcher should not interpret mean in isolation as the interpretation may be incomplete. If researcher considers both the values together then find the connections and the results can put up in more comprehensive manner.

The four measures are devised to indicate the variability (i) The range (ii) Average deviation (iii) Quartile deviation (iv) Standard deviation.

The range has been discussed earlier. Further we will calculate the standard deviation as we need it for further calculation of inferential statistics. The standard deviation or SD is the most stable index of variability therefore the researcher calculate it rather than other measures of variability. The conventional symbol for the SD is the Greek letter sigma (σ).

Calculation of the SD from ungrouped scores

The mean of the 5 scores 6, 8, 10, 12 and 14 is 10 the deviations of the separate scores from the mean are -4, -2, 0, 2 and 4, respectively. When each of these 5 deviations is squared up, it will be 16, 4, 0, 4 and 16; the sum is 40 and N is 5. The formula for σ when scores are ungrouped is as follows:

$$\sigma = \sqrt{\frac{\sum x^2}{N}}$$

In our example $\sum X^2$ is 40 & N is 5, so putting values in formula 40/5 and its under root is 2.38

Table 13.5: Calculation of the SD from grouped data

Class interval (C.I)	f	Mid-point C.I.	X′	fx′	fx'^2
127-129	1	128	4	4	16
124-126	2	125	3	6	18
121-123	3	122	2	6	12
118-120	1	119	1	1	1
115-117	6	116	0	0	0
112-114	4	113	-1	-4	4
109-111	3	110	-2	-6	12
106-108	2	107	-3	-6	18
103-105	1	104	-4	-4	16
100-102	1	101	-5	-5	25
	N = 24		$\sum fx' = -8$		$\sum fx'^2 = 122$

$SD = i\sqrt{\sum fx'^2/N - (\sum fx'/N)^2}$

i = class length = 3

$SD = 3 \times \sqrt{122/24 - (-8/24)^2}$

$= 3 \times \sqrt{5.08 - 0.111}$

$= 3 \times \sqrt{4.97 = 3 \times 2.229}$

SD = 6.68

MEASURES OF DISPERSION

In order to understand data and make decision about the inferential statistics the researcher try to understand the distribution of the data. Dispersion is the state of getting dispersed or spread. Statistical dispersion means the extent to which a numerical data is likely to vary about an average value. It is to measure divergence from the normal distribution. We will discuss two terms namely skewness & kurtosis.

Skewness

It is the degree of distortion from the symmetrical bell curve or the normal distribution. It measures the lack of symmetry in data distribution.

It differentiates extreme values in one versus the other tail. A symmetrical distribution will have a skewness of 0. In other words the normal probability has skewness zero.

The formula of skewness is $Sk = \frac{3\text{ (median-median)}}{\sigma}$

Fig. 13.4: Skewed distribution of data

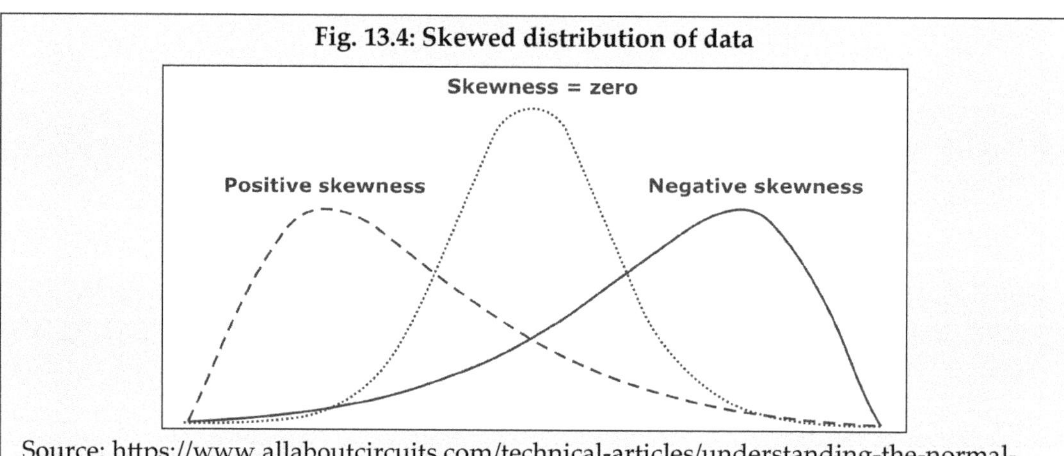

Source: https://www.allaboutcircuits.com/technical-articles/understanding-the-normal-distribution-parametric-tests-skewness-and-kurtosis/

A skewed data distribution can be either positive or negative. The data indicate positive skewness means when the tail on the right side of the distribution is longer or flatter. In such case the mean and median will be greater than the mode.

Negative Skewness is when the tail of the left side of the distribution is longer. In such case the mean and median will be less than the mode (Fig. 13.5).

Fig. 13.5: Negatively and Positively skewed distribution

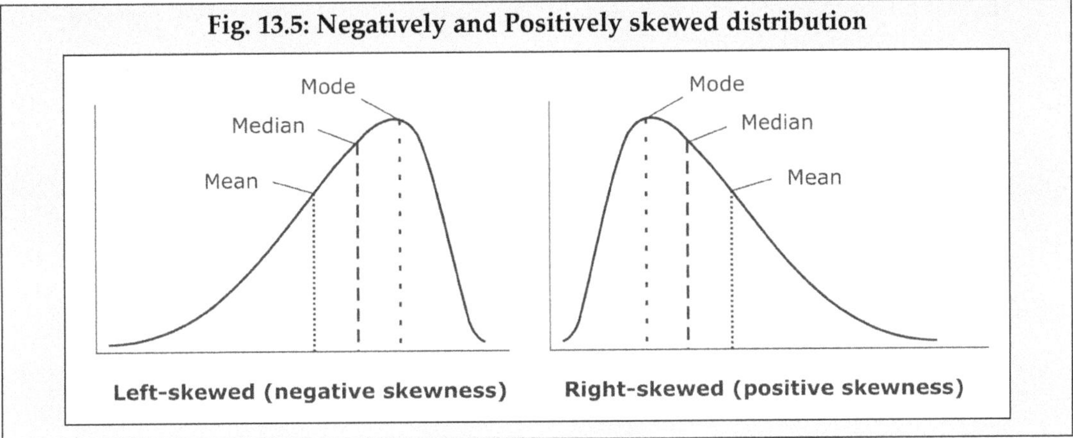

The value of skewness can be interpreted as follows :

If the skewness is between -0.5 & 0.5, the data are nearly symmetrical.

If the skewness is between -1 & -0.5 (negative skewed) or between 0.5 & 1 (positive skewed), the data are slightly skewed.

If the skewness is lower than -1 (negative skewed) or greater than 1 (positive skewed), the data are extremely skewed.

Kurtosis

The term kurtosis refers to the peakedness of frequency distribution. If frequency distribution is more peaked than the normal then it is said to be leptokurtic. When the distribution is flatter than normal then it is platykurtic. The normal probability curve is called as mesokurtic.

According to Garrett H. (pg 102) the kurtosis value of normal probability curve is 0.263. If the obtained kurtosis value is less than 0.263 then the distribution is said to be leptokurtic and if kurtosis value is greater than 0.263 then the distribution is said to be platykurtic.

Fig. 13.6: Understanding distribution in terms of peakedness of curve

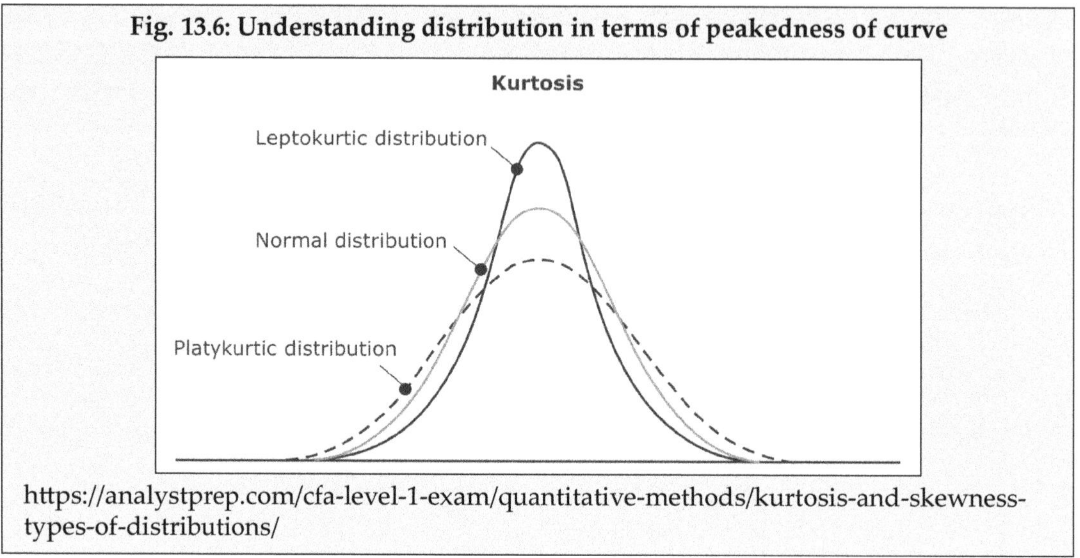

https://analystprep.com/cfa-level-1-exam/quantitative-methods/kurtosis-and-skewness-types-of-distributions/

Graphical Representation of Data

Researcher uses different type of data and present it in different forms. The graphical representation of data is one way of analysing and also presenting the information in a systematic way. A graph is a pictorial representation of data in an organized manner. Graphs are usually formed from various data points, which represent the relationship between two or more things. The different type of data are indicated by using different graphs. The graphs are used as it has many advantages as given below:

Facilitates and improves learning: Graphics make data easy to understand and eliminate language and literacy barriers

Understanding content: Visuals are more effective than text in human understanding

Flexibility of use: The different types of data can be used to present the information

Increases structured thinking: The visual provides stimuli and it is easy for reader to make connections in ideas. It supports creative, personalized reports for more engaging and stimulating visual presentations

Improves communication: Analysing graphs that highlight relevant themes is significantly faster than reading through a descriptive report line by line shows the comprehensive picture: The graphs provide the comprehensive picture of all variables, relationships etc. The comparative analysis can be understood quickly.

Some of the graphs used are as follows:

1. Bar Chart/Graph

   A bar chart is a graph represented by spaced rectangular bars that describe the data points in a set of data. It is usually used to plot discrete and categorical data.

   The horizontal axis of the chart represents categorical data while the vertical axis of the chart defines discrete data. Although the rectangular bars in a bar chart are mostly placed vertically, they can also be horizontal.

Fig. 13.7: Bar chart/graph

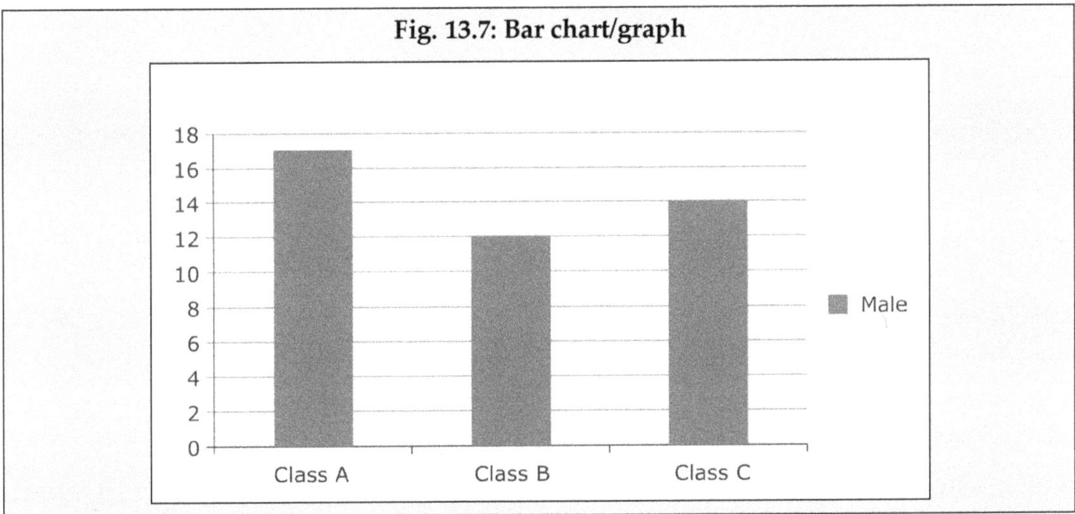

2. Pie Chart

   A pie chart is a circular graph used to illustrate numerical proportions in a dataset. This graph is usually divided into various sectors, where each sector represents the proportion of a particular numerical element in the set.

Fig. 13.8: Pie chart

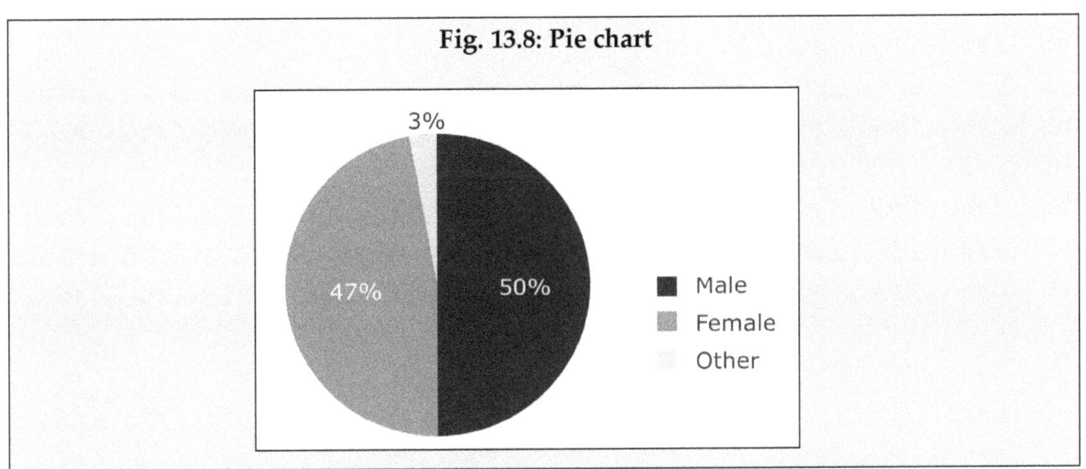

3. Line Graph or Chart

Line graphs are represented by a group of data points joined together by a straight line. Each of these data points describes the relationship between the horizontal and the vertical axis on the graph.

Fig. 13.9: Line graph

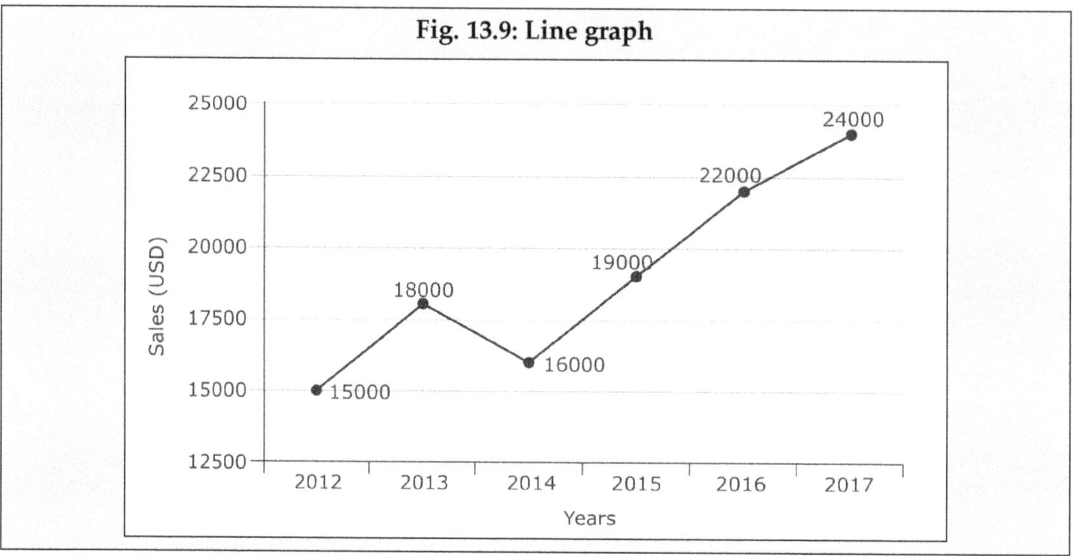

Types of Line Graph

- Simple Line Graph:

  In a simple line graph, only one line is plotted on the graph. One of the axes defines the independent variables while the other axis contains dependent variables.

- Multiple Line Graph (Fig 13.10):

  Multiple line graphs contain two or more lines representing more than one variable in a dataset. This type of graph can be used to study two or more variables over the same period of time.

4. Histogram (Fig 13.11)

The graph that uses bars to represent the frequency of numerical data that are organised into intervals. Since all the intervals are equal and continuous, all the bars have the same width.

5. Scatter Plot

Scatter plots are charts used to visualize random variables with dot-like markers that represent each data point. These markers are usually scattered across the chart area of the plot. It is widely used in relationship studies.

Types of Scatter Plot

Scatter plots are grouped into different types according to the correlation of the data points. These correlation types are highlighted in Fig. 13.12.

Fig. 13.10: Multiple line graph

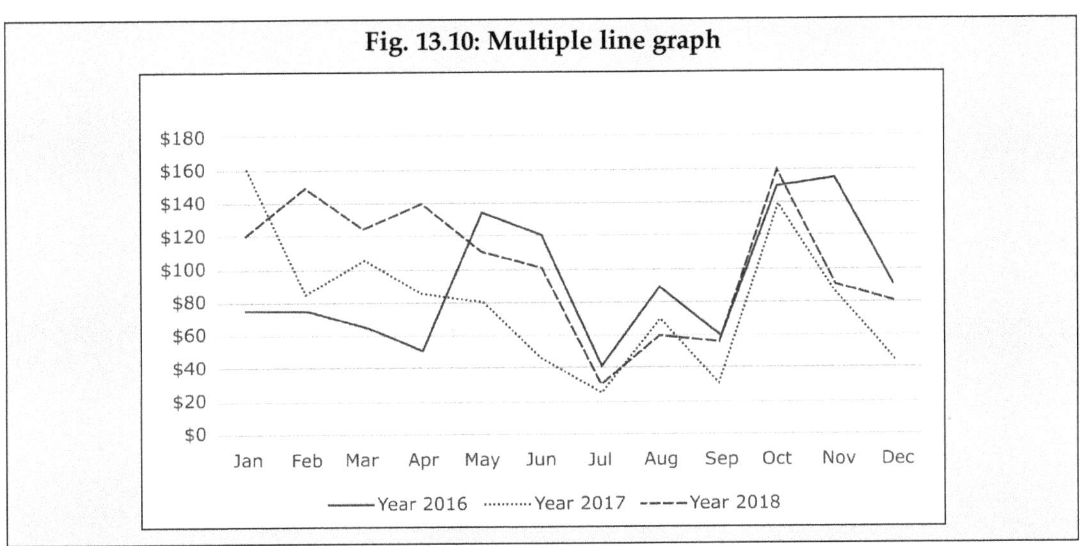

Fig. 13.11: Histogram

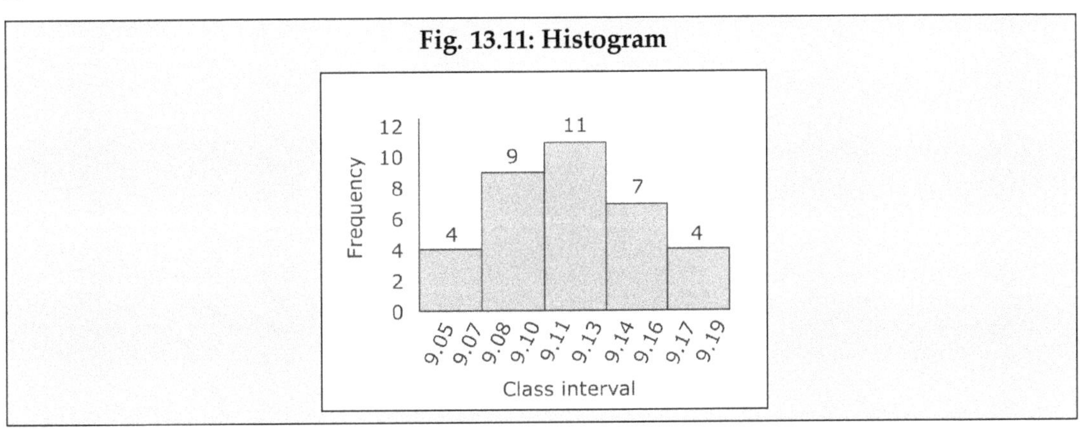

Fig. 13.12: Scatter diagram

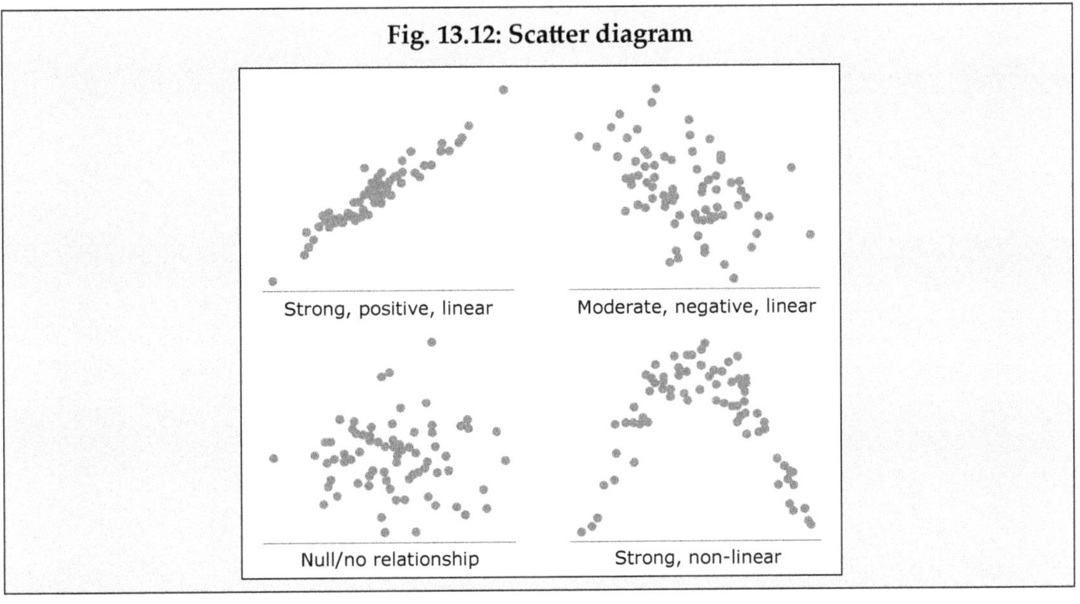

BIBLIOGRAPHY

- Best, J. W., & Kahn, J. V. (2006). Research in Education (10th ed.). Pearson Education Inc.
- Cohen, L., Manion, L., & Morrison, K. (2011). Research Methods in Education (7th ed.). Routledge.
- Gay, L. R., & Geoffrey E. Mills, P. A. (2011). Educational Research: Competencies for Analysis and Applications (10th ed.). Pearson.
- Garrett H. (2008) Statistics in Psychology and Education (First Indian reprint). Surjeet publication.

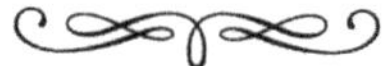

CHAPTER

14 Inferential Statistics

Pradnya Wakpainjan

Learning Objectives

This chapter helps the reader to –

- Explain various terms related to inferential analysis
- Select appropriate statistical test to analyse data
- Use appropriate statistical test
- Draw appropriate results using various statistical Tables
- Draw inferences and apply to relevant population.

Introduction

In the earlier chapter we discussed about descriptive analysis of data. The descriptive analysis help us to describe the characteristics of population and to take decision about the appropriate statistical test to be used. It is important to select appropriate statistical technique in order to draw the reliable inferences and conclusion that can be applied to the population through which the sample has been selected systematically.

The adjoining figure explain this relationship in a precise manner. It is not possible for researcher to collect data from every individual in population and therefore he/she has to select few individuals (sample) from the population and apply statistics and generalise result to population (Fig. 14.1).

Fig. 14.1: Application of inferential analysis from sample to population

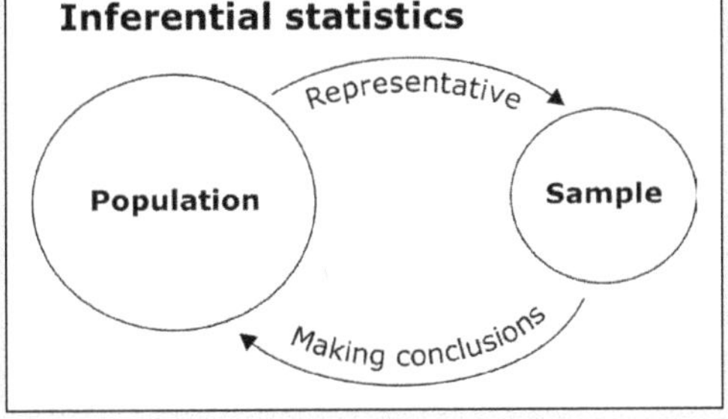

Understanding population and Sample

The main question that the researcher should ask while talking about sample is that who do you want to generalize the result? It should be to whom you want to generalize the findings. For example the researcher wants to know the organ donation awareness among 9th standard students in a city then he or she selects sample on the basis of sample and then generalize result to the population. Suppose there are two lac students of standard 9th in a city, then the researcher will select around 700-800 students, administer the tool take out the results and generalize about organ donation awareness among two lac students in a city. So here the researcher is likely to talk in general terms and does not want to be confined only to the people who are in the study. It is to be noted that there are times when researcher is not concerned about generalizing the result for population. For example, Ms. Sumathi is just evaluating a program in a local agency and interested in knowing whether this program is working well with this local people or not. Here the purview of research is very specific and limit to the specific community so the researcher will not generalize the results beyond that community.

What is inferential analysis?

Inferential analysis are techniques that allow us to use the samples to make generalizations about the populations from which the samples were drawn.

The word "inferential" is used because investigators and statisticians use data from samples to make inferences about the population-as-a-whole.

In short inferential analysis help–

To generalise the findings to population

To compare the attribute

To establish cause effect relationship

To predict the parameters in population

To provide information for designing strategies to overcome the problem/ situation (Policy formation)

Now we are clear on the difference is descriptive and inferential analysis of data. This difference in pointed out as follows.

Table 14.1

Descriptive analysis	Inferential analysis
It describes the characteristics of population	It draws inferences from the sample and apply to population
Organize, analyse and present data in meaningful manner	Test hypothesis and bring out conclusion (compare, predict)
Use of graphs, charts	Tables as per the statistical test used
Measures of central tendencies, variability and dispersion are the tools to describe the parameter	Statistical tests like t-test, ANOVA, ANCOVA and other are used
One describes what is seen through	Processes data statistically and draw conclusion about population

Terms in inferential Analysis

There are few terms we need to understand as it will help us to proceed with inferential analysis.

Standard Error of mean

In statistics, the standard error is the standard deviation of the sample distribution. The sample mean of a data is generally varied from the actual population mean. It is represented as SE. It is used to measure the amount of accuracy by which the given sample represents its population.

$$SE_{\bar{x}} = \frac{S}{\sqrt{n}}$$

Where S is the standard deviation and n is the number of observations.

Degrees of freedom

Degrees of Freedom refers to the maximum number of logically independent values that have the freedom to vary, in the data set. They are the number of values that are free to vary in a data set. In statistics, the degrees of freedom (df) indicate the number of independent values that can vary in an analysis without breaking any constraints.

Let's do some activity Give any five numbers Give any five numbers whose sum is 25 Give any five numbers and out of five one number should be 3 and sum of all numbers is 25
NOTE DOWN YOUR OBSERVATIONS IN THE FREEDOM YOU GET IN EACH CASE

The degrees of freedom for different test differs as it depends on the number of restriction imposed & applicable in a specific test. For example in case of t-test it is N_1-1 from group one and

N_2-1 from group two, so in all it is N-2.

Level of Significance

In Statistics, 'significance' means 'not by chance' or 'probably true'. We can say that if a statistician declares that some result is 'highly significant', then she indicates by stating that it might be very probably true. Whether a difference is to be taken as statistically significant depends upon the probability that the given difference could have arisen 'by chance'. When a finding is significant, it's simply means you can feel confident that it's real, not that you just got by chance. Before a judgment of significant or nonsignificant is made, some critical point or points must be designated along the probability scale which will serve to separate these two judgment categories. It must be stressed that judgments concerning differences are range over a scale of probability. The confidence level increases as the chances of a wrong judgment decreases. The 0.05 and 0.01 levels are most often used. The confidence with which an experimenter rejects/ retains a null hypothesis depends upon the level of significance adopted. The relationship between level of significance and level of confidence is depicted in the Figure 14.2.

The confidence with which an experimenter rejects-or retains-a null hypothesis depends upon the level of significance adopted. For example if the researcher compare the cultural competence of nurses working in private & government hospitals found that the t value obtained is greater than the tabulated t value at 0.01 level, then she will reject the null hypothesis at 0.01 level and with 99% confidence. It can be explained in a common man's language that if one repeats a study 100 times in a same population, 99 times the results will be same. It is only one time the result may differ. The 0.01 level of significance is more exact than the 0.05 level.

One tailed & two tailed test

A one-tailed test is a statistical test in which the critical area of a distribution is one-sided so that it is either greater than or less than a certain value, but not both. If the sample being tested falls into the one-sided critical area, the alternative hypothesis will be accepted instead of the null hypothesis. In case of experimental research, when the researcher intend to improve situation, the directional hypothesis is formulated (Fig. 14.3).

Fig. 14.2: Level of significance & level of confidence

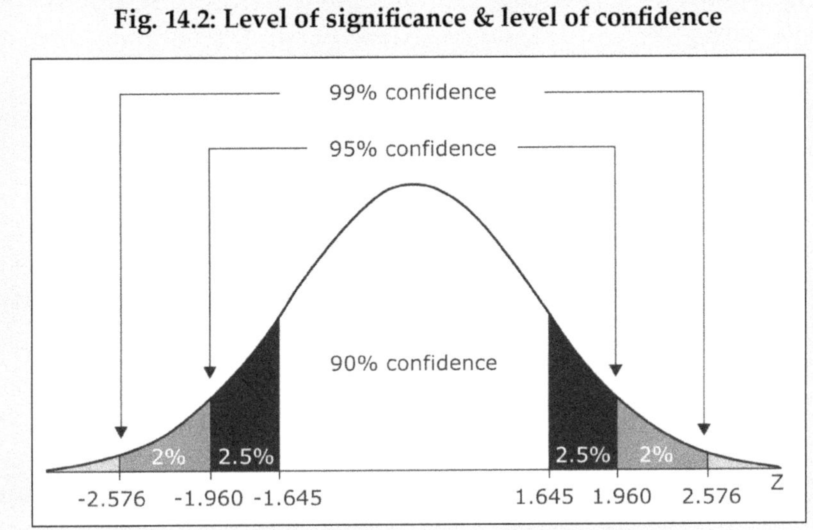

Level of significant and Level of confidence

Level of significance			Level of confidence	
0.01	1%	→	99%	0.99
0.05	5%	→	95%	0.95
0.10	10%	→	90%	0.90

Fig. 14.3: One-tailed tests

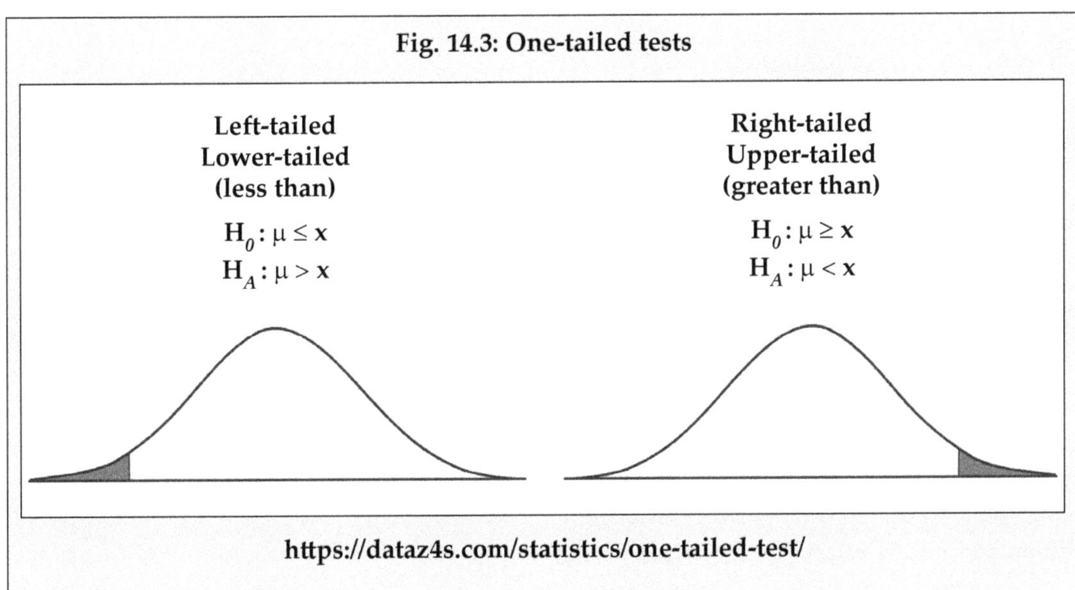

https://dataz4s.com/statistics/one-tailed-test/

When using a one-tailed test, one tests for the possibility of the relationship in one direction and completely disregard the possibility of a relationship in the other direction.

In statistics, a two-tailed test is a method in which the critical area of a distribution is two-sided and tests whether a sample is greater or less than a range of values. It is used in null-hypothesis testing and testing for statistical significance. If the sample being tested falls into either of the critical areas, the alternative hypothesis is accepted instead of the null hypothesis.

Type I & Type II error

Inferential analysis is about drawing conclusion and the researcher takes the decision of accepting or rejecting null hypothesis. In statistics, a Type I error is a false positive conclusion, while a Type II error is a false negative conclusion. Type I error is the false rejection of the null hypothesis and type II error is the false acceptance of the null hypothesis.

Type I error – occurs when researcher rejects H_0 when it is true

Type II error - occurs when researcher accepts H_0 when it is false

Example: Type I vs Type II error

You decide to get tested for COVID-19 based on mild symptoms. There are two errors that could potentially occur:

Type I error (false positive): the test result says you have coronavirus, but you actually don't.

Type II error (false negative): the test result says you don't have coronavirus, but you actually do.

In research when the researcher lower down the level of significance and reject the null hypothesis then the error occur is Type I, on the other hand the researcher maintains the high level of significance for rejecting the null hypothesis then the error occur is Type II. This type II error helps to maintain the standards so in a way it is beneficial to the field. The diagrammatic representation is given below.

Parametric & Non Parametric Tests

The researcher need to make a decision about the test to be used for the data analysis so that appropriate inferences can be drawn. There are two types of

Fig. 14.4: Type I & Type II errors

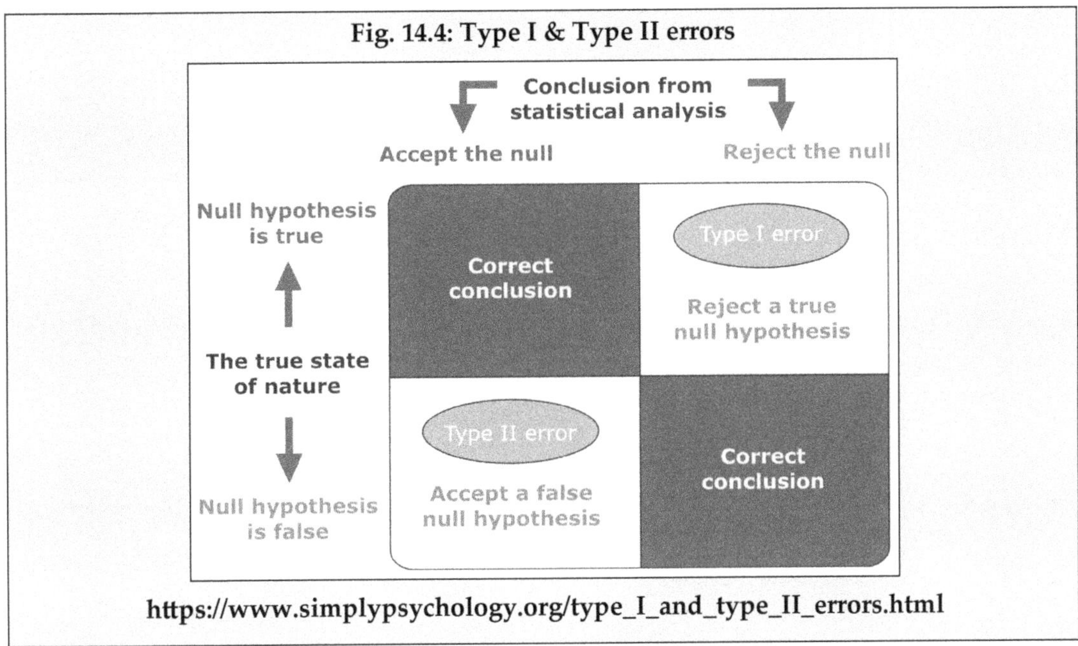

https://www.simplypsychology.org/type_I_and_type_II_errors.html

tests that can be used however there are few conditions the data need to follow to use the parametric test. If it does not fulfil any condition then one has to go for non-parametric test.

A parameter in statistics refers to an aspect of a population, while statistic refers to an aspect about a sample. For example, the population mean is a parameter, while the sample mean is a statistic. A parametric statistical test makes an assumption about the population parameters on the basis of sample. In other words, generalization of results to population that are drawn on sample.

When to use Parametric Tests

- When the sample is distributed normally
- When the variable measured are in interval or ratio scale
- When the observations are independent
- When the population have nearly same variance
- When the sample size is more than 30

Non-parametric Test

Non-parametric test are also known as distribution-free test. It is considered less powerful as it uses less information in its calculation and makes fewer assumption about the data set.

When non-parametric Tests are used?

- When the study is better represented by the median
- When the data has no normal distribution
- When the data is in ordinal or ranked form
- When the sample size is very small (less than 30)
- When the measurement scale used is nominal or ordinal

There are many tests available but the commonly used are indicated in the following figure.

Fig. 14.5
Calculated value of your data (t, F, r) Tabulated value of the concerned statistics Compare obtained value with tabulated value Make decision about rejection of hypothesis
https://keydifferences.com/difference-between-parametric-and-nonparametric-test.html

Fig. 14.6
If your obtained value is greater than tabulated value then reject null hypothesis (Rejection at 0.01 or 0.05 level) If your obtained value is less than tabulated value at 0.05 level then accept (retain) null hypothesis THE ACCEPTANCE & REJECTION OF NULL HYPOTHESIS DEPENDS ON YOUR LEVEL OF SIGNIFICANCE
https://keydifferences.com/difference-between-parametric-and-nonparametric-test.html

Let us understand few basic tests that are commonly used by the researchers

t-test:

It is a parametric test. The t-test is a type of inferential statistic used to determine if there is a significant difference between the means of two groups.

Calculating a t-test requires three key data values. The mean values of each group, the standard deviation of each group, and the number of data values of each group.

There are different types of t-test that can be performed depending on the data, research method and type of analysis required.

Formula for calculating t test (for Descriptive studies)

$$t = \frac{(X_1 - X_2)}{\sqrt{\frac{(S_1)^2}{n_1} + \frac{(S_2)^2}{n_2}}}$$

Where

X1 = Mean of first group n_1 = Size of first group

X2 = Mean of second group n_2 = Size of second group

S1 = SD of first group

S2 = SD of second group

For example: The null hypothesis stated by the researcher is as follows.

Ho: The null hypothesis states that there is no significant difference in the money

Planning ability of boys and girls.

The calculated values are displayed in a following table

Table 14.4: Gender difference in money planning ability of students

Gender	N	Mean	S.D.	't'	L.O.S.
Boys	274	42.00	5.65	4.11	0.01
Girls	178	44.55	6.05		
Total	452				

Interpretation

To interpret, the researcher will calculate df that is 452-2= 450. Enter in a Table of t test and check the value against in the Table. The sample is large and the researcher observe that the Table value of t is 2.58 at 0.01 level.

The obtained value is 4.11 that is greater than the tabulated value at 0.01 level, therefore the null hypothesis is rejected at 0.01 level. It means that there is a significant difference in the money planning ability of boys and girls. To understand who is having better money planning ability, look at the mean value (also note this tool measures higher is the value better is the money planning ability).

Conclusion

There is a significant difference in the money planning ability of boys and girls. The mean value indicates that the girls are found to be higher on money planning ability as compared to boys.

t -Test (Experimental study)

In some of the experimental studies a single group is tested in two different conditions & the observations are in pair. In these conditions, a modified formula of standard error of the difference of means is used. Therefore the formula for testing of the difference of two means of large correlated samples (sample more than 30) is as follows.

Sample 1 is pre-test and sample 2 is post test scores if you are using pre experimental single group pre test post-test design.

Example: The test on vocabulary is administered to student and the intervention strategy is used to enhance the vocabulary, so after intervention programme again the test is administered and the difference in pre and post is studied.

H_0: There is no significant difference in the pre and post test scores on vocabulary of students

Table 14.5: The following is the statistics obtained

Statistics	Pre-test	Post-test
Mean	52.5	58.7
SD (σ)	7.25	5.30
N	100	100
r	0.50	

$$t = \frac{M_1 - M_2}{\sqrt{\sigma M_1{}^2 + \sigma M_2{}^2\ 2r_{1.2}\sigma M_1\ \sigma M_2}}$$

Standard error of mean 1

$$\sigma M_1 = \frac{\sigma_1}{\sqrt{N_1}} = 7.25/\sqrt{100} = 7.25/10 = \mathbf{0.725}$$

Standard error of mean 2

$$\sigma M_2 = \frac{\sigma_2}{\sqrt{N_2}} = 5.30 / \sqrt{100} = 5.30 / 10 = \mathbf{0.53}$$

Correlation between pre & post test scores is 0.50

$$t = \frac{58.7 - 52.5}{\sqrt{(.725)\,2 + (0.53)\,2 - 2 \text{ X } 0.50 \text{ X}.725 \text{ X}.53}}$$

$$t = 9.54$$

Interpretation

To interpret, the researcher will calculate df that is 100-2=98. Enter in a Table of t test and check the value against in the table. The sample is large and the researcher observe that the Table value of t is 2.63 at 0.01 level.

The obtained value is 9.54 that is greater than the tabulated value at 0.01 level, therefore the null hypothesis is rejected at 0.01 level. It means that there is a significant difference in the vocabulary of students after the intervention programme. The mean score of post-test is higher than pre-test. It means the intervention programme is found to be effective to enhance the vocabulary of students.

Conclusion

There is a significant difference in the money planning ability of boys and girls. The mean value indicates that the girls are found to be higher on money planning ability as compared to boys.

Formula for t test (Pre-test-post -test design):

$$t = \frac{M1\text{-}M2}{\sqrt{\sigma M_1^{\,2} + \sigma M_2^{\,2} - 2r\,1.2\,\sigma M1\,\sigma M2}}$$

F-test (ANOVA) One way ANOVA

One way Analysis of Variance (ANOVA)

Analysis of Variance (ANOVA) is a statistical method used to test differences between means of more than two groups.

It helps to understand the difference within group and between groups.

The calculation of df depends on the number of conditions put (Number of groups and sample). (K-1) & (N-1) where k= number of groups.

Example: The null hypothesis states that there is no significant difference in financial literacy (FL) of the secondary school students on the basis of parental income. The following Table shows the necessary statistics for ANOVA.

Table 14.6 Statistics for fl on the basis of income

Statistics	25000 Below	25000- 50000	50000 –1, 00, 000	1, 00, 000 Above
N	39	153	126	63
Mean	115.79	125.87	131.99	136.29
SD	14.54	16.01	18.92	18.60

Table 14.7: Anova For Fl On The Basis Of Income

Sources of variance	df	SS	MSS	F ratio
Among the means of groups	3	13521.09	4507.3	18.76
Within groups	377	90529.42	240.1311	
Total	380	104050.5	4747.43	

From table F, for df = (3, 377) Critical F ratio at 0.05 level is = 2.63 and at 0.01 level is 3.83 The obtained F is = 18.76 which is greater than 4.63. This indicates that F s significant at 0.01 level and thus null hypothesis is rejected. **If the null hypothesis is rejected, further t-test is applied to test whether individual group differs from each other.**

Non-Parametric test

Chi-square test

Chi-square test is used to determine whether there is a statistically significant difference between the expected frequencies and the observed frequencies in one or more categories. It is used when the data is given in frequencies/ categories.

$$\chi^2 = \sum \frac{(f_O - f_E)^2}{f_E}$$

f_o = Observed frequencies

f_E = Expected frequencies

Example: There is no significant difference in the opinion of the people regarding introduction of grading system in schools

Table 14.8

Category of response	fo	fe	fo-fe	fo-fe ^{2}	fo-fe ^{2}/fe
Yes	13	20	-7	49	49/20 = 2.45
No	27	20	7	49	49/20 = 2.45
Indifferent	20	20	0	0	
Total	60	60			**4.90**

The obtained value of chi is to be compared with the Table value

df = (r-1) X (c-1)   LOS at 0.05–5.99

= (3-1) x (2-1)   LOS at 0.01–9.21

= (2) x (1)

= 2

The obtained value of chi is 4.90 that is less than the tabulated value at 0.05 level, therefore the null hypothesis is accepted.

Wilcoxon Signed Rank Test

Another popular nonparametric test for matched or paired data is called the Wilcoxon Signed Rank Test. Like the Sign Test, it is based on difference scores, but in addition to analysing the signs of the differences, it also takes into account the magnitude of the observed differences.

A researcher wants to assess the effectiveness of a new drug designed to reduce repetitive behaviors in children with autism. A total of 8 children with autism are involved in the study and the amount of time that each child is engaged in repetitive behavior during three hour observation periods are measured both before treatment and then again after taking the new medication for a period of 1 week. The data are shown below (Table 14.9).

Table 14.9

Child	Before Treatment	After 1 Week of Treatment
1	85	75
2	70	50
3	40	50
4	65	40
5	80	20
6	75	65
7	55	40
8	20	25

First, we compute difference scores for each child (Table 14.10).

Table 14.10

Child	Before Treatment	After 1 Week of Treatment	Difference
1	85	75	10
2	70	50	20
3	40	50	-10
4	65	40	25
5	80	20	60
6	75	65	10
7	55	40	15
8	20	25	-5

The next step is to rank the difference scores. Order the absolute values of the difference scores and assign rank from 1 through n to the smallest through largest absolute values of the difference scores, and assign the mean rank when there are ties in the absolute values of the difference scores (Table 14.11).

Table 14.11

Difference	Ordered absolute values of the difference	Rank
10	-5	1
20	10	3
-10	10	3
25	-10	3
60	15	5
10	20	6
15	25	7
-5	60	8

The final step is to attach the signs ("+" or "-") of the observed differences to each rank as shown below (Table 14.12).

Table 14.12

Difference	Ordered absolute values of the difference	Rank	Signed rank
10	-5	1	-1
20	10	3	3
-10	10	3	3
25	-10	3	-3
60	15	5	5
10	20	6	6
15	25	7	7
-5	60	8	8

The test statistic for the Wilcoxon Signed Rank Test is W, defined as the smaller of W+ (sum of the positive ranks) and W- (sum of the negative ranks). If the null hypothesis is true, we expect to see similar numbers of lower and higher ranks that are both positive and negative (i.e., W+ and W- would be similar). If the research hypothesis is true we expect to see more higher and positive ranks (in this example, more children with substantial improvement in repetitive behavior after treatment as compared to before, i.e., W+ much larger than W-).

In this example, W+ = 32 and W- = 4. Recall that the sum of the ranks (ignoring the signs) will always equal n (n+1)/2.In this example n=8, we have n (n+1)/2 = 8 (9)/2 = 36 which is equal to 32+4. The test statistic is W = 4.

Next we must determine whether the observed test statistic W supports the null or research hypothesis. This is done following the same approach used in parametric testing. Specifically, we determine a critical value of W such that if the observed value of W is less than or equal to the critical value, we reject H0 in favor of H1, and if the observed value of W exceeds the critical value, we do not reject H0.

To determine the appropriate one-sided critical value we need sample size (n=8) and our one-sided level of significance (α=0.05). For this example, the critical value of W is 6 and the decision rule is to reject H0 if W < 6. Thus, we reject H0, because 4 < 6. We have statistically significant evidence at α =0.05, to show that the median difference is positive (i.e., that repetitive behavior improves.)

Understanding association of variables

The correlation coefficient is a statistical measure of the strength of the relationship between the two variables and is widely used by the researcher Pearson's Coefficient of Correlation

The Pearson product-moment correlation coefficient (or Pearson correlation coefficient, for short) is a measure of the strength of a linear association between two variables and is denoted by r.

Correlation coefficients are used to measure how strong a relationship is between two variables.

It expresses the extent to which change in one variable are accompanied by changes in other variable.

It varies from -1 (indicating perfect negative correlation) to + 1 (indicating perfect positive correlation).

If coefficient of correlation is zero, it indicates zero correlation between variables.

$$r = \frac{N\Sigma xy - (\Sigma x)(\Sigma y)}{\sqrt{[N\Sigma x^2 - (\Sigma x)^2][N\Sigma y^2 - (\Sigma y)^2]}}$$

Spearman rank order correlation

The Spearman rank correlation is used to test the association between two ranked variables that exists between two variables measured on at least an ordinal scale.

$$R = 1 - \frac{6\Sigma d^2}{n(n^2 - 1)}$$

Where

$d = |R_1 - R_2|$

$\Rightarrow$ d = Difference in the ranks

We are interested in correlating the undergraduate marks and performance in the entrance test. We have a data of 10 individuals. But we only have ranks of these individuals in undergraduate examination, and merit list of the entrance performance. We want to find the correlation between rank in undergraduate examination and rank in entrance using spearman rho.

Table 14.13

Student	Undergraduate exam rank (X)	Entrance exam (Y)
A	1	4
B	5	6
C	3	2
D	6	7
E	9	10
F	2	1
G	4	3
H	10	9
I	8	8
J	7	5

List the names/serial number of subjects (students, in this case) in column

Write the scores of each subject on X variable (undergraduate examination in the column labeled as X (column 2), and write the scores of each subject on Y variable (Entrance test) in the column labeled as Y (column 3).

Rank the scores of X variable in ascending order. Give rank 1 to the lowest score, 2 to the next lowest score, and so on.

Table 14.14

Student	Undergraduate exam rank (X)	Entrance exam (Y)	Rx	Ry	D= Rx- Ry	D^2
A	1	4	1	4	-3	0
B	5	6	5	6	-1	1
C	3	2	3	2	1	1
D	6	7	6	7	-1	1
E	9	10	9	10	-1	1
F	2	1	2	1	1	1
G	4	3	4	3	1	1
H	10	9	10	9	1	1
I	8	8	8	8	0	0
J	7	5	7	5	2	4
n = 10						$\Sigma D^2 = 20$

Putting the values in the above formula
$= 1 - 6 \times 20/10\ (10^2-1)$
$= 1 - 180/990$
rho = 0.818

The value of rho is positive. It shows that the correlation between the rank in undergraduate examination & rank in entrance test is positive. The value is very close to 1.00 which indicates that the strength of association between the two set of rank is very high. The relationship should be interpreted considering the three aspects level of significance (refer Table for r), sign interpretation and the magnitude of association is as given below.

Table: 14.15

Range	Magnitude
+/- 0.00 to +/- 0.20	Negligible
+/- 0.21 to +/- 0.40	Low
+/- 0.41 to +/- 0.60	Moderate
+/- 0.61 to +/- 0.80	High
+/- 0.81 to +/- 1.00	Very high

Example: The null hypothesis states that there is no significant relationship between metacognition and achievement motivation of students.

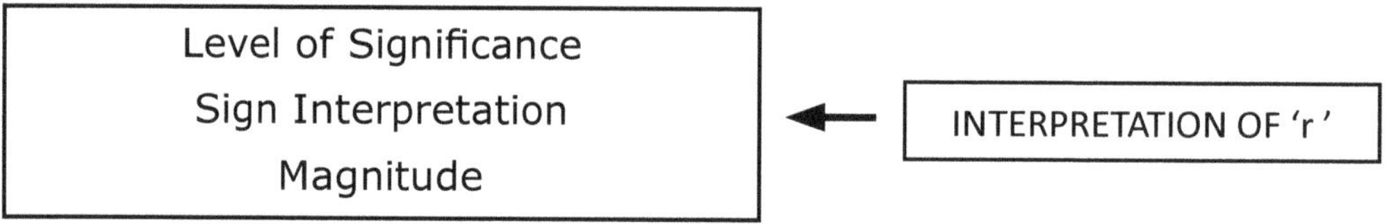

Table 14.16: Significance of 'r' For MC and AM of Students

N	df	r	l.o.s
259	257	0.924	0.01

Interpretation of 'r': The obtained 'r' for df 257 is 0.924 that is greater than the tabulated r at 0.01 level =0.115, Thus the null hypothesis is rejected at 0.01 level of significance. There is a significant relationship between metacognition and achievement motivation of students.

Conclusion: The coefficient of correlation between metacognition and achievement motivation of students is 0.924, which is positive, very high in magnitude and significant at 0.01 level. This implies that if the scores of metacognition of students is higher, then their scores of achievement motivation is likely to be higher.

Meta-analysis

Meta-analysis is a quantitative approach for systematically combining results of previous research to arrive at conclusions about the body of research. Quantitative: numbers

Systematic: methodical

Combining: putting together

Previous research: what is already done?

Conclusions: new knowledge

A study collects data from individual subjects (such as 100 subjects = 100 "data points")

A meta-analysis collects data from individual studies (such as 100 studies = 100 "data points")

Steps In Meta-Analysis (Fig. 14.12)

1. Define the research question and specific hypotheses
2. Define the criteria for including and excluding studies
3. Locate research studies
4. Determine which studies are eligible for inclusion
5. Classify and code important study characteristics (e.g., sample size; length of follow-up; definition of outcome; drug brand and dose)
6. Select or translate results from each study using a common metric
7. Aggregate findings across studies, generating weighted pooled estimates of effect size.
8. Evaluate the statistical homogeneity of pooled studies
9. Perform sensitivity analyses to assess the impact of excluding or down-weighting unpublished studies, studies of lower quality, out-of-date studies, etc.

Meta-analysis can be used as a guide to answer the question 'does what we are doing make a difference to X? 'even if 'X' has been measured using different instruments across a range of different people.

Meta-analysis provides a systematic overview of quantitative research which has examined a particular question.

Fig. 14.5: Steps in Meta-analysis

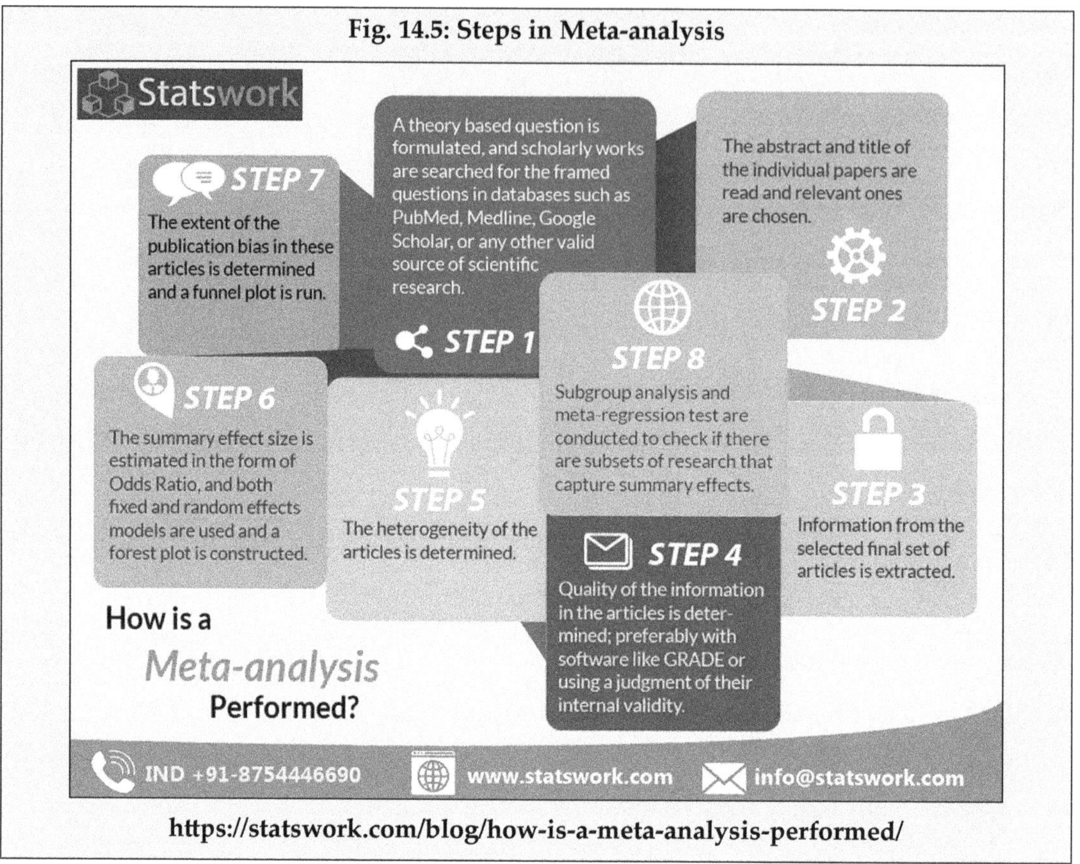

https://statswork.com/blog/how-is-a-meta-analysis-performed/

Meta-analysis has been used to give helpful insight into the effectiveness of interventions strategies, used in different fields (e.g. Psychotherapy, outdoor education), effect of independent variables and other strength of relationship between variables.

In statistics, a meta-analysis combines the results of several studies that address a set of related research hypotheses. This is normally done by identification of a common measure of effect size, which is modelled using a form of Meta regression.

Meta Synthesis

Meta-analysis is a quantitative, formal, epidemiological study design used to systematically assess the results of previous research to derive conclusions about that body of research. The study is based on randomized, controlled clinical trials. Meta-synthesis attempts to integrate results from a number of different but inter-related qualitative studies. The technique has an interpretative, rather than aggregating, intent, in contrast to meta-analysis of quantitative studies. Qualitative syntheses are now recognized as valuable tools for examining participants' meanings, experiences, and perspectives, both deeply (because of the qualitative approach) and broadly (because of the integration of studies from different healthcare contexts and participants).

According to Screiber et al. (1997, p.314), a metasynthesis "is bringing together and breaking down of findings, examining them, discovering essential features and, in some way, combining phenomena into a transformed whole" In basic terms, a meta-synthesis is the 'bringing together' of Qualitative data to form a new interpretation of the research field.

Fig. 14.6: Steps in Meta-synthesis

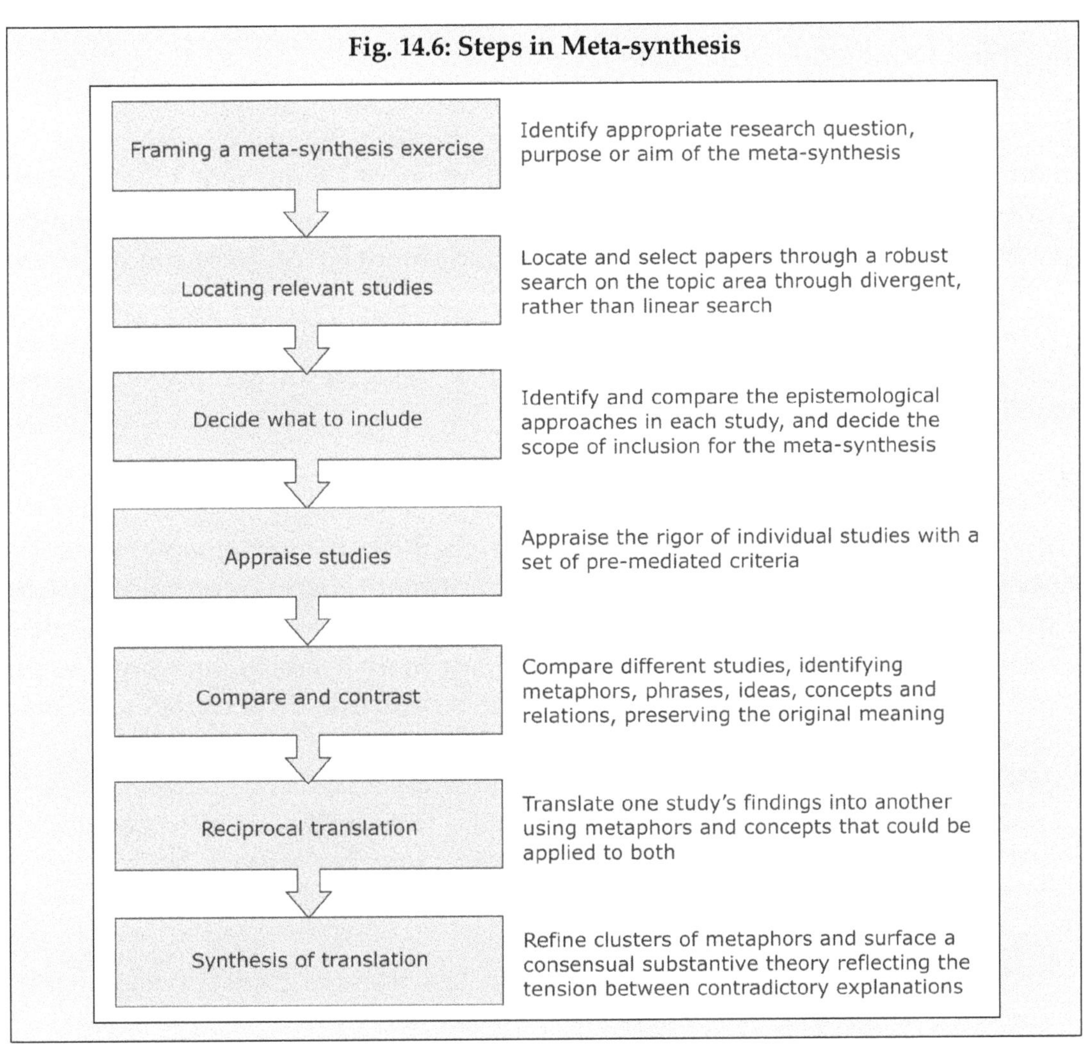

t-test

It is a parametric test. The t-test is a type of inferential statistic used to determine if there is a significant difference between the means of two groups.

F-test Or Analysis of Variance (ANOVA)

It is a parametric test. The F-test is a type of inferential statistic used to determine if there is a significant difference between the means of three or more groups.

Chi-square test: It is non parametric test & used to determine whether there is a statistically significant difference between the expected frequencies and the observed frequencies in one or more categories. It is used when the data is given in frequencies/categories.

Wilcoxon Signed Rank Test: Another popular nonparametric test for matched or paired data is called the Wilcoxon Signed Rank Test. Like the Sign Test, it is based on difference scores, but in addition to analysing the signs of the differences, it also takes into account the magnitude of the observed differences.

The correlation coefficient: It is a statistical measure of the strength of the relationship between the two variables.

Pearson's Coefficient of Correlation

The Pearson product-moment correlation coefficient (or Pearson correlation coefficient, for short) is a measure of the strength of a linear association between two variables and is denoted by r. Correlation coefficients are used to measure strength of relationship between two variables. It expresses the extent to which change in one variable are accompanied by changes in other variable. It varies from -1 (indicating perfect negative correlation) to + 1 (indicating perfect positive correlation). If coefficient of correlation is zero, it indicates zero correlation between variables. The coefficient of correlation to be interpreted with Level of Significance, Sign Interpretation & Magnitude of relationship.

The Spearman rank correlation is used to test the association between two ranked variables that exists between two variables measured on at least an ordinal scale.

Meta-analysis: It is a quantitative approach for systematically combining results of previous research to arrive at conclusions about the body of research. Quantitative: numbers, Systematic: Methodical, Combining: putting together, Previous research: what is already done, & Conclusions: new knowledge.

A study collects data from individual subjects (such as 100 subjects = 100 "data points").

A meta-analysis collects data from individual studies (such as 100 studies = 100 "data points").

Meta Synthesis

Meta-analysis is a quantitative, formal, epidemiological study design used to systematically assess the results of previous research to derive conclusions about that body of research. The study is based on randomized, controlled clinical trials. Meta-synthesis attempts to integrate results from a number of different but inter-related qualitative studies. The technique has an interpretative, rather than aggregating, intent, in contrast to meta-analysis of quantitative studies.

- **Data Analysis softwares** - Traditionally research data was handled manually involving laborious work. It was very much time consuming. Presently several computer packages are available, which can be used for statistical analysis in quantitative & qualitative research studies. There are a large numbers of tools used in health science research. These tools get the job done in similar ways, but differences lie in ease of use & presentation as differences in licensing, interface & cost. These tools handle the processes like collecting, organizing, analysing & interpreting statistical data. There are top ten tools used by various researchers. These are - **STATA, R, GRAPHPAD PRISM, SAS, IBM SPSS, MATLAB, JMP, MINITAB, STATISTICA,** EXCEL. (kolabtree.com/blog/top-10-statistical-tools-used in medical research cited on 2021-July-9)
- **SPSS** - Originally known as Statistical Package for Social Sciences, developed in 1960 at Stanford University. It is made & sold by IBM. It is comprehensive, flexible & can be used with almost any type of data file. It can be used to generate tabulated reports, charts, as well as generate descriptive statistics such as means, medians, modes & frequencies. In addition to more complex statistical analyses like regression models. It is also simple & easy to enter & edit data directly into program. Its

drawback is the limit on numbers of cases one can analyse (thought.com/ quantitative.analysis-softwarereview-3026539 cited on 2021-7-9). More information is available about it at the website www.spss.com.

- **SAS** - The Statistical Analysis System is developed by North Carolina State University. This system contains a very large variety of statistical methods. The more useful components of SAS are BASE SAS, SAS/STAT, SAS/GRAPH etc. More information about it is available at the website www.sas.com.
- **Minitab** - This package is designed to use it for teaching of statistical methods by using computer. It is very user friendly product. To get more information about it one need to visit the website www.minitab.com.
- **Ms Excel**- is very popular & useful spreadsheet program that can be used for data entry & analysis. It has a capacity to generate random numbers, & it can be used for the computation of many standard statistical applications like computation of mean, range, standard deviation etc. There are certain problems in the algorithms of some version of this program so it is better to use other packages like spss or sas for analysis purpose.
- There are **qualitative data analysis softwares** also available which help in the form of explanation, understanding or interpretation of the people & situations to help in the meaningful & symbolic content of qualitative data. The data in qualitative research can be analysed using some of the special soft wares as QSR'Sn6 & NVitro, WEFTQDA, Atlasti, Hyperresearch2.6.
- Discussion of findings, recommendations & summary - can be typed

SUMMARY

The main question the researcher should ask to whom you want to generalize the findings. The researcher selects sample, collect data and analyse it. The finding are drawn on the basis of sample and then generalize result to the population. Inferential analysis are techniques that allow us to use the samples to make generalizations about the populations from which the samples were drawn.

The word "inferential" is used because investigators and statisticians use data from samples to make inferences about the population-as-a-whole.

In short inferential analysis help

To generalise the findings to population

To compare the attribute

To establish cause effect relationship

To predict the parameters in population

To provide information for designing strategies to overcome the problem/ situation (Policy formation)

There are various statistical tests that are used for the data analysis. There are parametric and non-parametric tests that can be used for inferential analysis. The various terms are associated with inferential statistics.

The standard error of mean is the standard deviation of the sample distribution. The sample mean of a data is generally varied from the actual population mean. It is represented as SE. It is used to measure the amount of accuracy by which the given sample represents its population.

Degrees of Freedom refers to the maximum number of logically independent values that have the freedom to vary, in the data set.

In Statistics, 'significance' means 'not by chance' or 'probably true'. We can say that if a statistician declares that some result is 'highly significant', then she indicates by stating that it might be very probably true. The 0.01 & 0.05 are the level of significance commonly used. The confidence with which an experimenter rejects-or retains-a null hypothesis depends upon the level of significance adopted.

A one-tailed test is a statistical test in which the critical area of a distribution is one-sided so that it is either greater than or less than a certain value, but not both. If the sample being tested falls into the one-sided critical area, the alternative hypothesis will be accepted instead of the null hypothesis. In case of experimental research, when the researcher intend to improve situation, the directional hypothesis is formulated. A two-tailed test is a method in which the critical area of a distribution is two-sided. It is used in null-hypothesis testing and testing for statistical significance. If the sample being tested falls into either of the critical areas, the alternative hypothesis is accepted instead of the null hypothesis. In statistics, a Type I error is a false positive conclusion, while a Type II error is a false negative conclusion. Type I error is the false rejection of the null hypothesis and type II error is the false acceptance of the null hypothesis.

BIBLIOGRAPHY

- Kerlinger, F.N. (1986) Foundations of Behavioral research (third edition). New York: Holt, Rinehart & Winston
- Vockell E.& Asher J. (1995) Educational Research. New Jersey:Englewood cliff
- Wiersma, W. (1995) Research Methods in Education. Massachusetts: Allyn & Bacon.
- http://sphweb.bumc.bu.edu/otlt/MPHModules/BS/BS704_BiostatisticsBasics/BS704_BiostatisticsBasics2.html#
- https://www.statisticshowto.com/probability-and-statistics/hypothesis-testing/one-tailed-test-or-two/
- https://sphweb.bumc.bu.edu/otlt/mph-modules/bs/bs704_nonparametric/BS704_Nonparametric6.html
- https://www.statstutor.ac.uk/resources/uploaded/wilcoxonsignedranktest.pdf
- https://www.slideshare.net/RandelRoyRaluto/meta-synthesis

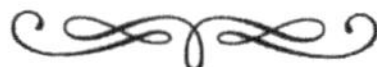

ANNEXURE

1 Evaluation Criteria of Research Report/Dissertition

1. **The problem Statement of the Study, Objectives & Hypotheses.**
   - Introduction : Interesting, relevance to study
   - The Problem Statement/question (well framed includes research area, setting, population and reflects the methodology)
   - Need for Study – supporting study with Primary & recent Sources of Literature and the researchers personal perspective why the need is felt by researcher
   - Objectives - relevance to study, clarity, specific & precise
   - Hypotheses - statistical, research - relevance to study, clarity
   - Permission letter from Institutional Ethical Committee
2. **Review of Literature**
   - Depth, Use of Primary Sources & Recent
   - Organization of the Literature Review
   - Adequate & Relevant to study
   - Inclusion of Studies from Nursing Literature
   - Appropriate use of referencing style.
3. **Conceptual/Theoretical Framework**
   - Use of Theory relevant to study Objectives, Hypotheses
   - Identifies /reflects the major Variables of the study
   - Relationship between Variables clearly identified
4. **Research Approach & Design**
   - Suitable to study
   - Control of factors affecting Internal & External Validity of Study
   - Control of Extraneous Variables
5. **Study Setting**
   - Selection justifying adequate availability of Sample
   - Availability of other Resources required for Study

6. **Sampling Process**
   - Identification of Target & Accessible Population
   - Description of Inclusion & Exclusion Criteria
   - Type of Sampling selected for Study
   - Sample size calculation : use of sources & formula
7. **Data Collection : Plan & Procedure**
   - Tool/Instrument used : Appropriateness
   - Self prepared or use of Standard/available tool
   - Prior permission for use of tool prepared by others
   - Detail description of tool
   - Description of Validity & Reliability of tool
   - Description of Pilot Study
   - Plan for Data Collection
   - Description of Actual Data Collection Procedure
8. **Data Analysis & Interpretation**
   - Organization of Data
   - Use of Descriptive & Inferential Analysis : Use of Appropriate Statistical Tests
   - Description of tests used
   - Tables & Graphs used
     - Clear Table titles
   - **Interpretations**
     - Addressing hypothesis
     - Level of probability & significance specified
     - Results are discussed with support from previous studies
9. **Summary & Recommendations to Nursing Practice/Education/Administration**
   - In Summary major findings are highlighted; Limitation if identified declared by the researcher, experience of the researcher end of the study.
10. **Abstract of the Study, References, Bibliography & Annexures**
    - Relevant & follows recommended style given by the institution.
11. **Overall Report**
    - Follows prescribed Standards & Principles

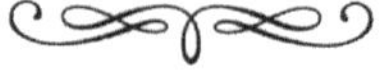

ANNEXURE

2 Journal Club Activity & Critiquing

Journal club presentations provide a forum through which the healthcare professionals/post-graduate learners of healthcare professionals get familiar with new developments in a particular field & engage in informal discussion & interaction. It also helps in developing presentation skills & mastering the ability to critically evaluate the research study. This is one of the learning experiences provided to postgraduate candidates in nursing.

Definition - An activity carried out by a group of individuals that meet to discuss & critique research that appears in professional journals.

Aim- A Journal club is aimed at improving the skills of critically appraising the journal article.

Practical tips in starting Journal Club

- Identification of purpose & goals.
- Identification of participants
- Development of guidelines for presentation
- Designating a leader who can plan journal club activity
- Deciding for length of meeting(not more than 60 minutes), venue & frequency of meeting
- Meeting agenda preparation

Contents to be included in Journal Club

- Introduction
- Brief information about author & journal
- Objectives & hypotheses
- Research approach & design
- Methodology

- Study results
- Discussion on implications to nursing practice/education/administration

Five steps to be followed by person who is presenting

- Get familiar with the research study to be presented
- Make presentation concise as per the above mentioned contents of journal club
- Simplify unfamiliar concepts
- Developing clarity about research study to be presented
- Developing questions for the members of journal club

Critiquing of Journal club presentation

The areas to be followed for critiquing are-

- Is there clear description of an introduction & problem statement?
- Are the objectives clearly stated & relevant to study?
- Are the hypotheses clearly stated & relevant to study?
- Is the literature review relevant & justifying need for study?
- Whether selection of research design & approach appropriate?
- Is the instrument used for data collection reliable & valid?
- What's the sampling size & characteristics of sample?
- Types of statistical tests used & appropriateness of the tests
- Are the conclusions appropriate & implications of the study to nursing practice, education & administration? Can study findings be generalized to the population from which sample is derived?

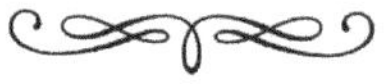

ANNEXURE

3 Critical Values for Pearson's Product-Moment Correlation (*r*)

n	α = **0.10**	α = **0.05**	α = **0.02**	α = **0.01**	*df*
3	0.988	0.997	0.9995	0.9999	1
4	0.900	0.950	0.980	0.990	2
5	0.805	0.8748	0.934	0.959	3
6	0.729	0.811	0.882	0.917	4
7	0.669	0.754	0.833	0.874	5
8	0.622	0.707	0.789	0.834	6
9	0.582	0.666	0.750	0.798	7
10	0.549	0.632	0.716	0.765	8
11	0.521	0.602	0.685	0.735	9
12	0.497	0.576	0.658	0.708	10
13	0.476	0.553	0.634	0.684	11
14	0.458	0.532	0.612	0.661	12
15	0.441	0.514	0.592	0.641	13
16	0.426	0.497	0.574	0.623	14
17	0.412	0.482	0.558	0.606	15
18	0.400	0.468	0.542	0.590	16
19	0.389	0.456	0.528	0.575	17
20	0.378	0.444	0.516	0.561	18
21	0.369	0.433	0.503	0.549	19
22	0.360	0.423	0.492	0.537	20
23	0.352	0.413	0.482	0.526	21
24	0.344	0.404	0.472	0.515	22
25	0.337	0.396	0.462	0.505	23
26	0.330	0.388	0.453	0.496	24
27	0.323	0.381	0.445	0.487	25

n	α = **0.10**	α = **0.05**	α = **0.02**	α = **0.01**	*df*
28	0.317	0.374	0.437	0.479	26
29	0.311	0.367	0.430	0.471	27
30	0.306	0.361	0.423	0.463	28
35	0.282	0.333	0.391	0.428	33
40	0.264	0.312	0.366	0.402	38
50	0.235	0.276	0.328	0.361	48
60	0.214	0.254	0.300	0.330	58
70	0.198	0.235	0.277	0.305	68
80	0.185	0.220	0.260	0.286	78
90	0.174	0.208	0.245	0.270	88
100	0.165	0.196	0.232	0.256	98
200	0.117	0.139	0.164	0.182	198
500	0.074	0.088	0.104	0.115	498
1000	0.052	0.062	0.074	0.081	998
10000	0.0164	0.0196	0.0233	0.0258	9998

* This table is abridged from Table 13 in *Biometrika Table for Statisticians*, Vol. 1, 2nd ed. New York: Cambridge, 1958. Edited by E.S. Pearson and H.O. Hartley. Reproduced with the kind permission of the editors and the trustees of Biometrika.

ANNEXURE

4 Statistical Tables

Table 4.1: Cumulative normal distribution
Table 4.2: Critical values of the t distribution
Table 4.3: Critical values of the F distribution
Table 4.4: Critical values of the chi-squared distribution

Table 4.1: Cumulative Standardized Normal Distribution

$A(z)$ is the integral of the standardized normal distribution from ∞–to z (in other words, the area under the curve to the left of z). It gives the probability of a normal random variable not being more than z standard deviations above its mean. Values of z of particular importance:

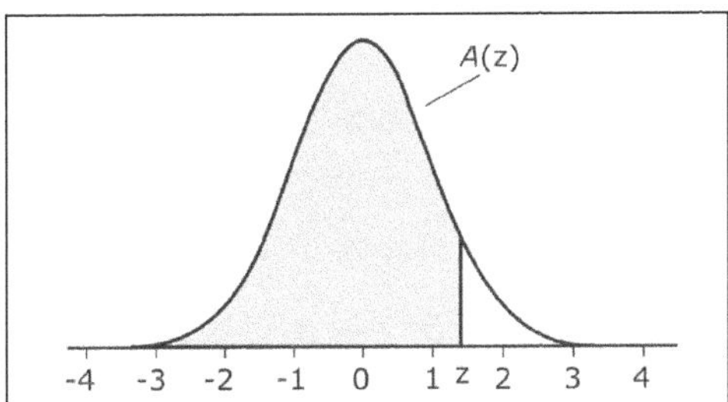

z	A(z)	
1.645	0.9500	Lower limit of right 5% tail
1.960	0.9750	Lower limit of right 2.5% tail
2.326	0.9900	Lower limit of right 1% tail
2.576	0.9950	Lower limit of right 0.5% tail
3.090	0.9990	Lower limit of right 0.1% tail
3.291	0.9995	Lower limit of right 0.05% tail

z	0.00	0.01	0.02	0.03	0.04	0.05	0.06	0.07	0.08	0.09
0.0	0.5000	0.5040	0.5080	0.5120	0.5160	0.5199	0.5239	0.5279	0.5319	0.5359
0.1	0.5398	0.5438	0.5478	0.5517	0.5557	0.5596	0.5636	0.5675	0.5714	0.5753
0.2	0.5793	0.5832	0.5871	0.5910	0.5948	0.5987	0.6026	0.6064	0.6103	0.6141
0.3	0.6179	0.6217	0.6255	0.6293	0.6331	0.6368	0.6406	0.6443	0.6480	0.6517
0.4	0.6554	0.6591	0.6628	0.6664	0.6700	0.6736	0.6772	0.6808	0.6844	0.6879
0.5	0.6915	0.6950	0.6985	0.7019	0.7054	0.7088	0.7123	0.7157	0.7190	0.7224
0.6	0.7257	0.7291	0.7324	0.7357	0.7389	0.7422	0.7454	0.7486	0.7517	0.7549
0.7	0.7580	0.7611	0.7642	0.7673	0.7704	0.7734	0.7764	0.7794	0.7823	0.7852
0.8	0.7881	0.7910	0.7939	0.7967	0.7995	0.8023	0.8051	0.8078	0.8106	0.8133

z	0.00	0.01	0.02	0.03	0.04	0.05	0.06	0.07	0.08	0.09
0.9	0.8159	0.8186	0.8212	0.8238	0.8264	0.8289	0.8315	0.8340	0.8365	0.8389
1.0	0.8413	0.8438	0.8461	0.8485	0.8508	0.8531	0.8554	0.8577	0.8599	0.8621
1.1	0.8643	0.8665	0.8686	0.8708	0.8729	0.8749	0.8770	0.8790	0.8810	0.8830
1.2	0.8849	0.8869	0.8888	0.8907	0.8925	0.8944	0.8962	0.8980	0.8997	0.9015
1.3	0.9032	0.9049	0.9066	0.9082	0.9099	0.9115	0.9131	0.9147	0.9162	0.9177
1.4	0.9192	0.9207	0.9222	0.9236	0.9251	0.9265	0.9279	0.9292	0.9306	0.9319
1.5	0.9332	0.9345	0.9357	0.9370	0.9382	0.9394	0.9406	0.9418	0.9429	0.9441
1.6	0.9452	0.9463	0.9474	0.9484	0.9495	0.9505	0.9515	0.9525	0.9535	0.9545
1.7	0.9554	0.9564	0.9573	0.9582	0.9591	0.9599	0.9608	0.9616	0.9625	0.9633
1.8	0.9641	0.9649	0.9656	0.9664	0.9671	0.9678	0.9686	0.9693	0.9699	0.9706
1.9	0.9713	0.9719	0.9726	0.9732	0.9738	0.9744	0.9750	0.9756	0.9761	0.9767
2.0	0.9772	0.9778	0.9783	0.9788	0.9793	0.9798	0.9803	0.9808	0.9812	0.9817
2.1	0.9821	0.9826	0.9830	0.9834	0.9838	0.9842	0.9846	0.9850	0.9854	0.9857
2.2	0.9861	0.9864	0.9868	0.9871	0.9875	0.9878	0.9881	0.9884	0.9887	0.9890
2.3	0.9893	0.9896	0.9898	0.9901	0.9904	0.9906	0.9909	0.9911	0.9913	0.9916
2.4	0.9918	0.9920	0.9922	0.9925	0.9927	0.9929	0.9931	0.9932	0.9934	0.9936
2.5	0.9938	0.9940	0.9941	0.9943	0.9945	0.9946	0.9948	0.9949	0.9951	0.9952
2.6	0.9953	0.9955	0.9956	0.9957	0.9959	0.9960	0.9961	0.9962	0.9963	0.9964
2.7	0.9965	0.9966	0.9967	0.9968	0.9969	0.9970	0.9971	0.9972	0.9973	0.9974
2.8	0.9974	0.9975	0.9976	0.9977	0.9977	0.9978	0.9979	0.9979	0.9980	0.9981
2.9	0.9981	0.9982	0.9982	0.9983	0.9984	0.9984	0.9985	0.9985	0.9986	0.9986
3.0	0.9987	0.9987	0.9987	0.9988	0.9988	0.9989	0.9989	0.9989	0.9990	0.9990
3.1	0.9990	0.9991	0.9991	0.9991	0.9992	0.9992	0.9992	0.9992	0.9993	0.9993
3.2	0.9993	0.9993	0.9994	0.9994	0.9994	0.9994	0.9994	0.9995	0.9995	0.9995
3.3	0.9995	0.9995	0.9995	0.9996	0.9996	0.9996	0.9996	0.9996	0.9996	0.9997
3.4	0.9997	0.9997	0.9997	0.9997	0.9997	0.9997	0.9997	0.9997	0.9997	0.9998
3.5	0.9998	0.9998	0.9998	0.9998	0.9998	0.9998	0.9998	0.9998	0.9998	0.9998
3.6	0.9998	0.9998	0.9999							

Table 4.2: *t* Distribution: Critical Values of *t*

		Significance level					
Degrees of freedom	Two-tailed test:	10%	5%	2%	1%	0.2%	0.1%
	One-tailed test:	5%	2.5%	1%	0.5%	0.1%	0.05%
1		6.314	12.706	31.821	63.657	318.309	636.619
2		2.920	4.303	6.965	9.925	22.327	31.599
3		2.353	3.182	4.541	5.841	10.215	12.924
4		2.132	2.776	3.747	4.604	7.173	8.610
5		2.015	2.571	3.365	4.032	5.893	6.869
6		1.943	2.447	3.143	3.707	5.208	5.959
7		1.894	2.365	2.998	3.499	4.785	5.408
8		1.860	2.306	2.896	3.355	4.501	5.041
9		1.833	2.262	2.821	3.250	4.297	4.781
10		1.812	2.228	2.764	3.169	4.144	4.587
11		1.796	2.201	2.718	3.106	4.025	4.437
12		1.782	2.179	2.681	3.055	3.930	4.318
13		1.771	2.160	2.650	3.012	3.852	4.221
14		1.761	2.145	2.624	2.977	3.787	4.140
15		1.753	2.131	2.602	2.947	3.733	4.073
16		1.746	2.120	2.583	2.921	3.686	4.015
17		1.740	2.110	2.567	2.898	3.646	3.965
18		1.734	2.101	2.552	2.878	3.610	3.922
19		1.729	2.093	2.539	2.861	3.579	3.883
20		1.725	2.086	2.528	2.845	3.552	3.850
21		1.721	2.080	2.518	2.831	3.527	3.819
22		1.717	2.074	2.508	2.819	3.505	3.792
23		1.714	2.069	2.500	2.807	3.485	3.768
24		1.711	2.064	2.492	2.797	3.467	3.745
25		1.708	2.060	2.485	2.787	3.450	3.725
26		1.706	2.056	2.479	2.779	3.435	3.707
27		1.703	2.052	2.473	2.771	3.421	3.690
28		1.701	2.048	2.467	2.763	3.408	3.674
29		1.699	2.045	2.462	2.756	3.396	3.659
30		1.697	2.042	2.457	2.750	3.385	3.646

		Significance level					
Degrees of freedom	Two-tailed test:	10%	5%	2%	1%	0.2%	0.1%
	One-tailed test:	5%	2.5%	1%	0.5%	0.1%	0.05%
32		1.694	2.037	2.449	2.738	3.365	3.622
34		1.691	2.032	2.441	2.728	3.348	3.601
36		1.688	2.028	2.434	2.719	3.333	3.582
38		1.686	2.024	2.429	2.712	3.319	3.566
40		1.684	2.021	2.423	2.704	3.307	3.551
42		1.682	2.018	2.418	2.698	3.296	3.538
44		1.680	2.015	2.414	2.692	3.286	3.526
46		1.679	2.013	2.410	2.687	3.277	3.515
48		1.677	2.011	2.407	2.682	3.269	3.505
50		1.676	2.009	2.403	2.678	3.261	3.496
60		1.671	2.000	2.390	2.660	3.232	3.460
70		1.667	1.994	2.381	2.648	3.211	3.435
80		1.664	1.990	2.374	2.639	3.195	3.416
90		1.662	1.987	2.368	2.632	3.183	3.402
100		1.660	1.984	2.364	2.626	3.174	3.390
120		1.658	1.980	2.358	2.617	3.160	3.373
150		1.655	1.976	2.351	2.609	3.145	3.357
200		1.653	1.972	2.345	2.601	3.131	3.340
300		1.650	1.968	2.339	2.592	3.118	3.323
400		1.649	1.966	2.336	2.588	3.111	3.315
500		1.648	1.965	2.334	2.586	3.107	3.310
600		1.647	1.964	2.333	2.584	3.104	3.307
∞		1.645	1.960	2.326	2.576	3.090	3.291

Table 4.3: *F* Distribution: Critical Values of *F* (5% significance level)

v_1 / v_2	1	2	3	4	5	6	7	8	9	10	12	14	16	18	20
1	161.45	199.50	215.71	224.58	230.16	233.99	236.77	238.88	240.54	241.88	243.91	245.36	246.46	247.32	248.01
2	18.51	19.00	19.16	19.25	19.30	19.33	19.35	19.37	19.38	19.40	19.41	19.42	19.43	19.44	19.45
3	10.13	9.55	9.28	9.12	9.01	8.94	8.89	8.85	8.81	8.79	8.74	8.71	8.69	8.67	8.66
4	7.71	6.94	6.59	6.39	6.26	6.16	6.09	6.04	6.00	5.96	5.91	5.87	5.84	5.82	5.80
5	6.61	5.79	5.41	5.19	5.05	4.95	4.88	4.82	4.77	4.74	4.68	4.64	4.60	4.58	4.56
6	5.99	5.14	4.76	4.53	4.39	4.28	4.21	4.15	4.10	4.06	4.00	3.96	3.92	3.90	3.87
7	5.59	4.74	4.35	4.12	3.97	3.87	3.79	3.73	3.68	3.64	3.57	3.53	3.49	3.47	3.44
8	5.32	4.46	4.07	3.84	3.69	3.58	3.50	3.44	3.39	3.35	3.28	3.24	3.20	3.17	3.15
9	5.12	4.26	3.86	3.63	3.48	3.37	3.29	3.23	3.18	3.14	3.07	3.03	2.99	2.96	2.94
10	4.96	4.10	3.71	3.48	3.33	3.22	3.14	3.07	3.02	2.98	2.91	2.86	2.83	2.80	2.77
11	4.84	3.98	3.59	3.36	3.20	3.09	3.01	2.95	2.90	2.85	2.79	2.74	2.70	2.67	2.65
12	4.75	3.89	3.49	3.26	3.11	3.00	2.91	2.85	2.80	2.75	2.69	2.64	2.60	2.57	2.54
13	4.67	3.81	3.41	3.18	3.03	2.92	2.83	2.77	2.71	2.67	2.60	2.55	2.51	2.48	2.46
14	4.60	3.74	3.34	3.11	2.96	2.85	2.76	2.70	2.65	2.60	2.53	2.48	2.44	2.41	2.39
15	4.54	3.68	3.29	3.06	2.90	2.79	2.71	2.64	2.59	2.54	2.48	2.42	2.38	2.35	2.33
16	4.49	3.63	3.24	3.01	2.85	2.74	2.66	2.59	2.54	2.49	2.42	2.37	2.33	2.30	2.28
17	4.45	3.59	3.20	2.96	2.81	2.70	2.61	2.55	2.49	2.45	2.38	2.33	2.29	2.26	2.23
18	4.41	3.55	3.16	2.93	2.77	2.66	2.58	2.51	2.46	2.41	2.34	2.29	2.25	2.22	2.19
19	4.38	3.52	3.13	2.90	2.74	2.63	2.54	2.48	2.42	2.38	2.31	2.26	2.21	2.18	2.16
20	4.35	3.49	3.10	2.87	2.71	2.60	2.51	2.45	2.39	2.35	2.28	2.22	2.18	2.15	2.12
21	4.32	3.47	3.07	2.84	2.68	2.57	2.49	2.42	2.37	2.32	2.25	2.20	2.16	2.12	2.10
22	4.30	3.44	3.05	2.82	2.66	2.55	2.46	2.40	2.34	2.30	2.23	2.17	2.13	2.10	2.07
23	4.28	3.42	3.03	2.80	2.64	2.53	2.44	2.37	2.32	2.27	2.20	2.15	2.11	2.08	2.05
24	4.26	3.40	3.01	2.78	2.62	2.51	2.42	2.36	2.30	2.25	2.18	2.13	2.09	2.05	2.03
25	4.24	3.39	2.99	2.76	2.60	2.49	2.40	2.34	2.28	2.24	2.16	2.11	2.07	2.04	2.01
26	4.22	3.37	2.98	2.74	2.59	2.47	2.39	2.32	2.27	2.22	2.15	2.09	2.05	2.02	1.99
27	4.21	3.35	2.96	2.73	2.57	2.46	2.37	2.31	2.25	2.20	2.13	2.08	2.04	2.00	1.97
28	4.20	3.34	2.95	2.71	2.56	2.45	2.36	2.29	2.24	2.19	2.12	2.06	2.02	1.99	1.96

v_1 / v_2	1	2	3	4	5	6	7	8	9	10	12	14	16	18	20
29	4.18	3.33	2.93	2.70	2.55	2.43	2.35	2.28	2.22	2.18	2.10	2.05	2.01	1.97	1.94
30	4.17	3.32	2.92	2.69	2.53	2.42	2.33	2.27	2.21	2.16	2.09	2.04	1.99	1.96	1.93
35	4.12	3.27	2.87	2.64	2.49	2.37	2.29	2.22	2.16	2.11	2.04	1.99	1.94	1.91	1.88
40	4.08	3.23	2.84	2.61	2.45	2.34	2.25	2.18	2.12	2.08	2.00	1.95	1.90	1.87	1.84
50	4.03	3.18	2.79	2.56	2.40	2.29	2.20	2.13	2.07	2.03	1.95	1.89	1.85	1.81	1.78
60	4.00	3.15	2.76	2.53	2.37	2.25	2.17	2.10	2.04	1.99	1.92	1.86	1.82	1.78	1.75
70	3.98	3.13	2.74	2.50	2.35	2.23	2.14	2.07	2.02	1.97	1.89	1.84	1.79	1.75	1.72
80	3.96	3.11	2.72	2.49	2.33	2.21	2.13	2.06	2.00	1.95	1.88	1.82	1.77	1.73	1.70
90	3.95	3.10	2.71	2.47	2.32	2.20	2.11	2.04	1.99	1.94	1.86	1.80	1.76	1.72	1.69
100	3.94	3.09	2.70	2.46	2.31	2.19	2.10	2.03	1.97	1.93	1.85	1.79	1.75	1.71	1.68
120	3.92	3.07	2.68	2.45	2.29	2.18	2.09	2.02	1.96	1.91	1.83	1.78	1.73	1.69	1.66
150	3.90	3.06	2.66	2.43	2.27	2.16	2.07	2.00	1.94	1.89	1.82	1.76	1.71	1.67	1.64
200	3.89	3.04	2.65	2.42	2.26	2.14	2.06	1.98	1.93	1.88	1.80	1.74	1.69	1.66	1.62
250	3.88	3.03	2.64	2.41	2.25	2.13	2.05	1.98	1.92	1.87	1.79	1.73	1.68	1.65	1.61
300	3.87	3.03	2.63	2.40	2.24	2.13	2.04	1.97	1.91	1.86	1.78	1.72	1.68	1.64	1.61
400	3.86	3.02	2.63	2.39	2.24	2.12	2.03	1.96	1.90	1.85	1.78	1.72	1.67	1.63	1.60
500	3.86	3.01	2.62	2.39	2.23	2.12	2.03	1.96	1.90	1.85	1.77	1.71	1.66	1.62	1.59
600	3.86	3.01	2.62	2.39	2.23	2.11	2.02	1.95	1.90	1.85	1.77	1.71	1.66	1.62	1.59
750	3.85	3.01	2.62	2.38	2.23	2.11	2.02	1.95	1.89	1.84	1.77	1.70	1.66	1.62	1.58
1000	3.85	3.00	2.61	2.38	2.22	2.11	2.02	1.95	1.89	1.84	1.76	1.70	1.65	1.61	1.58

Table 4.3 (Continued): *F* Distribution: Critical Values of *F* (5% significance level)

v_1 / v_2	25	30	35	40	50	60	75	100	150	200
1	249.26	250.10	250.69	251.14	251.77	252.20	252.62	253.04	253.46	253.68
2	19.46	19.46	19.47	19.47	19.48	19.48	19.48	19.49	19.49	19.49
3	8.63	8.62	8.60	8.59	8.58	8.57	8.56	8.55	8.54	8.54
4	5.77	5.75	5.73	5.72	5.70	5.69	5.68	5.66	5.65	5.65
5	4.52	4.50	4.48	4.46	4.44	4.43	4.42	4.41	4.39	4.39
6	3.83	3.81	3.79	3.77	3.75	3.74	3.73	3.71	3.70	3.69
7	3.40	3.38	3.36	3.34	3.32	3.30	3.29	3.27	3.26	3.25
8	3.11	3.08	3.06	3.04	3.02	3.01	2.99	2.97	2.96	2.95
9	2.89	2.86	2.84	2.83	2.80	2.79	2.77	2.76	2.74	2.73
10	2.73	2.70	2.68	2.66	2.64	2.62	2.60	2.59	2.57	2.56
11	2.60	2.57	2.55	2.53	2.51	2.49	2.47	2.46	2.44	2.43
12	2.50	2.47	2.44	2.43	2.40	2.38	2.37	2.35	2.33	2.32
13	2.41	2.38	2.36	2.34	2.31	2.30	2.28	2.26	2.24	2.23
14	2.34	2.31	2.28	2.27	2.24	2.22	2.21	2.19	2.17	2.16
15	2.28	2.25	2.22	2.20	2.18	2.16	2.14	2.12	2.10	2.10
16	2.23	2.19	2.17	2.15	2.12	2.11	2.09	2.07	2.05	2.04
17	2.18	2.15	2.12	2.10	2.08	2.06	2.04	2.02	2.00	1.99
18	2.14	2.11	2.08	2.06	2.04	2.02	2.00	1.98	1.96	1.95
19	2.11	2.07	2.05	2.03	2.00	1.98	1.96	1.94	1.92	1.91
20	2.07	2.04	2.01	1.99	1.97	1.95	1.93	1.91	1.89	1.88
21	2.05	2.01	1.98	1.96	1.94	1.92	1.90	1.88	1.86	1.84
22	2.02	1.98	1.96	1.94	1.91	1.89	1.87	1.85	1.83	1.82
23	2.00	1.96	1.93	1.91	1.88	1.86	1.84	1.82	1.80	1.79
24	1.97	1.94	1.91	1.89	1.86	1.84	1.82	1.80	1.78	1.77
25	1.96	1.92	1.89	1.87	1.84	1.82	1.80	1.78	1.76	1.75
26	1.94	1.90	1.87	1.85	1.82	1.80	1.78	1.76	1.74	1.73
27	1.92	1.88	1.86	1.84	1.81	1.79	1.76	1.74	1.72	1.71
28	1.91	1.87	1.84	1.82	1.79	1.77	1.75	1.73	1.70	1.69

29	1.89	1.85	1.83	1.81	1.77	1.75	1.73	1.71	1.69	1.67
30	1.88	1.84	1.81	1.79	1.76	1.74	1.72	1.70	1.67	1.66
35	1.82	1.79	1.76	1.74	1.70	1.68	1.66	1.63	1.61	1.60
40	1.78	1.74	1.72	1.69	1.66	1.64	1.61	1.59	1.56	1.55
50	1.73	1.69	1.66	1.63	1.60	1.58	1.55	1.52	1.50	1.48
60	1.69	1.65	1.62	1.59	1.56	1.53	1.51	1.48	1.45	1.44
70	1.66	1.62	1.59	1.57	1.53	1.50	1.48	1.45	1.42	1.40
80	1.64	1.60	1.57	1.54	1.51	1.48	1.45	1.43	1.39	1.38
90	1.63	1.59	1.55	1.53	1.49	1.46	1.44	1.41	1.38	1.36
100	1.62	1.57	1.54	1.52	1.48	1.45	1.42	1.39	1.36	1.34
120	1.60	1.55	1.52	1.50	1.46	1.43	1.40	1.37	1.33	1.32
150	1.58	1.54	1.50	1.48	1.44	1.41	1.38	1.34	1.31	1.29
200	1.56	1.52	1.48	1.46	1.41	1.39	1.35	1.32	1.28	1.26
250	1.55	1.50	1.47	1.44	1.40	1.37	1.34	1.31	1.27	1.25
300	1.54	1.50	1.46	1.43	1.39	1.36	1.33	1.30	1.26	1.23
400	1.53	1.49	1.45	1.42	1.38	1.35	1.32	1.28	1.24	1.22
500	1.53	1.48	1.45	1.42	1.38	1.35	1.31	1.28	1.23	1.21
600	1.52	1.48	1.44	1.41	1.37	1.34	1.31	1.27	1.23	1.20
750	1.52	1.47	1.44	1.41	1.37	1.34	1.30	1.26	1.22	1.20
1000	1.52	1.47	1.43	1.41	1.36	1.33	1.30	1.26	1.22	1.19

Table 4.3 (Continued): *F* Distribution: Critical Values of *F* (1% significance level)

v_1 / v_2	1	2	3	4	5	6	7	8	9	10	12	14	16
1	4052.18	4999.50	5403.35	5624.58	5763.65	5858.99	5928.36	5981.07	6022.47	6055.85	6106.32	6142.67	6170.10
2	98.50	99.00	99.17	99.25	99.30	99.33	99.36	99.37	99.39	99.40	99.42	99.43	99.44
3	34.12	30.82	29.46	28.71	28.24	27.91	27.67	27.49	27.35	27.23	27.05	26.92	26.83
4	21.20	18.00	16.69	15.98	15.52	15.21	14.98	14.80	14.66	14.55	14.37	14.25	14.15
5	16.26	13.27	12.06	11.39	10.97	10.67	10.46	10.29	10.16	10.05	9.89	9.77	9.68
6	13.75	10.92	9.78	9.15	8.75	8.47	8.26	8.10	7.98	7.87	7.72	7.60	7.52
7	12.25	9.55	8.45	7.85	7.46	7.19	6.99	6.84	6.72	6.62	6.47	6.36	6.28
8	11.26	8.65	7.59	7.01	6.63	6.37	6.18	6.03	5.91	5.81	5.67	5.56	5.48
9	10.56	8.02	6.99	6.42	6.06	5.80	5.61	5.47	5.35	5.26	5.11	5.01	4.92
10	10.04	7.56	6.55	5.99	5.64	5.39	5.20	5.06	4.94	4.85	4.71	4.60	4.52
11	9.65	7.21	6.22	5.67	5.32	5.07	4.89	4.74	4.63	4.54	4.40	4.29	4.21
12	9.33	6.93	5.95	5.41	5.06	4.82	4.64	4.50	4.39	4.30	4.16	4.05	3.97
13	9.07	6.70	5.74	5.21	4.86	4.62	4.44	4.30	4.19	4.10	3.96	3.86	3.78
14	8.86	6.51	5.56	5.04	4.69	4.46	4.28	4.14	4.03	3.94	3.80	3.70	3.62
15	8.68	6.36	5.42	4.89	4.56	4.32	4.14	4.00	3.89	3.80	3.67	3.56	3.49
16	8.53	6.23	5.29	4.77	4.44	4.20	4.03	3.89	3.78	3.69	3.55	3.45	3.37
17	8.40	6.11	5.18	4.67	4.34	4.10	3.93	3.79	3.68	3.59	3.46	3.35	3.27
18	8.29	6.01	5.09	4.58	4.25	4.01	3.84	3.71	3.60	3.51	3.37	3.27	3.19
19	8.18	5.93	5.01	4.50	4.17	3.94	3.77	3.63	3.52	3.43	3.30	3.19	3.12
20	8.10	5.85	4.94	4.43	4.10	3.87	3.70	3.56	3.46	3.37	3.23	3.13	3.05
21	8.02	5.78	4.87	4.37	4.04	3.81	3.64	3.51	3.40	3.31	3.17	3.07	2.99
22	7.95	5.72	4.82	4.31	3.99	3.76	3.59	3.45	3.35	3.26	3.12	3.02	2.94
23	7.88	5.66	4.76	4.26	3.94	3.71	3.54	3.41	3.30	3.21	3.07	2.97	2.89
24	7.82	5.61	4.72	4.22	3.90	3.67	3.50	3.36	3.26	3.17	3.03	2.93	2.85
25	7.77	5.57	4.68	4.18	3.85	3.63	3.46	3.32	3.22	3.13	2.99	2.89	2.81
26	7.72	5.53	4.64	4.14	3.82	3.59	3.42	3.29	3.18	3.09	2.96	2.86	2.78
27	7.68	5.49	4.60	4.11	3.78	3.56	3.39	3.26	3.15	3.06	2.93	2.82	2.75
28	7.64	5.45	4.57	4.07	3.75	3.53	3.36	3.23	3.12	3.03	2.90	2.79	2.72

v_1 / v_2	1	2	3	4	5	6	7	8	9	10	12	14	16
29	7.60	5.42	4.54	4.04	3.73	3.50	3.33	3.20	3.09	3.00	2.87	2.77	2.69
30	7.56	5.39	4.51	4.02	3.70	3.47	3.30	3.17	3.07	2.98	2.84	2.74	2.66
35	7.42	5.27	4.40	3.91	3.59	3.37	3.20	3.07	2.96	2.88	2.74	2.64	2.56
40	7.31	5.18	4.31	3.83	3.51	3.29	3.12	2.99	2.89	2.80	2.66	2.56	2.48
50	7.17	5.06	4.20	3.72	3.41	3.19	3.02	2.89	2.78	2.70	2.56	2.46	2.38
60	7.08	4.98	4.13	3.65	3.34	3.12	2.95	2.82	2.72	2.63	2.50	2.39	2.31
70	7.01	4.92	4.07	3.60	3.29	3.07	2.91	2.78	2.67	2.59	2.45	2.35	2.27
80	6.96	4.88	4.04	3.56	3.26	3.04	2.87	2.74	2.64	2.55	2.42	2.31	2.23
90	6.93	4.85	4.01	3.53	3.23	3.01	2.84	2.72	2.61	2.52	2.39	2.29	2.21
100	6.90	4.82	3.98	3.51	3.21	2.99	2.82	2.69	2.59	2.50	2.37	2.27	2.19
120	6.85	4.79	3.95	3.48	3.17	2.96	2.79	2.66	2.56	2.47	2.34	2.23	2.15
150	6.81	4.75	3.91	3.45	3.14	2.92	2.76	2.63	2.53	2.44	2.31	2.20	2.12
200	6.76	4.71	3.88	3.41	3.11	2.89	2.73	2.60	2.50	2.41	2.27	2.17	2.09
250	6.74	4.69	3.86	3.40	3.09	2.87	2.71	2.58	2.48	2.39	2.26	2.15	2.07
300	6.72	4.68	3.85	3.38	3.08	2.86	2.70	2.57	2.47	2.38	2.24	2.14	2.06
400	6.70	4.66	3.83	3.37	3.06	2.85	2.68	2.56	2.45	2.37	2.23	2.13	2.05
500	6.69	4.65	3.82	3.36	3.05	2.84	2.68	2.55	2.44	2.36	2.22	2.12	2.04
600	6.68	4.64	3.81	3.35	3.05	2.83	2.67	2.54	2.44	2.35	2.21	2.11	2.03
750	6.67	4.63	3.81	3.34	3.04	2.83	2.66	2.53	2.43	2.34	2.21	2.11	2.02
1000	6.66	4.63	3.80	3.34	3.04	2.82	2.66	2.53	2.43	2.34	2.20	2.10	2.02

Table 4.3 (Continued): *F* Distribution: Critical Values of *F* (1% significance level)

V_1 / V_2	18	20	25	30	35	40	50	60	75	100	150	200
1	6191.53	6208.73	6239.83	6260.65	6275.57	6286.78	6302.52	6313.03	6323.56	6334.11	6344.68	6349.97
2	99.44	99.45	99.46	99.47	99.47	99.47	99.48	99.48	99.49	99.49	99.49	99.49
3	26.75	26.69	26.58	26.50	26.45	26.41	26.35	26.32	26.28	26.24	26.20	26.18
4	14.08	14.02	13.91	13.84	13.79	13.75	13.69	13.65	13.61	13.58	13.54	13.52
5	9.61	9.55	9.45	9.38	9.33	9.29	9.24	9.20	9.17	9.13	9.09	9.08
6	7.45	7.40	7.30	7.23	7.18	7.14	7.09	7.06	7.02	6.99	6.95	6.93
7	6.21	6.16	6.06	5.99	5.94	5.91	5.86	5.82	5.79	5.75	5.72	5.70
8	5.41	5.36	5.26	5.20	5.15	5.12	5.07	5.03	5.00	4.96	4.93	4.91
9	4.86	4.81	4.71	4.65	4.60	4.57	4.52	4.48	4.45	4.41	4.38	4.36
10	4.46	4.41	4.31	4.25	4.20	4.17	4.12	4.08	4.05	4.01	3.98	3.96
11	4.15	4.10	4.01	3.94	3.89	3.86	3.81	3.78	3.74	3.71	3.67	3.66
12	3.91	3.86	3.76	3.70	3.65	3.62	3.57	3.54	3.50	3.47	3.43	3.41
13	3.72	3.66	3.57	3.51	3.46	3.43	3.38	3.34	3.31	3.27	3.24	3.22
14	3.56	3.51	3.41	3.35	3.30	3.27	3.22	3.18	3.15	3.11	3.08	3.06
15	3.42	3.37	3.28	3.21	3.17	3.13	3.08	3.05	3.01	2.98	2.94	2.92
16	3.31	3.26	3.16	3.10	3.05	3.02	2.97	2.93	2.90	2.86	2.83	2.81
17	3.21	3.16	3.07	3.00	2.96	2.92	2.87	2.83	2.80	2.76	2.73	2.71
18	3.13	3.08	2.98	2.92	2.87	2.84	2.78	2.75	2.71	2.68	2.64	2.62
19	3.05	3.00	2.91	2.84	2.80	2.76	2.71	2.67	2.64	2.60	2.57	2.55
20	2.99	2.94	2.84	2.78	2.73	2.69	2.64	2.61	2.57	2.54	2.50	2.48
21	2.93	2.88	2.79	2.72	2.67	2.64	2.58	2.55	2.51	2.48	2.44	2.42
22	2.88	2.83	2.73	2.67	2.62	2.58	2.53	2.50	2.46	2.42	2.38	2.36
23	2.83	2.78	2.69	2.62	2.57	2.54	2.48	2.45	2.41	2.37	2.34	2.32
24	2.79	2.74	2.64	2.58	2.53	2.49	2.44	2.40	2.37	2.33	2.29	2.27
25	2.75	2.70	2.60	2.54	2.49	2.45	2.40	2.36	2.33	2.29	2.25	2.23
26	2.72	2.66	2.57	2.50	2.45	2.42	2.36	2.33	2.29	2.25	2.21	2.19
27	2.68	2.63	2.54	2.47	2.42	2.38	2.33	2.29	2.26	2.22	2.18	2.16
28	2.65	2.60	2.51	2.44	2.39	2.35	2.30	2.26	2.23	2.19	2.15	2.13

v_1 / v_2	18	20	25	30	35	40	50	60	75	100	150	200
29	2.63	2.57	2.48	2.41	2.36	2.33	2.27	2.23	2.20	2.16	2.12	2.10
30	2.60	2.55	2.45	2.39	2.34	2.30	2.25	2.21	2.17	2.13	2.09	2.07
35	2.50	2.44	2.35	2.28	2.23	2.19	2.14	2.10	2.06	2.02	1.98	1.96
40	2.42	2.37	2.27	2.20	2.15	2.11	2.06	2.02	1.98	1.94	1.90	1.87
50	2.32	2.27	2.17	2.10	2.05	2.01	1.95	1.91	1.87	1.82	1.78	1.76
60	2.25	2.20	2.10	2.03	1.98	1.94	1.88	1.84	1.79	1.75	1.70	1.68
70	2.20	2.15	2.05	1.98	1.93	1.89	1.83	1.78	1.74	1.70	1.65	1.62
80	2.17	2.12	2.01	1.94	1.89	1.85	1.79	1.75	1.70	1.65	1.61	1.58
90	2.14	2.09	1.99	1.92	1.86	1.82	1.76	1.72	1.67	1.62	1.57	1.55
100	2.12	2.07	1.97	1.89	1.84	1.80	1.74	1.69	1.65	1.60	1.55	1.52
120	2.09	2.03	1.93	1.86	1.81	1.76	1.70	1.66	1.61	1.56	1.51	1.48
150	2.06	2.00	1.90	1.83	1.77	1.73	1.66	1.62	1.57	1.52	1.46	1.43
200	2.03	1.97	1.87	1.79	1.74	1.69	1.63	1.58	1.53	1.48	1.42	1.39
250	2.01	1.95	1.85	1.77	1.72	1.67	1.61	1.56	1.51	1.46	1.40	1.36
300	1.99	1.94	1.84	1.76	1.70	1.66	1.59	1.55	1.50	1.44	1.38	1.35
400	1.98	1.92	1.82	1.75	1.69	1.64	1.58	1.53	1.48	1.42	1.36	1.32
500	1.97	1.92	1.81	1.74	1.68	1.63	1.57	1.52	1.47	1.41	1.34	1.31
600	1.96	1.91	1.80	1.73	1.67	1.63	1.56	1.51	1.46	1.40	1.34	1.30
750	1.96	1.90	1.80	1.72	1.66	1.62	1.55	1.50	1.45	1.39	1.33	1.29
1000	1.95	1.90	1.79	1.72	1.66	1.61	1.54	1.50	1.44	1.38	1.32	1.28

Table 4.3 (Continued): *F* Distribution: Critical Values of *F* (0.1% significance level)

v_1 / v_2	1	2	3	4	5	6	7	8	9	10	12	14	16
1	4.05e05	5.00e05	5.40e05	5.62e05	5.76e05	5.86e05	5.93e05	5.98e05	6.02e05	6.06e05	6.11e05	6.14e05	6.17e05
2	998.50	999.00	999.17	999.25	999.30	999.33	999.36	999.37	999.39	999.40	999.42	999.43	999.44
3	167.03	148.50	141.11	137.10	134.58	132.85	131.58	130.62	129.86	129.25	128.32	127.64	127.14
4	74.14	61.25	56.18	53.44	51.71	50.53	49.66	49.00	48.47	48.05	47.41	46.95	46.60
4	74.14	61.25	56.18	53.44	51.71	50.53	49.66	49.00	48.47	48.05	47.41	46.95	46.60
5	47.18	37.12	33.20	31.09	29.75	28.83	28.16	27.65	27.24	26.92	26.42	26.06	25.78
6	35.51	27.00	23.70	21.92	20.80	20.03	19.46	19.03	18.69	18.41	17.99	17.68	17.45
7	29.25	21.69	18.77	17.20	16.21	15.52	15.02	14.63	14.33	14.08	13.71	13.43	13.23
8	25.41	18.49	15.83	14.39	13.48	12.86	12.40	12.05	11.77	11.54	11.19	10.94	10.75
9	22.86	16.39	13.90	12.56	11.71	11.13	10.70	10.37	10.11	9.89	9.57	9.33	9.15
10	21.04	14.91	12.55	11.28	10.48	9.93	9.52	9.20	8.96	8.75	8.45	8.22	8.05
11	19.69	13.81	11.56	10.35	9.58	9.05	8.66	8.35	8.12	7.92	7.63	7.41	7.24
12	18.64	12.97	10.80	9.63	8.89	8.38	8.00	7.71	7.48	7.29	7.00	6.79	6.63
13	17.82	12.31	10.21	9.07	8.35	7.86	7.49	7.21	6.98	6.80	6.52	6.31	6.16
14	17.14	11.78	9.73	8.62	7.92	7.44	7.08	6.80	6.58	6.40	6.13	5.93	5.78
15	16.59	11.34	9.34	8.25	7.57	7.09	6.74	6.47	6.26	6.08	5.81	5.62	5.46
16	16.12	10.97	9.01	7.94	7.27	6.80	6.46	6.19	5.98	5.81	5.55	5.35	5.20
17	15.72	10.66	8.73	7.68	7.02	6.56	6.22	5.96	5.75	5.58	5.32	5.13	4.99
18	15.38	10.39	8.49	7.46	6.81	6.35	6.02	5.76	5.56	5.39	5.13	4.94	4.80
19	15.08	10.16	8.28	7.27	6.62	6.18	5.85	5.59	5.39	5.22	4.97	4.78	4.64
20	14.82	9.95	8.10	7.10	6.46	6.02	5.69	5.44	5.24	5.08	4.82	4.64	4.49
21	14.59	9.77	7.94	6.95	6.32	5.88	5.56	5.31	5.11	4.95	4.70	4.51	4.37
22	14.38	9.61	7.80	6.81	6.19	5.76	5.44	5.19	4.99	4.83	4.58	4.40	4.26
23	14.20	9.47	7.67	6.70	6.08	5.65	5.33	5.09	4.89	4.73	4.48	4.30	4.16
24	14.03	9.34	7.55	6.59	5.98	5.55	5.23	4.99	4.80	4.64	4.39	4.21	4.07
25	13.88	9.22	7.45	6.49	5.89	5.46	5.15	4.91	4.71	4.56	4.31	4.13	3.99
26	13.74	9.12	7.36	6.41	5.80	5.38	5.07	4.83	4.64	4.48	4.24	4.06	3.92
27	13.61	9.02	7.27	6.33	5.73	5.31	5.00	4.76	4.57	4.41	4.17	3.99	3.86
28	13.50	8.93	7.19	6.25	5.66	5.24	4.93	4.69	4.50	4.35	4.11	3.93	3.80

v_1 / v_2	1	2	3	4	5	6	7	8	9	10	12	14	16
29	13.39	8.85	7.12	6.19	5.59	5.18	4.87	4.64	4.45	4.29	4.05	3.88	3.74
30	13.29	8.77	7.05	6.12	5.53	5.12	4.82	4.58	4.39	4.24	4.00	3.82	3.69
35	12.90	8.47	6.79	5.88	5.30	4.89	4.59	4.36	4.18	4.03	3.79	3.62	3.48
40	12.61	8.25	6.59	5.70	5.13	4.73	4.44	4.21	4.02	3.87	3.64	3.47	3.34
50	12.22	7.96	6.34	5.46	4.90	4.51	4.22	4.00	3.82	3.67	3.44	3.27	3.41
60	11.97	7.77	6.17	5.31	4.76	4.37	4.09	3.86	3.69	3.54	3.32	3.15	3.02
70	11.80	7.64	6.06	5.20	4.66	4.28	3.99	3.77	3.60	3.45	3.23	3.06	2.93
80	11.67	7.54	5.97	5.12	4.58	4.20	3.92	3.70	3.53	3.39	3.16	3.00	2.87
90	11.57	7.47	5.91	5.06	4.53	4.15	3.87	3.65	3.48	3.34	3.11	2.95	2.82
100	11.50	7.41	5.86	5.02	4.48	4.11	3.83	3.61	3.44	3.30	3.07	2.91	2.78
120	11.38	7.32	5.78	4.95	4.42	4.04	3.77	3.55	3.38	3.24	3.02	2.85	2.72
150	11.27	7.24	5.71	4.88	4.35	3.98	3.71	3.49	3.32	3.18	2.96	2.80	2.67
200	11.15	7.15	5.63	4.81	4.29	3.92	3.65	3.43	3.26	3.12	2.90	2.74	2.61
250	11.09	7.10	5.59	4.77	4.25	3.88	3.61	3.40	3.23	3.09	2.87	2.71	2.58
300	11.04	7.07	5.56	4.75	4.22	3.86	3.59	3.38	3.21	3.07	2.85	2.69	2.56
400	10.99	7.03	5.53	4.71	4.19	3.83	3.56	3.35	3.18	3.04	2.82	2.66	2.53
500	10.96	7.00	5.51	4.69	4.18	3.81	3.54	3.33	3.16	3.02	2.81	2.64	2.52
600	10.94	6.99	5.49	4.68	4.16	3.80	3.53	3.32	3.15	3.01	2.80	2.63	2.51
750	10.91	6.97	5.48	4.67	4.15	3.79	3.52	3.31	3.14	3.00	2.78	2.62	2.49
1000	10.89	6.96	5.46	4.65	4.14	3.78	3.51	3.30	3.13	2.99	2.77	2.61	2.48

Table 4.3 (Continued): *F* Distribution: Critical Values of *F* (0.1% significance level)

v_1 / v_2	18	20	25	30	35	40	50	60	75	100	150	200
1	6.19e05	6.21e05	6.24e05	6.26e05	6.28e05	6.29e05	6.30e05	6.31e05	6.32e05	6.33e05	6.35e05	6.35e05
2	999.44	999.45	999.46	999.47	999.47	999.47	999.48	999.48	999.49	999.49	999.49	999.49
3	126.74	126.42	125.84	125.45	125.17	124.96	124.66	124.47	124.27	124.07	123.87	123.77
4	46.32	46.10	45.70	45.43	45.23	45.09	44.88	44.75	44.61	44.47	44.33	44.26
5	46.32	46.10	25.08	24.87	24.72	24.60	24.44	24.33	24.22	24.12	24.01	23.95
6	25.57	25.39	16.85	16.67	16.54	16.44	16.31	16.21	16.12	16.03	15.93	15.89
7	17.27	17.12	12.69	12.53	12.41	12.33	12.20	12.12	12.04	11.95	11.87	11.82
8	13.06	12.93	10.26	10.11	10.00	9.92	9.80	9.73	9.65	9.57	9.49	9.45
9	10.60	10.48	8.69	8.55	8.46	8.37	8.26	8.19	8.11	8.04	7.96	7.93
10	9.01	8.90	7.60	7.47	7.37	7.30	7.19	7.12	7.05	6.98	6.91	6.87
11	7.91	7.80	6.81	6.68	6.59	6.52	6.42	6.35	6.28	6.21	6.14	6.10
12	7.11	7.01	6.22	6.09	6.00	5.93	5.83	5.76	5.70	5.63	5.56	5.52
13	6.51	6.40	5.75	5.63	5.54	5.47	5.37	5.30	5.24	5.17	5.10	5.07
14	6.03	5.93	5.38	5.25	5.17	5.10	5.00	4.94	4.87	4.81	4.74	4.71
15	5.66	5.56	5.07	4.95	4.86	4.80	4.70	4.64	4.57	4.51	4.44	4.41
16	5.35	5.25	4.82	4.70	4.61	4.54	4.45	4.39	4.32	4.26	4.19	4.16
17	5.09	4.99	4.60	4.48	4.40	4.33	4.24	4.18	4.11	4.05	3.98	3.95
18	4.87	4.78	4.42	4.30	4.22	4.15	4.06	4.00	3.93	3.87	3.80	3.77
19	4.68	4.59	4.26	4.14	4.06	3.99	3.90	3.84	3.78	3.71	3.65	3.61
20	4.52	4.43	4.12	4.00	3.92	3.86	3.77	3.70	3.64	3.58	3.51	3.48
21	4.38	4.29	4.00	3.88	3.80	3.74	3.64	3.58	3.52	3.46	3.39	3.36
22	4.26	4.17	3.89	3.78	3.70	3.63	3.54	3.48	3.41	3.35	3.28	3.25
23	4.15	4.06	3.79	3.68	3.60	3.53	3.44	3.38	3.32	3.25	3.19	3.16
24	4.05	3.96	3.71	3.59	3.51	3.45	3.36	3.29	3.23	3.17	3.10	3.07
25	3.96	3.87	3.63	3.52	3.43	3.37	3.28	3.22	3.15	3.09	3.03	2.99
26	3.88	3.79	3.56	3.44	3.36	3.30	3.21	3.15	3.08	3.02	2.95	2.92
27	3.81	3.72	3.49	3.38	3.30	3.23	3.14	3.08	3.02	2.96	2.89	2.86
28	3.75	3.66	3.43	3.32	3.24	3.18	3.09	3.02	2.96	2.90	2.83	2.80

v_1 / v_2	18	20	25	30	35	40	50	60	75	100	150	200
29	3.69	3.60	3.38	3.27	3.18	3.12	3.03	2.97	2.91	2.84	2.78	2.74
30	3.63	3.54	3.33	3.22	3.13	3.07	2.98	2.92	2.86	2.79	2.73	2.69
35	3.58	3.49	3.13	3.02	2.93	2.87	2.78	2.72	2.66	2.59	2.52	2.49
40	3.38	3.29	2.98	2.87	2.79	2.73	2.64	2.57	2.51	2.44	2.38	2.34
50	3.23	3.14	2.79	2.68	2.60	2.53	2.44	2.38	2.31	2.25	2.18	2.14
60	3.04	2.95	2.67	2.55	2.47	2.41	2.32	2.25	2.19	2.12	2.05	2.01
70	2.91	2.83	2.58	2.47	2.39	2.32	2.23	2.16	2.10	2.03	1.95	1.92
80	2.83	2.74	2.52	2.41	2.32	2.26	2.16	2.10	2.03	1.96	1.89	1.85
90	2.76	2.68	2.47	2.36	2.27	2.21	2.11	2.05	1.98	1.91	1.83	1.79
100	2.71	2.63	2.43	2.32	2.24	2.17	2.08	2.01	1.94	1.87	1.79	1.75
120	2.68	2.59	2.37	2.26	2.18	2.11	2.02	1.95	1.88	1.81	1.73	1.68
150	2.62	2.53	2.32	2.21	2.12	2.06	1.96	1.89	1.82	1.74	1.66	1.62
200	2.56	2.48	2.26	2.15	2.07	2.00	1.90	1.83	1.76	1.68	1.60	1.55
250	2.51	2.42	2.23	2.12	2.03	1.97	1.87	1.80	1.72	1.65	1.56	1.51
300	2.48	2.39	2.21	2.10	2.01	1.94	1.85	1.78	1.70	1.62	1.53	1.48
400	2.43	2.34	2.18	2.07	1.98	1.92	1.82	1.75	1.67	1.59	1.50	1.45
500	2.41	2.33	2.17	2.05	1.97	1.90	1.80	1.73	1.65	1.57	1.48	1.43
600	2.40	2.32	2.16	2.04	1.96	1.89	1.79	1.72	1.64	1.56	1.46	1.41
750	2.39	2.31	2.15	2.03	1.95	1.88	1.78	1.71	1.63	1.55	1.45	1.40
1000	2.38	2.30	2.14	2.02	1.94	1.87	1.77	1.69	1.62	1.53	1.44	1.38

Table 4.4: χ^2 (Chi-Squared) Distribution: Critical Values of χ^2

	Significance level		
Degrees of freedom	5%	1%	0.1%
1	3.841	6.635	10.828
2	5.991	9.210	13.816
3	7.815	11.345	16.266
4	9.488	13.277	18.467
5	11.070	15.086	20.515
6	12.592	16.812	22.458
7	14.067	18.475	24.322
8	15.507	20.090	26.124
9	16.919	21.666	27.877
10	18.307	23.209	29.588

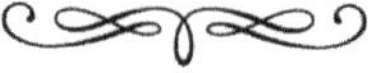

ANNEXURE

5 Critical Value for Wilcoxon Ranked Sign Test

Two-Sided Test	0.1	0.05	0.02	0.01
One-Sided Test	0.05	0.025	, 01	0.005
n				
5	1			
6	2	1		
7	4	2	0	
8	6	4	2	0
9	8	6	3	2
10	11	8	5	3
11	14	11	7	5
12	17	14	19	7
13	21	117	13	10
14	26	21	16	13
15	30	25	20	16
16	36	30	24	19
17	41	35	28	23
18	47	40	33	28
19	54	46	38	32
20	60	52	43	37
21	68	59	49	43
22	75	66	56	49
23	83	73	62	55
24	92	81	69	61
25	101	90	77	68
26	110	98	85	76
27	120	107	93	84
28	130	112	102	92
29	141	127	111	100
30	152	137	120	109

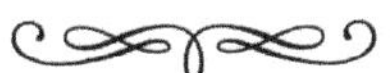

Annotated Bibliography

Introduction

It is a list of citations to books, articles and documents. Each citation includes a short write up giving description and evaluating not exceeding 100 to 150 words.

An annotation is critical and descriptive giving the point of view of the author their clarity, expression and indicates their authority on the topic. Annotated bibliography appears more like a reference page but includes annotation after each source cited. It is often found as a part of a larger research project, it can be also a stand-alone report by itself.

Purpose

The purpose of an annotated bibliography is to make readers aware of the relevance, quality and accuracy of the material cited.

How to go about Preparing Annotated Bibliography

It requires application of intellectual skill and critical thinking to concise and for exposition and the individual should have excellent library searching skill to trace relevant documents. As they have to locate material from books, journals, periodicals and relevant documents on a select topic of interest. Then study the material located to identify and review, next choose content/material which provide adequate dimension to the topic of interest.

When citing a book, article or literature materials use appropriate style so that it's well concise annotation which includes the essence of the subject /theme/ idea and its scope. Highlight on the following aspects i.e. about the author and his/ her background i.e. credentials and qualifications, who the interested readers would be or target group. It's important to draw focus on the work of the author and compare and contrast with other authors who have done similar work that it being cited. Indicted how the work enhances your topic that is helps the work to shine and its support to your reviewed bibliography.

Points to keep in mind while preparing annotated bibliography:

1. Make brief summary of the source (reputed journals preferred and how current is the material or research work).
2. Identify strength and weakness.
3. Relevance of the source in the study area or to the topic.
4. Its relationship to other studies in your area/field.
5. Research methodology should be evaluated to see if its applicable in your work
6. Conclusions drawn.
7. About the author's background.(as reputed author adds weightage)
8. Be aware of errors, omissions of facts or bias look for truth.

Use the appropriate style like API style or others which best suite or is accepted. Keep in mind the three parts of annotated bibliography i.e. title, citation and annotation as the format may vary based on the style which one uses while annotation can include a summary, evaluation and reflection. Annotations could be descriptive or indicative, i.e. a descriptive describes while indicative provides a quick summary, describe main points and make an argument. Evaluative annotations may stop at summarizations and enrich it by pointing reliability of source. One need not use a fixed method but a combination that best suits the work being done.

Annotated bibliography enhances skill in critical reading evaluation and drawing key points.

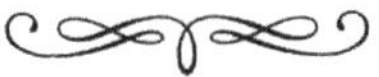

Nursing Research Glossary

Abstract	A brief description of a study, approximately limited to 100 or 250 words.
Accessible population	Part of target population, which is available to the researcher & which will be participating in the study.
Alpha	(1) In tests of statistical significance, the level indicating the possibility of a Type l error, possibly set at 0.05, 0.01, 0.001 level. (2) In assessment of reliability, a reliability co-efficient, Cronhbach's alpha.
Analysis	The process of organizing & synthesizing the data so as to answer research questions & test hypotheses.
Analysis of Covariance (ANCOVA)	A statistical procedure used to test mean differences among groups on a dependent variable, while controlling for one or more covariates.
Analysis of Variance	A statistical procedure for testing mean differences among three or more groups by comparing variability between groups to variability within groups.
Anonymity	Protection of participant's confidentiality such that even the researcher cannot link individuals with information provided.
Ambispective cohort design	This design moves both forward & backward in time. The exposure is measured twice i.e. historical & in real time during the study period.
Applied research	Research conducted to generate knowledge that will directly influence clinical practice.
Assent	An affirmative agreement of a child to participate in a research study.
Associative hypothesis	Hypothesis that identifies variables that occur or exist together in real world, such that when one variable changes, the other also changes.

Assumptions	A statement/principle accepted as being true based on logic or reason, without verification or scientific testing.
Authority	A person with expertise & power, who is able to influence the opinions & behavior of others.
Basic research	Research conducted for the pursuit of knowledge's sake or for finding truth.
Benchmark	An identified standard an agency wants to achieve in the provision of healthcare.
Beneficence principle	One of the principles to be followed by researcher so that subjects are benefitted.
Bias	Influence or action in a study that distorts or deviates findings from the true/expected.
Block randomization	A more advanced method for random assignment of subjects to experimental group, where size of block depends on number of treatments.
Case study	A qualitative research method involving a thorough, in depth analysis of an individual, group or other social unit.
Causal hypothesis	Hypothesis that states the relationship between two variables, in which one variable (independent variable) is thought to cause or determine the presence of the other variable (dependent variable).
Chi-square test	A statistical test used to assess nominal data to determine significant differences between observed frequencies within the data & frequencies that were expected.
Citation	Information to locate a reference. Citation of a journal article includes the author's name, year of publication, title, journal name, volume number, issue number & page numbers.
Cluster sampling	Sampling in which a frame is developed that includes a list of all the states, cities, institutions, or organizations (clusters) that could be used in a study; a randomized sample is drawn from this list.
Code	Symbol or abbreviation used to classify words or phrases in qualitative data.
Cohorts	Samples in time-dimensional studies within the field or epidemiology.
Concept	An abstraction based on observations of behaviors or characteristics.

Conceptual definition	The abstract or theoretical meaning of the concept being studied.
Conceptual map	A schematic representation of a theory or conceptual model that graphically represent key concepts & linkages among them.
Conceptual model	A set of highly abstract, related constructs that broadly explains phenomena of interest, expresses assumptions & reflects a philosophical stance.
Confidence Interval (CI)	The range of values within which a population parameter is estimated to lie, at a specified probability.
Confounding variable	An extraneous variable that confounds or obscures the relationship between the central variables of a study.
Consent form	An agreement signed by a study participant & a researcher concerning the terms & conditions of voluntary participation in a study.
Constructs	Concepts at very high levels of abstraction that have general meanings.
Content validity	The degree to which the items in an instrument adequately represent the universe of content for the concept being measured.
Content Validity Index	(CVI) An index of the degree to which an instrument is content valid, based on aggregated ratings of a panel of experts, both items (I-CVI) & the overall scale content validity (S-CVI) can be assessed.
Control	The process of holding constant confounding influences on the dependent variable under study.
Control group	The group which is not exposed to the experimental treatment in a study in which the sample is randomly selected.
Convenience sampling	Selection of the most readily available persons as participants in the study, also called as an accidental sampling.
Correlational co-efficient	Statistical term used to indicate the degree of relationship between two variables; the co-efficients range in value from +1.00 (perfect positive relationship to 0.00 (no relationship) to -1.00 (perfect negative to inverse relationship).

Correlational design	A study design that explores the interrelationships among variables of interest without researcher's intervention.
Crammer's V	Analysis technique for nominal data, a modification of phi for contingency Tables.
Critical incident technique	A method of obtaining data from study participants by in-depth exploration of specific incidents & behaviors related to the topic under study.
Critically appraised topic	A quick summary of a clinical question & an appraisal of the best evidence (best practice recommendation).
Cross sectional designs	Designs used to examine groups of subjects in various stages of development simultaneously, with the intent of inferring trends over time.
Culture	Way of life belonging to a designated group of people.
Data	Information that is collected during a research study.
Data analysis	Technique used to organize, summarize & give meaning to data.
Data triangulation	Collection of data from multiple sources in the same study, for the purpose of validating the conclusions.
Declaration of Helsinki	An ethical code that distinguishes therapeutic from non-therapeutic research, based on the Nuremberg code.
Deductive reasoning	The process of reasoning from general principles to specific predictions.
Degrees of freedom (df)	A statistical concept referring to the number of sample values free to vary (df = n-1 in paired t test).
Delimitations	Pre-determined restrictions or boundaries for the particular study, by researcher with regard to location, setting, sample size, variables studied, the instruments, generalizability etc.
Demographic variables	Characteristics or attributes of subjects that are collected to describe the sample.
Dependent variable	The response or outcome that is predicted or explained in research & caused by independent variable.
Descriptive correlational design	Design used to describe variables & examine relationships that exist in a situation.
Descriptive design	Design used to identify a phenomenon of interest, identify variables within phenomenon, operationally define & describe variables

Descriptive statistics	Statistics used to describe & summarize data (e.g. percentages, means etc.).
Design	Blueprint for conducting study; maximizes control over factors that could interfere with the validity of the findings.
Dialectic reasoning	Reasoning that involves a holistic perspective, in which the whole is greater than the sum of the parts; examining factors that are opposites & making sense of them by merging them into a single unit.
Dichotomous variable	A variable having only two values or categories (e.g. gender).
Directional hypothesis	A hypothesis that makes a specific prediction about the direction of the relationship between two variables.
Discrete variable	A variable with a finite number of values between two points.
Ecological studies	Ecological studies are epidemiological research design, which compares measurements in groups rather than individuals.
Effect size	The degree to which the phenomenon studied is present in the population or to which the null hypothesis is false.
Ethics	A system of moral values that is concerned with the degree to which research procedures adhere to professional, legal & social obligations to the study participants.
Ethical principles	Principles of respect for persons, beneficence & justice that are relevant to the conduct of research.
Ethnographic research	A kind of a qualitative research methodologies. The research involves collection, description & analysis of data to develop a theory of cultural behavior.
Evidence based practice (EBP)	The conscientious integration of best research evidence with clinical expertise, patient's values & needs in the delivery of high quality, cost-effective health care.
Exclusion sample criteria	Sampling criteria or characteristics that can cause a person or element to be excluded from the target population.
Experiment	A study in which subjects are randomly selected & independent variable is manipulated. Also there is good control of extraneous variables.

Experimental research	An objective, systematic, controlled investigation to examine probability & causality among selected variables for the purpose of predicting & controlling phenomena.
External validity	Extent to which the study findings can be generalized beyond the sample used in the study.
Extraneous variables	Variables that confounds the relationship between the independent & dependent variables & that needs to be controlled either in research design or through statistical procedures.
Factor analysis	A statistical procedure for reducing a large set of variables into a smaller set of variables with common underlying dimensions.
Factorial analysis of variance	Analysis technique that is mathematically a special version of multiple regression; various types of factorial ANOVAs have been developed to analyse data from specific experimental designs.
Fair treatment	Ethical principle that promotes fair selection & treatment of subjects during the course of a study.
Falsification of research	A type of scientific misconduct that involves manipulating research materials, equipment or processes or changing or omitting data or results, such that the research is not accurately represented in the research record.
Focus groups	These are the groups assembled to obtain the participant's perceptions in focused areas in settings that are permissive & nonthreatening in a qualitative study.
Framework	An abstract, logical structure of meaning, such as a portion of a theory, that guides the development of the study, is tested in the study & enables the researcher to link the findings to the theory or specific knowledge.
Frequency distribution	Statistical procedure that lists all possible measures of variables & tallies each datum on the listing.
Generalization	Findings from the sample that was studied & applied to the population.
General proposition	A highly abstract statement of the relationship between two or more concepts that is found in a conceptual model.
Grounded theory	A qualitative type of research approach to discover the problems that exist in a social science & process that persons involved to handle them, leading to a theory development process.

Hawthorne effect	Psychological response in which subjects change their behavior simply because they are participating in a study & not because of the research treatment.
Heterogeneous sample	In which subjects have a broad range of attributes to be studied which increases the representativeness of the sample & ability to generalize findings to target population.
Historical cohort design	Also known as retrospective cohort design where one can undertake a cohort study by using information collected in the past & kept in records or file.
Historical research	Studies designed to discover facts & relationships about past events.
Homogenous sample	Sample in which subjects score selected measurement methods in a study are similar, resulting in a limited or narrow distribution or spread of scores.
Hypothesis	A statement of predicted relationships between variables in a specified population.
Independent (treatment or experimental) variable	The variable which is manipulated & has effect on dependent variable; is also called as treatment or experimental variable.
Index	A library resource that can be used to identify journal articles & other publications relevant to a topic.
Inductive reasoning	It is a reasoning from specific to the general, in which specific events or situations are observed & then combined into a larger whole or general treatment.
Inference	Conclusion drawn from a research study, applicable from specific case to general truth, from part to whole.
Inferential statistics	Statistics that permit inferences on whether results observed in a sample are likely to occur in the larger population.
Informed consent	Willingness given by the subjects to participate in a research study voluntarily, after getting all necessary information of risks & benefits of the study.
Internal validity	The degree to which two raters or observers, operating independently, assign the same ratings or values for an attribute being measured or observed.

Interval	scale measurement - Has equal numerical distances between intervals of the scale & an attribute of a variable is rank ordered.
Intervention	Treatment or independent variable that is manipulated during the conduct of a study which has an effect on the dependent or outcome variables.
	Interview structured or unstructured oral communication between the researcher & the subject for the purpose of seeking information essential for a study.
Invasion of privacy	Sharing personal information with others without a person's knowledge or against his/her will.
Investigator triangulation	When two or more trained investigators with different backgrounds explore the same phenomenon using different methods.
Justice principle	An ethical principle, emphasizing a fair treatment to all subjects participating in the study.
Kendall's tau	Non-parametric test used to determine correlations among variables that have been measured at the ordinal level.
Keywords	Major concepts or variables of a research problem or topic that are used to begin a search of a database.
Kolmogorov	Smirnov two - sample test - non-parametric test used to determine whether two independent samples have been drawn from the same population.
Kurtosis	Degree of peakedness (platykurtic, mesokurtic, or leptokurtic) of the curve that is related to the spread or variance of the scores.
Leptokurtik	An extremely peaked shape distribution of a curve, which means that the scores in the distribution are similar & have limited variance.
Lickert scale	An instrument designed to determine the opinion on or attitude towards a particular subject; contains a number of declarative statements with a scale after each statement.
Limitations	Theoretical or methodological restrictions in a study that may be seen in the last chapter of research report.
Literature review	Summary of theoretical & research studies related to sources on a topic of interest, often prepared to justify & focus on research under investigation.

Log	In participant observation studies, the observers daily record of events & conversations.
Logistic regression	It is also known as binary logistic regression, which is used to predict relationship between one dependent binary variable & one or more nominal, ordinal, interval or ratio level independent variable.
Longitudinal designs	Designs used to identify changes in the same subjects over an extended period of time.
Manipulation	An intervention or treatment introduced by the researcher in an experimental, quasi-experimental, or pre-experimental study to identify its effect on dependent variable.
Mann-Whitney U test	Test used to analyse ordinal data (with 95% of the power of the t test) to detect the difference between groups of normally distributed populations.
Maturation effect	Natural changes the subject experiences during the course of the study e.g. growing older, wiser etc that can have effect on the findings of the study.
McNemar test	Non-parametric test used to analyse the changes that occur in dichotomous variables.
Mean	A measure of central tendency, computed by totalling all scores & dividing by the total number of subjects.
Measurement	To characterize quantities of some attribute, the numbers are assigned to objects as per the specified rules.
Measures of central tendency	Statistical procedures which include mode, median & mean for determining the center of a distribution of scores.
Measures of dispersion	Statistical procedures like range, difference scores, variance & standard deviation for examining how scores are dispersed or deviated from mean.
Median	A measure of central tendency, representing the exact middle value in a score distribution, the value above & below which 50% of the scores lie.
Memoing	A method to record insights or ideas related to notes, transcripts or codes during qualitative data analysis.
Mesokurtik	Term that describes a normal curve with an intermediate degree of kurtosis & intermediate variance of scores.

Meta-analysis	A technique for integration of results of multiple quantitative similar research studies addressing the same research question.
Meta-synthesis	The grand narratives or interpretative translations produced from the integration or comparison of findings from qualitative studies.
Methodological designs	Studies conducted to develop the validity & reliability of instruments to measure research concepts & variables.
Methodological triangulation	Use of two or more research methods or procedures such as different designs, instruments & data collection procedures in a study.
Middle range theories	Theories which are not covering broad areas but specific in nature & have limited number of concepts & propositions & tested by empirical research.
Minimal risks	Anticipated risks during research study are no greater than those ordinarily encountered in daily life ordering the performance of routine tests or procedures.
Mixed method research	In which both qualitative & quantitative data are collected & analysed.
Mode	Numerical value or score that occurs with the greatest frequency in a distribution but does not necessarily indicate the center of the data set.
Mortality threat	A threat to the internal validity of a study, referring to the differential loss of participants (attrition) from different groups.
Multiple triangulation	Use of two or more types of triangulation i.e. theoretical, data, methodological, investigator & analysis, in a study.
Multistage sampling	A sampling strategy that proceeds through a set of stages from larger to smaller sampling units.
Multivariate analysis of variance (MANOVA)	A statistical procedure used to test the significance of differences between the means of two or more groups on two or more dependent variables, considered simultaneously.
Multivariate statistics	Statistical procedures designed to analyse the relationships among three or more variables (e.g. multiple regression, ANCOVA).

Narrative analysis	An approach in qualitative research that focuses on the story as the object of the inquiry.
Natural setting	Real life setting with no or minimum control where research is conducted, such as subject's home, work sites & schools.
Network or snowball sampling	The sampling of participants based on referrals from others already in the sample.
Nominal scale measurement	The lowest level of measurement involving the assignment of characteristics into categories (e.g. males – category 1, females – category -2)
Non-directional hypothesis	Hypothesis that does not predict the exact nature of the relationship but states that relationship between variables exist.
Non-equivalent control group designs	Designs in which the control group is not selected randomly. e.g. one group post-test only design, or post-test only design & one group pre-test, post-test design.
Non-parametric statistics	Statistical techniques used when the assumptions of parametric statistics are not met; most commonly used to analyse nominal & ordinal data.
Non-probability sampling	The selection of sampling units (participants/subjects) from a population using non-random procedures (purposive, convenience sampling).
Normal curve	A theoretical distribution that is bell-shaped & symmetrical, also called as Gaussian distribution.
Null (statistical) hypothesis	Hypothesis stating that no relationship exists between the variables being studied, a hypothesis used for statistical testing & for interpreting statistical outcomes.
Nuremberg code	Ethical code of conduct to guide researcher in conducting research ethically.
Operational definition	Concepts or variables are defined in measurable terms.
Ordinal scale measurement	Measurement level that rank orders phenomena along some dimension.
Outcome research	Research designed to document the effectiveness of healthcare services & the end results of patient care.

Parametric tests	A class of statistical tests that involve assumptions about the distribution of the variables & the estimation of a parameter.
Participant observation	A special form of observation in which the researcher is a part of the environment/setting & so he/she can observe the participants of the study.
Pearson product moment correlation	Parametric test used to determine relationships among variables.
Peer reviewer	A researcher who reviews & critics a research report or proposal & who makes a recommendation about publishing or funding the research.
Periodicals	Literature sources such as journals that are published over time & are numbered sequentially for years published.
Person triangulation	The collection of data from different levels of persons, with the aim of validating data through multiple perspectives on the phenomenon.
Phenomenology	A qualitative research design based on a philosophy for the purpose of describing lived experiences of study participants.
Phenomenon (pleural – phenomena)	An abstract concept under study or any circumstance that influences researcher.
Phi coefficient	A statistical index describing the magnitude of relationship between two dichotomous variables.
Pilot study	A rehearsal or small trial of proposed study, conducted to develop & refine the methodology, such as the treatment, instrument, or data collection process to be used in the larger study.
Placebo	A placebo is a pseudo intervention or a substance that has no pharmacological or therapeutic property, used for control group & it is compared with effect of independent variable.
Plagiarism	A type of scientific misconduct, by copying/using another person's ideas, processes, results, or words without acknowledging or without giving appropriate credit to the author.

Population	All elements (people, objects, events or substances that have common characteristics of a sample. Also called as universe/target population.
Power analysis	Techniques used to determine the risk of a Type - ll error so the study can be modified to decrease the risk if necessary or sample size requirements.
Practice theories	Specific theories, developed to explain particular element of practice. These theories can be developed or tested through research.
Primary source	First hand study reports in research, the original report published by researcher who conducted the study.
Principal investigator	The person who will have primary responsibility for overseeing the projects.
Probability sampling	Random sampling technique in which each element has equal chance to be selected as a sample.
Problem solving process	It is scientific in nature & there are definite steps to be followed, from problem identification till evaluation of goal achievement.
Problem statement	A statement with justification of gap in knowledge & provides a basis for research study to be conducted.
Propositions	In relation to theories, statements expressed at various levels of abstraction.
Projective techniques	A method in which respondents are exposed to unstructured stimuli to measure psychological attributes like values, attitudes & personality.
Prospective cohort study	A design that begins with an examination of presumed causes & then moves forward in time to observe presumed effects.
Purposive sampling	A non-probability sampling technique in which selection of participants is based on personal judgment, so that they provide more information. This technique is also called as judgmental sampling & mostly used in qualitative research.
Q plots	Displays of scores or data in a distribution by quartile for exploratory data analysis.
Q sorts	A data collection method in which participants sorts cards with statements into a number of piles i.e. 7 to 11 piles those might range from best to worst.

Qualitative research	An indepth & holistic investigation of phenomena through the systematic & subjective methodological approach.
Quantitative research	A research process used to measure or quantify & test cause & effect relationship between variables.
Quasi-experimental design	An interventional design in which there is non-random selection of subjects.
Questionnaire	A document used to gather self-report data via written or verbal responses of the subjects.
Quota sampling	A non-probability sampling technique in which certain sample characteristics are established to increase the representativeness of the sample.
Random assignment	Subjects are assigned randomly to treatment conditions. Subjects have an equal probability of being assigned to either group.
Random sampling	Technique in which every member of the population has an equal chance to be selected as a sample, which increases the sample's representativeness of the target population.
Randomized Controlled Trial	Most effective research method where effect of various treatments/interventions is examined in randomly assigned experimental & control groups.
Range	A simplest measure of dispersion by subtracting the lowest value from the highest value in a distribution of scores.
Rating scale	A scale that requires ratings of an object or concept along a continuum.
Ratio scale measurement	A measurement level with equal distances between scores & an absolute zero.
Referencing	Subjects scores are compared against a standard. Used in norm referenced & criterion referenced testing.
Regression analysis	A statistical procedure for predicting values of a dependent variable based on one or more independent variables.
Reliability	The degree of consistency or dependability with which an instrument measures an attribute.
Representative-ness	Degree to which the sample, accessible population & target population are alike.

Research	Systematic investigation to validate & refine existing knowledge & generating new knowledge.
Research design	Blueprint for conducting study, maximizes control over factors that could interfere with the validity of findings, guides the planning & implementation of a study in a way that most likely to achieve intended goal.
Research hypothesis	Alternative hypothesis to null hypothesis; stating the relationship existing between two or more variables.
Research objective	A clear, precise, declarative statement of identification of variables to direct research study.
Research study	An interrogative statement of the specific question the researcher wants to answer to address a research problem.
Research report	A summary of the main features of a study, including research problem, the methods used, the findings & interpretation of the findings.
Research tradition	Related to a particular phenomena & body of knowledge is developed based on a particular conceptual model.
Research utilization	Use of research generated knowledge to affect or change the existing practices in the healthcare system.
Results	The answers to research questions, obtained through an analysis of the collected data.
Retrospective design	A study conducted on group of people who have experienced a particular event, followed by a search for presumed cause.
Sample	Portion of the population that is selected for a study to represent the entire population.
Sample characteristics	Analysis of demographic variables to provide a picture of the sample.
Sampling	A process of selecting a group of people, events, behaviors, or other elements that are representative of the population being studied.
Sampling bias	Distortions that arise when a sample is not representative of the population from which it was drawn.
Sampling criteria	List of characteristics essential for inclusion or exclusion in the target population.
Sampling error	The variations in the values of a statistic from one sample to another drawn from the same population.

Sampling frame	A list of all elements in the population from which the sample is drawn.
Sampling plan	The strategy or plan to select sample & determine sample size.
Saturation of data	The collection of data in qualitative study, to the point where sampling provides no new information. Thus sample size in a qualitative study is determined when saturation of data occurs.
Secondary analysis design	Design for studying data previously collected in another study; data are re-examined using different organizations of the data & different statistical analysis.
Semantic differential scale	The scale with two opposite bipolar testing scale & subject selects a point on the scale that best describes his/her view of the concept being examined.
Setting	Place & conditions in which data collection takes place, can be natural, partially controlled or highly controlled.
Significance level	The probability that an observed relationship could be caused by chance; significance at the .05 level indicates the probability that a relationship of the observed magnitude would be found by chance only 5 times out of 100.
Simple random sampling	Probability sampling involving random selection of elements from the sampling frame for inclusion in a study.
Split body design	A true experimental research design, in which the body is divided into left & right half, one side serve as an experimental arm & another side serve as control arm.
Split half reliability	Technique used to determine the homogeneity of an instrument's items, in which items are split in half & a correlational procedure is performed between the two halves.
Standard deviation	Measure of dispersion that is calculated by taking the square root of the variance.
Statistics	An estimate of the parameter, calculated from sample data.
Statistical inference	The process of inferring attributes about the population based on information from a sample, using laws of probability.
Statistical significance	A term indicating that the results from an analysis of sample data are unlikely to have been caused by chance, at a specified level of probability.

Stratified random sampling	The probability technique in which the random selection of study participants from two or more strata of the population done independently.
Subjects	Individuals participating in a study (those being studied).
Survey design	Design used to describe a phenomenon by collecting data using questionnaires or personal interviews.
Systematic review of research	Specifically focused synthesis of the findings from quantitative studies focused on a particular practice intervention or problem.
Target population	The entire population in which a researcher is interested & to which he or she would like to generalize the study results.
Theory	An abstract generalization that presents a systematic explanation about the relationships among phenomena.
Triangulation	Use of two or more theories, methods, data sources, investigations, or analysis methods in a study.
t-test	Parametric statistical test for analysing the difference between two means.
Type l error	An error created by rejecting the null hypothesis when it is true (the researcher concludes that no relationship exists when in fact it does - a false negative)
Type ll error	An error created by accepting the null hypothesis when it is false (i.e. the researcher concludes that no relationship exists when in fact it does - a false negative).
Unstructured interview	An interview in which subjects are encouraged to express freely on particular dimensions of a topic.
Validity	An extent to which an instrument accurately reflects the abstract construct (or concept) being examined.
Variables	A quality, property or characteristics of persons, things or situations that change or vary & are manipulated or measured in research.
Visual analogue scale	A 100 mm scale used to measure certain clinical symptoms e.g. pain, fatigue etc., which indicates the intensity of the symptom.
Wilcoxon matched	Pairs signed - ranks test - non parametric analysis of changes that occur in pre-test post-test measures or matched - pairs measures.

World Wide Web (www)	Information services for access to Internet resources by content rather than file names.
X-axis	The horizontal scale of a scatter plot.
Y-axis	The vertical scale of a scatter plot.
Z score	Standardized score of the normal curve that is equivalent to the standard deviation of the normal curve.

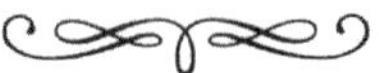

www.ingramcontent.com/pod-product-compliance
Ingram Content Group UK Ltd.
Pitfield, Milton Keynes, MK11 3LW, UK
UKHW061952290726
14090UKWH00021B/1184